Helicobacter pylori Infection and Related Diseases: Clinical Updates and Perspectives

Helicobacter pylori Infection and Related Diseases: Clinical Updates and Perspectives

Editors

Tamaki Ikuse
Mariko Hojo

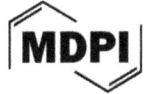

Basel • Beijing • Wuhan • Barcelona • Belgrade • Novi Sad • Cluj • Manchester

Editors
Tamaki Ikuse
Department of Pediatrics
Juntendo University Faculty of Medicine
Tokyo
Japan

Mariko Hojo
Department of Gastroenterology
Juntendo University Faculty of Medicine
Tokyo
Japan

Editorial Office
MDPI
St. Alban-Anlage 66
4052 Basel, Switzerland

This is a reprint of articles from the Special Issue published online in the open access journal *Journal of Clinical Medicine* (ISSN 2077-0383) (available at: https://www.mdpi.com/journal/jcm/special_issues/Helicobacter_Pylori_Infection_Diseases).

For citation purposes, cite each article independently as indicated on the article page online and as indicated below:

Lastname, A.A.; Lastname, B.B. Article Title. *Journal Name* **Year**, *Volume Number*, Page Range.

ISBN 978-3-0365-9554-2 (Hbk)
ISBN 978-3-0365-9555-9 (PDF)
doi.org/10.3390/books978-3-0365-9555-9

© 2023 by the authors. Articles in this book are Open Access and distributed under the Creative Commons Attribution (CC BY) license. The book as a whole is distributed by MDPI under the terms and conditions of the Creative Commons Attribution-NonCommercial-NoDerivs (CC BY-NC-ND) license.

Contents

Luigi Basso, Gaetano Gallo, Daniele Biacchi, Maria Vittoria Carati, Giuseppe Cavallaro,
Luca Esposito, et al.
Role of New Anatomy, Biliopancreatic Reflux, and Helicobacter Pylori Status in
Postgastrectomy Stump Cancer
Reprinted from: *J. Clin. Med.* **2022**, *11*, 1498, doi:10.3390/jcm11061498 1

Olga P. Nyssen, Dino Vaira, Ilaria Maria Saracino, Giulia Fiorini, María Caldas,
Luis Bujanda, et al.
Experience with Rifabutin-Containing Therapy in 500 Patients from the European Registry on
Helicobacter pylori Management (Hp-EuReg)
Reprinted from: *J. Clin. Med.* **2022**, *11*, 1658, doi:10.3390/jcm11061658 13

Junichi Uematsu, Mitsushige Sugimoto, Mariko Hamada, Eri Iwata, Ryota Niikura,
Naoyoshi Nagata, et al.
Efficacy of a Third-Generation High-Vision Ultrathin Endoscope for Evaluating Gastric Atrophy
and Intestinal Metaplasia in *Helicobacter pylori*-Eradicated Patients
Reprinted from: *J. Clin. Med.* **2022**, *11*, 2198, doi:10.3390/jcm11082198 27

Elena Resina, María G. Donday, Samuel J. Martínez-Domínguez,
Emilio José Laserna-Mendieta, Ángel Lanas, Alfredo J. Lucendo, et al.
Evaluation of a New Monoclonal Chemiluminescent Immunoassay Stool Antigen Test for the
Diagnosis of *Helicobacter pylori* Infection: A Spanish Multicentre Study
Reprinted from: *J. Clin. Med.* **2022**, *11*, 5077, doi:10.3390/jcm11175077 39

Malek Shatila and Anusha Shirwaikar Thomas
Current and Future Perspectives in the Diagnosis and Management of
Helicobacter pylori Infection
Reprinted from: *J. Clin. Med.* **2022**, *11*, 5086, doi:10.3390/jcm11175086 53

Shotaro Oki, Tsutomu Takeda, Mariko Hojo, Ryota Uchida, Nobuyuki Suzuki,
Daiki Abe, et al.
Comparative Study of *Helicobacter pylori*-Infected Gastritis in Okinawa and Tokyo Based on the
Kyoto Classification of Gastritis
Reprinted from: *J. Clin. Med.* **2022**, *11*, 5739, doi:10.3390/jcm11195739 71

Yingchao Sun, Mengjia Zhu, Lei Yue and Weiling Hu
Multiple Bismuth Quadruple Therapy Containing Tetracyclines Combined with Other
Antibiotics and *Helicobacter pylori* Eradication Therapy
Reprinted from: *J. Clin. Med.* **2022**, *11*, 7040, doi:10.3390/jcm11237040 83

Seiichi Kato, Benjamin D. Gold and Ayumu Kato
Helicobacter pylori-Associated Iron Deficiency Anemia in Childhood and
Adolescence-Pathogenesis and Clinical Management Strategy
Reprinted from: *J. Clin. Med.* **2022**, *11*, 7351, doi:10.3390/jcm11247351 93

Shotaro Nakamura and Mariko Hojo
Diagnosis and Treatment for Gastric Mucosa-Associated Lymphoid Tissue (MALT) Lymphoma
Reprinted from: *J. Clin. Med.* **2023**, *12*, 120, doi:10.3390/jcm12010120 107

Takahisa Furuta, Mihoko Yamade, Tomohiro Higuchi, Satoru Takahashi, Natsuki Ishida,
Shinya Tani, et al.
Expectations for the Dual Therapy with Vonoprazan and Amoxicillin for the Eradication
of *H. pylori*
Reprinted from: *J. Clin. Med.* **2023**, *12*, 3110, doi:10.3390/jcm12093110 119

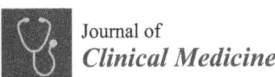

Review

Role of New Anatomy, Biliopancreatic Reflux, and Helicobacter Pylori Status in Postgastrectomy Stump Cancer

Luigi Basso [1,*], **Gaetano Gallo** [2,*], **Daniele Biacchi** [1], **Maria Vittoria Carati** [1], **Giuseppe Cavallaro** [1], **Luca Esposito** [1], **Andrea Giuliani** [1], **Luciano Izzo** [1], **Paolo Izzo** [1], **Antonietta Lamazza** [1], **Andrea Polistena** [1], **Mariarita Tarallo** [1], **Alessandro Micarelli** [3,4] and **Enrico Fiori** [1]

1. "Pietro Valdoni" Department of Surgery, Policlinico "Umberto I", "Sapienza" University of Rome, 00161 Rome, Italy; daniele.biacchi@uniroma1.it (D.B.); mariavittoria.carati@uniroma1.it (M.V.C.); giuseppe.cavallaro@uniroma1.it (G.C.); lcu.esposito@gmail.com (L.E.); andrea.giuliani@uniroma1.it (A.G.); luciano.izzo@uniroma1.it (L.I.); p_izzo@hotmail.it (P.I.); antonietta.lamazza@uniroma1.it (A.L.); andrea.polistena@uniroma1.it (A.P.); mariarita.tarallo@uniroma1.it (M.T.); enrico.fiori@uniroma1.it (E.F.)
2. Department of Medicine, Surgery and Neurosciences, Operative Unit of General Surgery and Surgical Oncology, University of Siena, 53100 Siena, Italy
3. ITER Center for Balance and Rehabilitation Research (ICBRR), 02032 Rome, Italy; alessandromicarelli@yahoo.it
4. Eurac Research, Institute of Mountain Emergency Medicine, 39100 Bolzano, Italy
* Correspondence: luigi.basso@uniroma1.it (L.B.); gaetano.gallo@unisi.it (G.G.)

Abstract: Distal gastrectomy for benign gastroduodenal peptic disease has become rare, but it still represents a widely adopted procedure for advanced and, in some countries, even for early distal gastric cancer. Survival rates following surgery for gastric malignancy are constantly improving, hence the residual mucosa of the gastric stump is exposed for a prolonged period to biliopancreatic reflux and, possibly, to Helicobacter pylori (HP) infection. Biliopancreatic reflux and HP infection are considered responsible for gastritis and metachronous carcinoma in the gastric stump after oncologic surgery. For gastrectomy patients, in addition to eradication treatment for cases that are already HP positive, endoscopic surveillance should also be recommended, for prompt surveillance and detection in the residual mucosa of any metaplastic-atrophic-dysplastic features following surgery.

Keywords: gastric cancer; biliopancreatic reflux; gastritis; carcinoma; endoscopic surveillance; Helicobacter pylori infection; gastric stump cancer

1. Introduction

In 1881, the Viennese surgeon Theodor Billroth and his colleagues, following previous experimental studies, successfully performed the first distal gastrectomy on a 43-year-old patient with cancer of the pylorus. Surgical reconstruction of the continuity between the residual stomach and the duodenum (gastroduodenostomy) was called "Billroth 1" (B1); three years later, Billroth experimented another technique involving anastomosis of the residual stomach to one of the first loops of the jejunum (gastrojejunostomy, Billroth 2 or B2) [1]. Both procedures were not widely adopted until the end of the 19th century: while Billroth never published his own results, these were released by one of his scholars, Wolfler, who is considered the inventor of the gastrojejunostomy antecolic technique [2]. In the following years, both techniques became universally adopted, with some geographical differences, to treat both benign and malignant gastroduodenal conditions of the distal stomach. In Asia, B1 was preferred to B2 [3], whereas in the West, and especially in Europe, B2 became more popular [4]. Since the mid-1970s, particularly in more developed countries, gastric resection has progressively become less common to cure gastroduodenal peptic ulcer disease, except for complicated cases, thanks to the diffusion of effective anti-ulcer drugs (such as H-2 receptor antagonists and, later, proton pump inhibitors). More recently, with the identification of Helicobacter pylori (HP) as a pathogen for gastroduodenal peptic disorders [5] and the introduction of specific medical treatments, surgical intervention has become even less indicated [6–8]. The present study is a non-systematic, narrative review of the fate of gastric resected patients, examining the role of gastric stump and of new anatomy, enteric reflux, and HP status. In non-systematic reviews there is always a risk of selection bias, including arbitrary weighing, choice and inclusion of the reported research, the way these studies are emphasized, assessed and presented, and the difficulty in integrating complex results. Nevertheless, the following is still meant to be an exhaustive and informative, albeit non-systematic, review, certainly not covering every aspect, yet still important for definition of the problem and for stressing the role of HP and of the new local environment toward the development of further malignancy, which is of potentially tremendous beneficial clinical impact.

1.1. Gastric Stump Cancer after Partial Gastrectomy: Role of Time

In 1922, Donald C. Balfour first noted that one of the factors which reduced life expectancy after gastric resection for peptic ulcer was later development of cancer in the residual gastric stump [9]. Since the 1950s the number of observations of "gastric stump cancer" (GSC) following B1 or B2 gastric resection increased progressively [10,11]. Thanks to the success of medical treatment of benign peptic conditions, GSC following benign situations has been decreasing, while an increase in GSC has been observed, especially in Asia, due to a larger number of gastric carcinomas operated in the early stage (early gastric cancer or EGC), translating into longer life expectancy [12,13]. In a series of 108 cases of GSC following distal gastrectomy for gastric cancer, 7 were diagnosed between 1970–1980, 28 between 1981–1991, and 73 between 1992–2002 [12]. Originally, GSC was defined as cancer arising from the remnant stomach five years after distal gastrectomy for benign disease, while later, this definition included cancers arising up to 10 years following distal gastrectomy for malignancy. This broader interval was due to the prolonged life expectancy of patients operated on for stomach cancer, and it was established that GSC is a metachronous occurrence, thus excluding the possibility of a locally recurring malignancy [14,15]. Indeed, it has been demonstrated that GSC is, on average, found 300 months after resection for benign gastroduodenal diseases and 100 months following resection for gastric cancer [12,16–23]. The type of reconstructive surgery also influences the interval of development of GSC, which occurs 84 months (mean) after B1, and 276 months (mean) after B2 ($p < 0.01$) [18]. There are, however, conflicting observations. For instance, Tokudome et al. [24] found that the ratio between observed and expected deaths from GSC was <1, and no difference was found in the cause of death in relation to the type of reconstruction performed. Asano et al. followed up for 13.1 years (mean) 6662 gastric-resected patients, finding a lower risk of death from carcinoma than in the general population, regardless of the primary disease and of the adopted surgical procedure [25]. Despite these data, distal gastrectomy is considered a precancerous condition and it represents a model to be used to study gastric carcinogenesis. In addition to time from surgery, other features have also been shown to play some role and are still investigated.

1.2. Gastric Stump Cancer: Role of Type of Reconstruction and of Biliopancreatic Reflux

Following distal gastrectomy, the ideal reconstruction of the intestinal continuity should not create immediate or long-term post-operative problems, nor should it alter quality of life, although alterations of the natural anatomic and functional gastric conditions cannot be avoided. B2 reconstruction is the most popular surgical procedure, but it involves a greater risk of carcinoma. Caygill et al. [26] and Toftgaard [27] in two different studies on 4466 and on 4131 patients, respectively, receiving partial gastrectomy for peptic ulcer, found that the risk of GSC was greater in those with a B2 reconstruction compared to B1 patients. In another study, the incidence of GSC in male patients younger than 40 years was four times higher after B2 than a after B1 [28]. B2 implies close exposure of the anastomosis and of the residual gastric mucosa to biliopancreatic secretions and favors gastroesophageal reflux. B1, on the other hand, preserves the physiological continuity of the duodenum, but suppression of the pyloric function may cause reflux of biliopancreatic secretions into the gastric stump, even if at a lower degree than in B2. In order to minimize reflux, B2 has been modified by connecting the afferent and the efferent loops of the jejunum (Braun's anastomosis), a few centimeters away from the gastro-jejunal anastomosis. However, functional studies [29,30] have shown that B2 associated with Braun's anastomosis is ineffective in preventing biliopancreatic reflux into the gastric stump, both in fasting conditions and after fatty meals. Further surgical procedures were later proposed and performed: gastro-jejunal reconstruction Roux-en-Y (R-Y), and reconstruction involving the interposition of a jejunal loop between the gastric and the duodenal stumps (jejunal interposition bilio-duodenal anastomosis, J-I). Both the R-Y and J-I procedures significantly decrease biliopancreatic reflux, which, however, to some extent still persists [31]. In any case, a 50–60 cm long R-Y loop is considered the most effective solution to reduce this problem [32]. Indeed, experimental and clinical studies have consistently demonstrated the role of reflux of duodenal contents (both bile and pancreatic juice) in the carcinogenesis of GSC [33–37] or, at least, as a cause of histological alterations considered to be precursors of cancer [38,39]. The carcinogenic effect of biliopancreatic reflux on the residual gastric mucosa is also indirect, due to: (1) increased alkalinity of the gastric stump caused by atrophy of the mucosa (following absence of the trophic action of antral gastrin), (2) surgical suppression of the vagal intramucosal innervation, and (3) alkaline reflux which favors growth of anaerobic nitrate-reducing bacteria. As a result, the nitrites produced by these bacteria can form cancerogenic substances when in contact with alimentary proteins [4,40]. All these changes in the microenvironment of the stump trigger chronic inflammation in the remnant mucosa, its severity gradually decreasing away from the anastomosis [41]. According to some authors, this mechanism seems to be particularly significant in carcinogenesis after B2 reconstruction, as precancerous lesions and cancer are often found at the anastomosis [19,42]. Hammar [43] analyzed the primary location of gastric carcinoma and precancerous alterations in the gastric stump of 56 B2 and 5 B1 patients. The most frequent site of GSC following B2 was right at the anastomosis. Regardless of the adopted technique of reconstruction, however, the location of GSC was often not at the anastomosis but at a site between the lesser curve and the posterior wall of the stump, corresponding to the location of the primary carcinoma of the proximal third of the stomach (PUGC) [18]. These findings suggest that pre-existing atrophic-metaplastic alterations of the mucosa, rather than biliopancreatic reflux, are the most likely cause of GSC [12]. As suggested by Kondo [44], GSC after gastrectomy for cancer, in addition to arising earlier after surgery, is non-anastomotic when compared to GSC after resection for benign diseases.

1.3. Gastric Stump Cancer: The Issue of Synchronous Multiple Gastric Cancers

Patients receiving surgical treatment for cancer already harbor, at the time of their surgery, alterations in the residual gastric mucosa which can have some relationship with primary cancer. The importance of synchronous multiple gastric cancers has also been highlighted. Fujita et al. [13] noted a higher incidence of GSC in patients with less differentiated synchronous multiple gastric cancers at primary surgery, compared to patients with single well-differentiated tumors (respectively $p < 0.05$ and $p < 0.05$). Nevertheless, in two series of 639 patients with distal EGC, secondary lesions were rarely found and no patient with distal EGC showed a secondary synchronous cancer in the upper third of the stomach [45,46]. Once again, although there are similar features in PUGC and GSC, both arising in the same gastric mucosa area, the incidence of PUGC decreases parallel to the incidence of gastric carcinoma in general, although PUGC represents only 3–4% of all gastric malignancies [47–50]. Some authors have shown that a few genetic alterations cause gastric metaplastic lesions, which are considered precursors of cancer, while others influence the proliferation and aggressiveness of gastric cancer [51–55]. It has been hypothesized that the onset of GSC can be related to these genetic predispositions [13]. Matsui et al. suggested that reflux is the major cause of GSC in patients receiving hemigastrectomy for benign disease, whereas, in those operated for cancer, if GSC appears ≥ 10 years later, this could be related to genetic factors (such as p53), responsible for multiple metachronous carcinogenesis, while if GSC occurs <10 years, this new cancer could be caused by diffuse metaplastic lesions of the residual mucosa [56]. Molecular studies [57,58] have shown an incidence of micro satellite instability in patients with GSC higher than in those with PUGC. It is impossible to verify the existence of residual malignant cells or potentially malignant mucosal fields at the time of gastric resection. It can be hypothesized that these pathways of carcinogenesis could have remained silent and inactive if the anatomic and functional alterations produced by surgery had not occurred.

1.4. Gastric Stump Cancer: Role of HP Infection

The residual post-gastrectomy mucosa is considered hostile to HP; hence HP infection progressively decreases following surgery. This is due to at least three reasons: (1) the antrum, which is the HP natural environment, has been removed; (2) the increased pH due to biliopancreatic reflux inhibits HP proliferation [59–61]; (3) the residual mucosa is replaced by an infection-resistant atrophic-metaplastic epithelium [62]. Some authors think that the spontaneous decrease in the infection starts at the anastomosis, where the gastric mucosa changes from the characteristics of infective chronic active gastritis to those of reflux gastritis (foveolar hyperplasia, congestion, paucity of inflammatory infiltrate, glandular cystic dilatation) [43]. Suh et al. have shown the spontaneous disappearance of infection in 38.6% of 70 patients within 18 months from distal gastrectomy [63], while in another study [60], the prevalence of HP infection varied over time following surgery, being 29.5% less than 25 years after gastric resection, 13.6% from 16 to 30 years after surgery, and 10% > 30 years later. In the published literature, however, the rates of gastric stump infection fall within a broad range. Indeed, according to some authors, overall HP infection occurs in 50–68.2% of distal-gastrectomy patients, in 55–72% of B1 patients, in 58–66% of B2, and in 26% of patients reconstructed by R-Y surgery [31,60,62,64]. In a review of 36 studies on partial gastrectomy for gastric ulcer, HP infection occurred in 50% of cases after surgery (range from 19% to 73%) [65]. In another research, HP infection rate was 71% after B1, and 46% after B2 [66]. Other authors have confirmed HP infection rates in patients treated by B2 lower than those observed in subjects treated by B1 or R-Y reconstruction [66,67]. Chan et al. [31] showed that R-Y reconstruction causes less reflux during fasting and in the postprandial period, and a lower incidence of HP gastric stump infection than B2 reconstruction, even when B2 is associated with Braun's anastomosis. These conflicting results can be explained by differences in HP infection diagnostic methods in resected stomachs. In these instances, diagnosis of HP infection is less accurate with the urease breath test (UBT) than histology, while the rapid urease test (RUT) is more accurate than histology [68]. However, it should also be considered that the accuracy of biopsies is altered by patchy and uneven distribution of HP infection in the gastric mucosa [69] and by the number of biopsies taken. As reported by Chun et al. [70], following partial gastrectomy for cancer, UBT was comparable to RUT in terms of accuracy (UBT 87%, RUT 72%). High levels of anti-HP antibodies can be found in the serum, even when infection is not detected by microscopic examination or by culture methods [64]. Diagnosis of infection using enzyme immunoassay for HP antigen in stools appears to be a highly reliable test in gastrectomy patients, capable of detecting both the presence of infection and the success of post-treatment HP eradication [71]. Furthermore, based on the accepted role of HP infection in gastric carcinogenesis [72–74] (HP infection being found in 54–71% of cases of primitive gastric carcinoma), it has been hypothesized that HP eradication in gastrectomy patients could prevent the development of GSC. The Maastricht IV/ Florence Consensus Report and the Second Asia-Pacific Consensus Guidelines both recommend eradication of HP infection from the gastric stump [75,76]. However, it has also been highlighted that the role of the microorganism in the development of GSC is different from primitive gastric cancer in the intact stomach, where HP promotes carcinogenesis through the cytotoxin-associated gene A or CagA protein, which acts as a growth factor for the cells of the gastric mucosa [77,78]. Due to the reduced levels of the microorganism in the partial-gastrectomy patients, it is unlikely that HP plays here the same carcinogenic role as in the intact stomach [59,79–82]. There are data, however, confirming the importance of HP infection also in the development of gastritis in the gastric stump. Our research group has shown that in 151 partial-gastrectomy peptic ulcer patients, after a mean interval of 25 years from surgery, there was a 10-fold increase in the prevalence of normal mucosa in HP-negative (22.0%) vs. HP-positive (2.4%) patients, and the prevalence of intestinal metaplasia was four times higher in HP-positive than in HP-negative patients (19.6% vs 4.6%) [83]. In another endoscopic study assessing 187 peptic ulcer hemi-gastrectomy patients (mean interval from surgery = 27.8 years) or distal gastric cancer patients (mean interval from surgery = 7.6 years), we observed that chronic atrophic gastritis, intestinal metaplasia, and dysplasia are more common in the HP-positive group (OR 2.37, $p = 0.007$) [84]. However, HP-positive patients resected for cancer showed a higher risk of atrophic/metaplastic/dysplastic lesions compared to both HP-negative cancer patients (OR 4.20) and to HP-negative and HP-positive patients resected for peptic ulcer (OR 1.59). The concentration of interleukin (IL)-8, a marker for inflammation, in the residual gastric mucosa three months after surgery, was significantly higher in B1-B2 than in R-Y reconstruction and in HP-positive compared to HP-negative patients.

1.5. Gastric Stump Cancer: Combined and Synergic Role of HP Infection and of Biliopancreatic Reflux

Biliopancreatic reflux and HP infection are considered independent risk factors for the development of gastritis-metaplastic lesions of the gastric stump [85]. Hamaguchi et al. [86] studied 12 cases of gastrectomy with B1 reconstruction for EGC resulting HP-positive after resection; one- and six-months after eradication, significant improvements of the mucosal erythema at endoscopy ($p = 0.038$) and of the gastritis activity at histology ($p < 0.0001$) were observed compared to pre-eradication findings. In another study on eight patients with B1 reconstruction for carcinoma, following confirmed UBT eradication, the microscopic features of chronic inflammation improved progressively over a period of 9 years in both greater and lesser curves of the gastric stump. The improvement of these potentially precancerous alterations might inhibit the development of metachronous cancer [87]. However, in resected patients, there is a possible synergic role of both biliopancreatic reflux and HP infection in the development of lesions of gastric mucosa. The relative importance of each of them in the development of metaplastic-atrophic lesions has not yet been established, and it is likely that these mucosal alterations, representing a morphological point of no return, may not be repaired by eradication alone [88]. In HP-positive patients, infection is one of the risk factors contributing to carcinogenesis, and its eradication decreases the damage to the gastric mucosa, mainly by reducing inflammation. There is no guarantee of a similar positive effects for metaplastic-atrophic lesions [89–92], and simple improvement of some features of mucosal inflammation might not suffice to prevent metachronous carcinoma [93]. Johannesson et al. [81] studied 29 partial gastrectomy patients (5 B1 and 24 B2). These patients were re-resected with a R-Y reconstruction, due to reflux gastritis or to severe dysplasia/EGC, at a median interval of 19 years from index surgery. The aim of this research was to investigate the effect of bile diversion and of HP infection on histological features of anastomotic biopsies taken 5–17 years after re-operation. Regarding the surgical specimen of re-resection, the follow-up biopsies showed an unchanged prevalence of infection but an increase in active chronic gastritis, atrophy, intestinal metaplasia, and dysplasia. The HP status, however, had no effect on the progression of active chronic gastritis, atrophy, and intestinal metaplasia. A significant increase in dysplasia as such was observed in HP-positive patients, while prevalence of both moderate and severe grades of dysplasia were not related to HP status. In any case, a significant reduction of gastric carcinoma was achieved in non-operated stomachs by the eradication of HP infection, as long as metaplastic-atrophic-dysplastic lesions were absent [88]. Therefore, eradication should be completed rapidly to inhibit the development and progression of pre-cancerous lesions [94,95]. GSC may occur even in patients with resected stomachs as part of pancreatoduodenectomy for malignant disease. Pflüger et al. found six cases of GSC out of

4414 cases treated at their institution from 2000 until 2015 for pancreatic malignancy [96]. Nevertheless, GSC in these situations is rare, simply because of the grim prognosis and short life expectancy of these patients.

1.6. HP Infection and Metachronous Carcinoma following Endoscopic Resection of EGC

There are no data confirming the beneficial role of HP eradication when comparing metachronous gastric cancer in eradicated vs. non-eradicated HP-positive partial-gastrectomy cancer patients, while there are interesting data on the impact of eradication of HP infection on the incidence of metachronous gastric cancer following endoscopic resection of EGC. After endoscopic resection, the residual gastric mucosa represents a potential site for metaplastic-atrophic lesions. In these circumstances, metachronous carcinomas may occur more frequently, while it cannot be ruled out that undetected synchronous cancers, already present, are left untreated. In a non-randomized study on 132 HP-seropositive patients after endoscopic resection of EGC, Uemura et al. [97] completed oral HP eradication therapy on 65 of these 132. In the treated group, endoscopic biopsies from the antrum and the greater curvature 6 months after eradication showed a significant reduction of neutrophilic infiltration ($p < 0.01$) and of the severity of metaplasia ($p < 0.05$), while in the non-treated group (67 patients), there were six cases of metachronous gastric cancer over a period of 48 months, compared to no cases in the treated group ($p < 0.01$). In a retrospective multicenter study, Nakagawa et al. [98] analyzed the incidence of metachronous gastric carcinoma in 2835 patients endoscopically resected for EGC. At a mean follow-up of 2 years, metachronous carcinoma was found in 5% of 2469 non-HP eradicated patients and in 2% of 356 successfully eradicated subjects ($p = 0.021$). In a series of 176 patients with EGC endoscopically treated [99], nine cases of metachronous gastric carcinoma were detected after a mean period of 30 months following treatment. In the univariate analysis, age >70 years ($p = 0.015$) and the presence of severe mucosal atrophy of the gastric body ($p = 0.031$) and antrum ($p = 0.008$) were significantly linked to metachronous malignancy. In the multivariate analysis, the degree of antrum atrophy was confirmed as an independent risk factor for metachronous carcinoma ($p = 0.011$). In relation to HP infection, four metachronous gastric cancers were found in 94 patients to have been successfully eradicated after endoscopic resection, and in 2 of 22 non-treated patients (p = not significant). In a multicenter, open label, randomized controlled trial [100], Fukase et al. analyzed the prophylactic role of HP eradication on the incidence of metachronous gastric carcinoma following endoscopic resection for EGC. In the studied population of 505 patients, 255 belonged to the eradication group (203 of whom had their cancer successfully eradicated), and 250 patients were controls. During a 3-year follow-up after endoscopic resection, metachronous carcinoma developed in 9 of the 203 eradicated patients and in 24 of the 250 controls (HR 0.399 $p = 0.003$). Similar trends were reported by Maehata et al. [93] in 268 patients followed-up for a mean period of 3 years after endoscopic resection for EGC. Over an 11-year term, metachronous gastric carcinomas were detected in 13 of 91 non-successfully eradicated patients, and in 15 of 177 successfully eradicated subjects (p = not significant). In 10 of the 15 eradicated patients who developed metachronous gastric cancer, this developed more than 5 years after endoscopic resection of the primary malignancy. In the multivariate analysis, in addition to the post-treatment interval, an independent risk factor for metachronous gastric carcinoma was represented by severe gastric atrophy at the time of endoscopic resection. These results suggest that HP eradication delays but does not completely protect against later development of a malignancy if the residual mucosa already suffers from atrophic lesions. Besides, another study on patients endoscopically resected for EGC, found no significant differences in metachronous carcinoma between 263 eradicated and 105 non-eradicated patients, over a period of 60 months [101]. More recently, Li and Yu, reviewing 15 years of literature, suggested that eradication of HP infection after endoscopic resection of EGC could reduce the incidence of metachronous precancerous lesions and of metachronous gastric cancer [102]. Hence, the role of HP in chronic gastritis, peptic ulcer disease and gastric cancer is, once again, confirmed, while its importance for many types of extra-gastric disease still remains poorly researched [103].

2. Conclusions

Following distal gastric resection, the microenvironment of the gastric stump changes dramatically, due to both the new anatomy and to the consequences of surgery on the residual gastric stump, which favor biliopancreatic reflux. The presence of HP infection gradually decreases following surgery but contributes, together with reflux, to damage the residual gastric mucosa. Under these influences, the gastric epithelium becomes a site for metaplastic-atrophic lesions, referable to either the pre- or the post-operative phases, which can be considered as precursors for cancer. Eradication of HP infection can prevent or delay both the development of precancerous lesions and their favoring role on carcinogenesis. There is a lack of studies evaluating the effect of eradication therapy in preventing GSC in hemi-gastrectomy cancer patients, HP-positives after surgery. As we have already emphasized, ours is only a non-systematic, narrative review of the local outcome of gastric resected patients, and, therefore, our research is probably biased, at least to some extent. Nevertheless, we would like to stress that our purpose was to provide an exhaustive and informative review, still important for definition of the problem and for stressing the role of HP and of the new local environment in the development of further malignancy, which has important clinical implications.

Author Contributions: All of the above authors have substantially contributed to the conception, design, and acquisition of data. All of the above authors drafted the article and revised it critically for important intellectual content. All authors have read and agreed to the published version of the manuscript.

Funding: This research received no external funding.

Institutional Review Board Statement: Not applicable.

Informed Consent Statement: Not applicable.

Conflicts of Interest: The authors declare no conflict of interest.

References

1. Busman, D.C. Theodor Billroth 1829–1894. *Acta Chir. Belg.* **2006**, *106*, 743–752. [CrossRef] [PubMed]
2. Nagayo, T. *Histogenesis and Precursors of Human Gastric Cancer: Research and Practice*; Springer: Berlin, Germany, 1986.
3. Yoshino, K. History of gastric cancer surgery. *J. Jpn. Surg. Soc.* **2000**, *101*, 855–860.
4. Safatle-Ribeiro, A.V.; Ribeiro, U.; Reynolds, J.C. Gastric stump cancer: What is the risk? *Dig. Dis.* **1998**, *16*, 159–168. [CrossRef] [PubMed]
5. Marshall, B.J.; Warren, J.R. Unidentified curved bacilli in the stomach of patients with gastritis and peptic ulceration. *Lancet* **1984**, *1*, 1311–1315. [CrossRef]
6. Ishikawa, M.; Ogata, S.; Harada, M.; Sakakihara, Y. Changes in surgical strategies for peptic ulcers before and after the introduction of H2-receptor antagonists and endoscopic hemostasis. *Surg. Today* **1995**, *25*, 318–323. [CrossRef]
7. Wyllie, J.H.; Clark, C.G.; Alexander-Williams, J.; Bell, P.R.; Kennedy, T.L.; Kirk, R.M.; MacKay, C. Effect of cimetidine on surgery for duodenal ulcer. *Lancet* **1981**, *1*, 1307–1308. [CrossRef]
8. Kleeff, J.; Friess, H.; Büchler, M.W. How *Helicobacter pylori* changed the life of surgeons. *Dig. Surg.* **2002**, *20*, 93–102. [CrossRef]
9. Balfour, D.C. Factors influencing the life expectancy of patients operated on for gastric ulcer. *Ann. Surg.* **1922**, *76*, 405–408. [CrossRef]
10. Freedman, M.A.; Berne, C.J. Gastric carcinoma of gastrojejunal stoma. *Gastroenterology* **1954**, *27*, 210–217. [CrossRef]
11. Heinzel, J.; Laqua, H. Magencarcinom Enachfruherner Resektion Wegen Ulcus Ventriculi Bzw. duodeni. *Langenbecks Arch. Chir.* **1954**, *278*, 87–95. [CrossRef]
12. Ohashi, H.; Katai, H.; Fukagawa, T.; Gotoda, T.; Sano, T.; Sasako, M. Cancer of the gastric stump following distal gastrectomy for cancer. *Br. J. Surg.* **2007**, *94*, 92–95. [CrossRef] [PubMed]
13. Fujita, T.; Gotohda, N.; Takahashi, S.; Nakagohri, T.; Konishi, M.; Kinoshita, T. Relationship between the histological type of initial lesions and the risk for the development of remnant gastric cancers after gastrectomy for synchronous multiple gastric cancers. *World J. Surg.* **2010**, *34*, 296–302. [CrossRef] [PubMed]
14. Japanese Research Society for Gastric Cancer and Japanese Gastric Cancer Association. *(1972–2001) Statistical Report of Nationwide Registry of Gastric Carcinoma*; National Cancer Center: Tokyo, Japan, No. 1-54. (In Japanese)
15. Japanese Gastric Cancer Association Registration Committee; Maruyama, K.; Hayashi, K.; Isobe, Y. Gastric cancer treated in 1991 in Japan: Analysis of nationwide registry. *Gastric Cancer* **2006**, *9*, 51–66. [PubMed]

16. Msika, S.; Benhamiche, A.M.; Jouve, J.L.; Rat, P.; Faivre, J. Prognostic factors after curative resection for gastric cancer. A population-based study. *Eur. J. Cancer* **2000**, *36*, 390–396. [CrossRef]
17. Kaneko, K.; Kondo, H.; Saito, D.; Shirao, K.; Yamaguchi, H.; Yokota, T.; Yamao, G.; Sano, T.; Sasako, M.; Yoshida, S. Early gastric stump cancer following distal gastrectomy. *Gut* **1998**, *43*, 342–344. [CrossRef]
18. Takeno, S.; Noguchi, T.; Kimura, Y.; Fujiwara, S.; Kubo, N.; Kawahara, K. Early and late gastric cancer arising in the remnant stomach after distal gastrectomy. *Eur. J. Surg. Oncol.* **2006**, *32*, 1191–1194. [CrossRef]
19. Ahn, H.S.; Kim, J.W.; Yoo, M.W.; Park, D.J.; Lee, H.J.; Lee, K.U.; Yang, H.K. Clinicopathological features and surgical outcomes of patients with remnant gastric cancer after a distal gastrectomy. *Ann. Surg. Oncol.* **2008**, *15*, 1632–1639. [CrossRef]
20. Tanigawa, N.; Nomura, E.; Lee, S.W.; Kaminishi, M.; Sugiyama, M.; Aikou, T.; Kitajima, M. Current state of gastric stump carcinoma in Japan: Based on the results of a nationwide survey. *World J. Surg.* **2010**, *34*, 1540–1547. [CrossRef]
21. Ojima, T.; Iwahashi, M.; Nakamori, M.; Nakamura, M.; Naka, T.; Katsuda, M.; Iida, T.; Tsuji, T.; Hayata, K.; Takifuji, K.; et al. Clinicopathological characteristics of remnant gastric cancer after a distal gastrectomy. *J. Gastrointest. Surg.* **2010**, *14*, 277–281. [CrossRef]
22. Komatsu, S.; Ichikawa, D.; Okamoto, K.; Ikoma, D.; Tsujiura, M.; Nishimura, Y.; Murayama, Y.; Shiozaki, A.; Ikoma, H.; Kuriu, Y. Progression of remnant gastric cancer is associated with duration of follow-up following distal gastrectomy. *World J. Gastroenterol.* **2012**, *18*, 2832–2836. [CrossRef]
23. Li, F.; Zhang, R.; Liang, H.; Zhao, J.; Liu, H.; Quan, J.; Wang, X.; Xue, Q. A retrospective clinicopathologic study of remnant gastric cancer after distal gastrectomy. *Am. J. Clin. Oncol.* **2013**, *36*, 244–249. [CrossRef] [PubMed]
24. Tokudome, S.; Kono, S.; Ikeda, M.; Kuratsune, M.; Sano, C.; Inokuchi, K.; Kodama, Y.; Ichimiya, H.; Nakayama, F.; Kaibara, N.; et al. A prospective study on primary gastric stump cancer following partial gastrectomy for benign gastroduodenal diseases. *Cancer Res.* **1984**, *44*, 2208–2212. [PubMed]
25. Asano, A.; Mizuno, S.; Sasaki, R.; Aoki, K.; Yokoyama, H.; Yokoyama, Y. The long term prognosis of patients gastrectomized for benign gastroduodenal diseases. *Jpn. J. Cancer Res.* **1987**, *78*, 337–348. [PubMed]
26. Caygill, C.P.J.; Kirkhama, J.S.; Hilla, M.J.; Northfielda, T.C. Mortality from gastric cancer following gastric surgery for peptic ulcer. *Lancet* **1986**, *327*, 929–931. [CrossRef]
27. Toftgaard, C. Gastric cancer after peptic ulcer surgery. A historic prospective cohort investigation. *Ann. Surg.* **1989**, *210*, 159–164. [CrossRef]
28. Kondo, K.; Yamauchi, M.; Sasaki, R.; Akiyama, S.; Watanabe, T.; Yokoyama, Y.; Takagi, H. Statistical and pathological study of carcinoma in the gastric remnant. *Nippon Shoukaigeka Gakkai Zasshi Jpn. J. Gastroenterol. Surg.* **1991**, *24*, 2105–2112. (In Japanese with English abstract) [CrossRef]
29. O'Connor, H.J.; Dixon, M.F.; Wyatt, J.I.; Axon, A.T.; Ward, D.C.; Dewar, E.P. Effect of duodenal ulcer surgery and enterogastric reflux on Campylobacter pyloridis. *Lancet* **1986**, *2*, 1178–1181. [CrossRef]
30. Vogel, S.B.; Drane, W.E.; Woodward, E.R. Clinical and radionuclide evaluation of bile diversion by Braun enteroenterostomy: Prevention and treatment of alkaline reflux gastritis. An alternative to Roux-en-Y diversion. *Ann. Surg.* **1994**, *219*, 458–466. [CrossRef]
31. Chan, D.C.; Fan, Y.M.; Lin, C.K.; Chen, C.J.; Chen, C.Y.; Chao, Y.C. Roux-en-Y Reconstruction after Distal Gastrectomy to Reduce Enterogastric Reflux and Helicobacter pylori infection. *J. Gastrointest. Surg.* **2007**, *11*, 1732–1740. [CrossRef]
32. Hollands, M.J.; Filipe, I.; Edwards, S.; Brame, K.; Maisey, M.; Owen, W.J. Clinical and histological sequelae of Roux-en-Y diversion. *Br. J. Surg.* **1989**, *76*, 481–484. [CrossRef]
33. Kondo, K.; Suzuki, H.; Nagayo, T. The influence of gastro-jejunal anastomosis on gastric carcinogenesis in rats. *Jpn. J. Cancer Res.* **1984**, *75*, 362–369.
34. Salmon, R.J.; Merle, S.; Zafrani, B.; Decosse, J.J.; Sherloch, P.; Deschner, E.E. Gastric carcinogenesis induced by N-methyl-N-nitrosoguanidine: Role of gastrectomy and duodenal reflux. *Jpn. J. Cancer Res.* **1985**, *76*, 167–172. [PubMed]
35. Mason, R.C. Duodenogastric reflux in rat gastric carcinoma. *Br. J. Surg.* **1986**, *73*, 801–803. [CrossRef] [PubMed]
36. Mason, R.C.; Filipe, I. The aetiology of gastric stump carcinoma in the rat. *Scand. J. Gastroenterol.* **1990**, *25*, 961–965. [CrossRef] [PubMed]
37. Kojima, H.; Kondo, K.; Takagi, H. The influence of reflux of bile and pancreatic juice on gastric carcinogenesis in rats. *Nippon Geka Gakkai Zasshi (J. Jpn. Surg. Soc.)* **1990**, *91*, 818–826. (In Japanese with English abstract)
38. Sinning, C.; Schaefer, N.; Standop, J.; Hirner, A.; Wolff, M. Gastric stump carcinoma—Epidemiology and current concepts in pathogenesis and treatment. *Eur. J. Surg. Oncol.* **2007**, *33*, 133–139. [CrossRef]
39. Uchiyama, K.; Onishi, H.; Tani, M.; Kinoshita, H.; Kawai, M.; Ueno, M.; Yamaue, H. Long-term prognosis after treatment of patients with choledocholithiasis. *Ann. Surg.* **2003**, *238*, 97–102. [CrossRef]
40. Muscroft, T.J.; Deane, S.A.; Youngs, D.; Burdon, D.W.; Keighley, M.R. The microflora of the postoperative stomach. *Br. J. Surg.* **1981**, *68*, 560–564. [CrossRef]
41. Bechi, P.; Amorosi, A.; Mazzanti, R.; Romagnoli, P.; Tonelli, L. Gastric histology and fasting bile reflux after partial gastrectomy. *Gastroenterology* **1987**, *93*, 335–343. [CrossRef]
42. Sitarz, R.; Maciejewski, R.; Polkowski, W.P.; Offerhaus, G.J. A Gastroenterostoma after Billroth antrectomy as a premalignant condition. *World J. Gastroenterol.* **2012**, *18*, 3201–3206.
43. Hammar, E. The localization of precancerous changes and carcinoma after previous gastric operation for benign condition. *Acta Pathol. Microbiol. Scand. A* **1976**, *84*, 495–507. [CrossRef] [PubMed]
44. Kondo, K. Duodenogastric reflux and gastric stump carcinoma. *Gastric Cancer* **2002**, *5*, 16–22. [CrossRef] [PubMed]
45. Morgagni, P.; Marfisi, C.; Gardini, A.; Marrelli, D.; Saragoni, L.; Roviello, F.; Vittimberga, G.; Garcea, D. Subtotal gastrectomy as treatment for distal multifocal early gastric cancer. *J. Gastrointest. Surg.* **2009**, *13*, 2239–2244. [CrossRef] [PubMed]

46. Morgagni, P.; Gardini, A.; Marrelli, D.; Vittimberga, G.; Marchet, A.; de Manzoni, G.; Di Cosmo, M.A.; Rossi, G.M.; Garcea, D.; Roviello, F. Gastric stump carcinoma after distal subtotal gastrectomy for early gastric cancer: Experience of 541 patients with long-term follow-up. *Am. J. Surg.* **2015**, *209*, 1063–1068. [CrossRef] [PubMed]
47. Ferretti, S.; Gafa, L. Upper gastrointestinal tract cancers: Oesophagus, stomach, liver, gallbladder and biliary ducts, pancreas. *Epidemiol. Prev.* **2004**, *28* (Suppl. S2), 34–42.
48. Corley, D.A.; Kubo, A. Influence of site classification on cancer incidence rates: An analysis of gastric cardia carcinomas. *J. Natl. Cancer Inst.* **2004**, *96*, 1383–1387. [CrossRef]
49. Bottcher, K.; Roder, J.D.; Busch, R. Epidemiologie des magenkarzinomsauschirurgischersicht. Ergebnisse der Deutschen Magenkarzinom-Studie von 1992. *Dtsch. Med. Wochenschr.* **1993**, *118*, 729–736. [CrossRef]
50. Fuchs, C.S.; Mayer, R.J. Gastric carcinoma. *N. Engl. J. Med.* **1995**, *333*, 32–41. [CrossRef]
51. Hamamoto, T.; Yokozaki, H.; Semba, S.; Yasui, W.; Yunotani, S.; Miyazaki, K.; Tahara, E. Altered microsatellites in incomplete-type intestinal metaplasia adjacent to primary gastric cancers. *J. Clin. Pathol.* **1997**, *50*, 841–846. [CrossRef]
52. Zhe, J.; Gen, T.; Michiko, S.; Toru, M.; Takayuki, M.; Masahiro, H.; Mitsumasa, O.; Kiyonari, O.; Shin-ya, O.; Yasushi, E.; et al. Absence of BAT-26 instability in gastric intestinal metaplasia. *Pathol. Int.* **2001**, *51*, 473–475.
53. Choi, S.W.; Choi, J.R.; Chung, Y.J. Prognostic implications of microsatellite genotypes in gastric carcinoma. *Int. J. Cancer* **2000**, *89*, 378–383. [CrossRef]
54. Candusso, M.E.; Luinetti, O.; Villani, L.; Alberizzi, P.; Klersy, C.; Fiocca, R.; Ranzani, G.N.; Solcia, E. Loss of heterozygosity at 18q21 region in gastric cancer involves a number of cancer-related genes and correlates with stage and histology, but lacks independent prognostic value. *J. Pathol.* **2002**, *197*, 44–50. [CrossRef]
55. Sepulveda, A.R.; Santos, A.C.; Yamaoka, Y.; Wu, L.; Gutierrez, O.; Kim, J.G.; Graham, D.Y. Marked differences in the frequency of microsatellite instability in gastric cancer from different countries. *Am. J. Gastroenterol.* **1999**, *94*, 3034–3038. [CrossRef]
56. Matsui, N.; Yao, T.; Akazawa, K.; Nawata, H.; Tsuneyoshi, M. Different characteristics of carcinoma in the gastric remnant: Histochemical and immunohistochemical studies. *Oncol. Rep.* **2001**, *8*, 17–26. [CrossRef] [PubMed]
57. Nakachi, A.; Miyazato, H.; Shimoji, H.; Hiroyasu, S.; Isa, T.; Shiraishi, M.; Muto, Y. Microsatellite instability in patients with gastric remnant cancer. *Gastric Cancer* **1999**, *2*, 210–214. [CrossRef] [PubMed]
58. Aya, M.; Yashiro, M.; Nishioka, N.; Onoda, N.; Hirakawa, K. Carcinogenesis in the remnant stomach following distal gastrectomy with Billroth II reconstruction is associated with high-level microsatellite instability. *Anticancer Res.* **2006**, *26*, 1403–1411.
59. Fukuhara, K.; Osugi, H.; Takada, N.; Takemura, M.; Lee, S.; Taguchi, S.; Kaneko, M.; Tanaka, Y.; Fujiwara, Y.; Nishizawa, S.; et al. Duodenogastric reflux eradicates Helicobacter pylori after distal gastrectomy. *Hepatogastroenterology* **2004**, *51*, 1548–1550.
60. Bair, M.J.; Wu, M.S.; Chang, W.H.; Shih, S.C.; Wang, T.E.; Chen, C.J.; Lin, C.C.; Liu, C.Y.; Chen, M.J. Spontaneous clearance of Helicobacter pylori colonization in patients with partial gastrectomy: Correlates with operative procedures and duration after operation. *J. Formos. Med. Assoc.* **2009**, *108*, 13–19. [CrossRef]
61. Abe, H.; Murakami, K.; Satoh, S.; Sato, R.; Kodama, M.; Arita, T.; Fujioka, T. Influence of bile reflux and Helicobacter pylori infection on gastritis in the remnant gastric mucosa after distal gastrectomy. *J. Gastroenterol.* **2005**, *40*, 563–569. [CrossRef]
62. Onoda, N.; Maeda, K.; Sawada, T.; Wakasa, K.; Arakawa, T.; Chung, K.H. Prevalence of Helicobacter pylori infection in gastric remnant after distal gastrectomy for primary gastric cancer. *Gastric Cancer* **2001**, *4*, 87–92. [CrossRef]
63. Suh, S.; Nah, J.C.; Uhm, M.S.; Jung, Y.M.; Kim, N.; Lee, D.H.; Jung, H.C.; Song, I.S. Changes in prevalence of Helicobacter pylori infection after subtotal gastrectomy. *Hepatogastroenterology* **2012**, *59*, 646–648. [PubMed]
64. Matsukura, N.; Tajiri, T.; Kato, S.; Togashi, A.; Masuda, G.; Fujita, I.; Tokunaga, A.; Yamada, N. Helicobacter pylori eradication therapy for the remnant stomach after gastrectomy. *Gastric Cancer* **2003**, *6*, 100–107. [CrossRef] [PubMed]
65. Danesh, J.; Appleby, P.; Peto, R. How often does surgery for peptic ulceration eradicate Helicobacter pylori? Systematic review of 36 studies. *BMJ* **1998**, *316*, 746–747. [CrossRef] [PubMed]
66. Tomtitchong, P.; Onda, M.; Matsukura, N.; Tokunaga, A.; Kato, S.; Matsuhisa, T.; Yamada, N.; Hayashi, A. Helicobacter pylori infection in the remnant stomach after gastrectomy: With special reference to the difference between Billroth I and II anastomoses. *J. Clin. Gastroenterol.* **1998**, *27*, 154–158. [CrossRef]
67. Offerhaus, G.J.; Rieu, P.N.; Jansen, J.B.; Joosten, H.J.; Lamers, C.B. Prospective comparative study of the influence of postoperative bile reflux on gastric mucosal histology and Campylobacter pylori infection. *Gut* **1989**, *30*, 1552–1557. [CrossRef]
68. Adamopoulos, A.B.; Stergiou, G.S.; Sakizlis, G.N.; Tiniakos, D.G.; Nasothimiou, E.G.; Sioutis, D.K.; Achimastos, A.D. Diagnostic value of rapid urease test and urea breath test for Helicobacter pylori detection in patients with Billroth II gastrectomy: A prospective controlled trial. *Dig. Liver Dis.* **2009**, *41*, 4–8. [CrossRef]
69. Morris, A.; Ali, M.R.; Brown, P.; Lane, M.; Patton, K. Campylobacter pylori infection in biopsy specimens of gastric antrum: Laboratory diagnosis and estimation of sampling error. *J. Clin. Pathol.* **1989**, *42*, 727–732. [CrossRef]
70. Chun, H.J.; Park, S. Helicobacter pylori infection following partial gastrectomy for gastric cancer. *World J. Gastroenterol.* **2014**, *20*, 2765–2770.
71. Nakagawara, H.; Miwa, K.; Nakamura, S.; Hattori, T. Duodenogastric reflux sustains Helicobacter pylori infection in the gastric stump. *Scand. J. Gastroenterol.* **2003**, *38*, 931–937.
72. Uemura, N.; Okamoto, S.; Yamamoto, S.; Matsumura, N.; Yamaguchi, S.; Yamakido, M.; Taniyama, K.; Sasaki, N.; Schlemper, R.J. Helicobacter pylori infection and the development of gastric cancer. *N. Engl. J. Med.* **2001**, *345*, 784–789. [CrossRef]

73. Forman, D.; Newell, D.G.; Fullerton, F.; Yarnell, J.W.; Stacey, A.R.; Wald, N.; Sitas, F. Association between infection with Helicobacter pylori and risk of gastric cancer: Evidence from a prospective investigation. *BMJ* **1991**, *302*, 1302–1305. [CrossRef] [PubMed]
74. Parsonnet, J.; Friedman, G.D.; Vandersteen, D.P.; Chang, Y.; Vogelman, J.H.; Orentreich, N.; Sibley, R.K. Helicobacter pylori infection and the risk of gastric carcinoma. *N. Engl. J. Med.* **1991**, *325*, 1127–1131. [CrossRef] [PubMed]
75. Malfertheiner, P.; Megraud, F.; O'Morain, C.A.; Atherton, J.; Axon, A.T.; Bazzoli, F.; Gensini, G.F.; Gisbert, J.P.; Graham, D.Y.; Rokkas, T. Management of Helicobacter pylori infection—The Maastricht IV/Florence Consensus Report. *Gut* **2012**, *61*, 646–664. [CrossRef]
76. Fock, K.M.; Talley, N.; Moayyedi, P.; Hunt, R.; Azuma, T.; Sugano, K.; Xiao, S.D.; Lam, S.K.; Goh, K.L.; Chiba, T.; et al. Asia-Pacific consensus guidelines on gastric cancer prevention. *J. Gastroenterol. Hepatol.* **2008**, *23*, 351–365. [CrossRef] [PubMed]
77. Asaka, M.; Dragosics, B.A. Helicobacter pylori and gastric malignancies. *Helicobacter* **2004**, *9*, 35–41. [CrossRef] [PubMed]
78. Sugiyama, T. Development of gastric cancer associated with Helicobacter pylori infection. *Cancer Chemother. Pharmacol.* **2004**, *54*, 12–20. [CrossRef] [PubMed]
79. Baas, I.O.; van Rees, B.P.; Musler, A.; Craanen, M.E.; Tytgat, G.N.; van den Berg, F.M.; Offerhaus, G.J. Helicobacter pylori and Epstein–Barr virus infection and the p53 tumor suppressor pathway in gastric stump cancer compared with carcinoma in the non-operated stomach. *J. Clin. Pathol.* **1998**, *51*, 662–666. [CrossRef]
80. van Rees, B.P.; Musler, A.; Caspers, E.; Drillenburg, P.; Craanen, M.E.; Polkowski, W.; Chibowski, D.; Offerhaus, G.J. K-Ras mutations in gastric stump carcinomas and in carcinomas from the non-operated stomach. *Hepatogastroenterology* **1999**, *46*, 2063–2068.
81. Johannesson, K.A.; Hammar, E.; Staël von Holstein, C. Mucosal changes in the gastric remnant: Long-term effects of bile reflux diversion and Helicobacter pylori infection. *Eur. J. Gastroenterol. Hepatol.* **2003**, *15*, 35–40. [CrossRef]
82. Katsube, T.; Ogawa, K.; Hamaguchi, K.; Murayama, M.; Konnno, S.; Shimakawa, T.; Naritaka, Y.; Yagawa, H.; Kajiwara, T.; Aiba, M. Prevalence of Helicobacter pylori in the residual stomach after gastrectomy for gastric cancer. *Hepatogastroenterology* **2002**, *49*, 128–132.
83. Giuliani, A.; Caporale, A.; Demoro, M.; Benvenuto, E.; Scarpini, M.; Spada, S.; Angelico, F. Gastric cancer precursor lesions and helicobacter pylori infection in patients with partial gastrectomy for peptic ulcer. *World J. Surg.* **2005**, *29*, 1127–1130. [CrossRef] [PubMed]
84. Giuliani, A.; Galati, G.; Demoro, M.; Scimò, M.; Pecorella, I.; Basso, L. Screening of Helicobacter pylori infection after gastrectomy for cancer or peptic ulcer. *Arch. Surg.* **2010**, *145*, 962–967. [CrossRef] [PubMed]
85. Fukuhara, K.; Osugi, H.; Takada, N.; Takemura, M.; Ohmoto, Y.; Kinoshita, H. Quantitative determinations of duodenogastric reflux, prevalence of Helicobacter pylori infection, and concentrations of interleukin-8. *World J. Surg.* **2003**, *27*, 567–570. [CrossRef] [PubMed]
86. Hamaguchi, K.; Ogawa, K.; Katsube, T.; Konno, S.; Aiba, M. Does eradication of Helicobacter pylori reduce the risk of carcinogenesis in the residual stomach after gastrectomy for early gastric cancer? *Langenbecks Arch. Surg.* **2004**, *389*, 83–91. [CrossRef] [PubMed]
87. Sakakibara, M.; Ando, T.; Ishiguro, K.; Maeda, O.; Watanabe, O.; Hirayama, K.; Nakamura, M.; Miyhara, R.; Goto, H. Usefulness of Helicobacter pylori eradication for precancerous lesions of the gastric remnant. *J. Gastroenterol. Hepatol.* **2014**, *29*, 60–64. [CrossRef] [PubMed]
88. Wong, B.C.Y.; Lam, S.K.; Wong, W.M.; Chen, J.S.; Zheng, T.T.; Feng, R.E.; Lai, K.C.; Hu, W.H.C.; Yuen, S.T.; Leung, S.Y.; et al. Helicobacter pylori eradication to prevent gastric cancer in a high-risk region of China: A randomized controlled trial. *JAMA* **2004**, *291*, 187–194. [CrossRef]
89. Zhou, L.Y.; Lin, S.R.; Ding, S.G.; Huang, X.B.; Zhang, L.; Meng, L.M. The changing trends of the incidence of gastric cancer after Helicobacter pylori eradication in Shandong area. *Chin. J. Dig. Dis.* **2005**, *6*, 114–115. [CrossRef]
90. Mer, R.; Fontham, E.T.H.; Bravo, L.E.; Bravo, J.C.; Piazuelo, M.B.; Camargo, M.C.; Correa, P. Long term follow up of patients treated for Helicobacter pylori infection. *Gut* **2005**, *54*, 1536–1540. [CrossRef]
91. Ito, M.; Haruma, K.; Kamada, T.; Mihara, M.; Kim, S.; Kitadai, Y.; Sumii, M.; Tanaka, S.; Yoshihara, M.; Chayama, K. Helicobacter pylori eradication therapy improves atrophic gastritis and intestinal metaplasia: A 5-year prospective study of patients with atrophic gastritis. *Aliment. Pharmacol. Ther.* **2002**, *16*, 1449–1456. [CrossRef]
92. Sung, J.J.Y.; San-Rin, L.; Ching, J.Y.L.; Li-Ya, Z.; Kar, F.T.; Ren-Ten, W.; Wai, K.L.; Enders, K.W.; James, Y.W.L.; Yuk, T.L.; et al. Atrophy and intestinal metaplasia one year after cure of H. pylori infection: A prospective, randomized study. *Gastroenterology* **2000**, *119*, 7–14. [CrossRef]
93. Maehata, Y.; Nakamura, S.; Fujisawa, K.; Esaki, M.; Moriyama, T.; Asano, K.; Fuyuno, Y.; Yamaguchi, K.; EgashiraIssei Kim, H.; Kanda, M.; et al. Long-term effect of metachronous gastric cancer after endoscopic resection of early gastric cancer. *Gastrointest. Endosc.* **2012**, *75*, 39–46. [CrossRef] [PubMed]
94. Nozaki, K.; Shimizu, N.; Ikehara, Y.; Inoue, M.; Tsukamoto, T.; Inada, K.; Tanaka, H.; Kumagai, T.; Kaminishi, M.; Tatematsu, M. Effect of early eradication on Helicobacter pylori-related gastric carcinogenesis in Mongolian gerbils. *Cancer Sci.* **2003**, *94*, 235–239. [CrossRef]
95. Wu, C.Y.; Kuo, K.N.; Wu, M.S.; Chen, Y.J.; Wang, C.B.; Lin, J.T. Early Helicobacter pylori eradication decreases risk of gastric cancer in patients with peptic ulcer disease. *Gastroenterology* **2009**, *137*, 1641–1648. [CrossRef] [PubMed]
96. Pflüger, M.J.; Felsenstein, M.; Schmocker, R.; Wood, L.D.; Hruban, R.; Fujikura, K.; Rozich, N.; van Oosten, F.; Weiss, M.; Burns, W.; et al. Gastric cancer following pancreaticoduodenectomy: Experience from a high-volume center and review of existing literature. *Surg. Open Sci.* **2020**, *2*, 32–40. [CrossRef] [PubMed]
97. Uemura, N.; Mukai, T.; Okamoto, S.; Yamaguchi, S.; Mashiba, H.; Taniyama, K.; Sasaki, N.; Haruma, K.; Sumii, K.; Kajiyama, G. Effect of Helicobacter pylori eradication on subsequent development of cancer after endoscopic resection of early gastric cancer. *Cancer Epidemiol. Biomarkers Prev.* **1997**, *6*, 639–642. [CrossRef]

98. Nakagawa, S.; Asaka, M.; Kato, M.; Nakamura, M.; Kato, C.; Fujioka, T.; Tatsuta, M.; Keida, K.; Terao, S.; Takahashi, S.; et al. Helicobacter pylori eradication and metachronous gastric cancer after endoscopic mucosal resection of early gastric cancer. *Aliment. Pharmacol. Ther. Symp.* **2006**, *24* (Suppl. S4), 214–218. [CrossRef]
99. Han, J.S.; Jang, J.S.; Choi, S.R.; Kwon, H.C.; Kim, M.C.; Jeong, J.S.; Kim, S.J.; Sohn, Y.J.; Lee, E.J. A study of metachronous cancer after endoscopic resection of early gastric cancer. *Scand. J. Gastroenterol.* **2011**, *46*, 1099–1104. [CrossRef]
100. Fukase, K.; Kato, M.; Kikuchi, S.; Inoue, K.; Uemura, N.; Okamoto, S.; Terao, S.; Amagai, K.; Hayashi, S.; Asaka, M. Effect of eradication of Helicobacter pylori on incidence of metachronous gastric carcinoma after endoscopic resection of early gastric cancer: An open-label, randomised controlled trial. *Lancet* **2008**, *372*, 392–397. [CrossRef]
101. Kato, M.; Nishida, T.; Yamamoto, K.; Hayashi, S.; Kitamura, S.; Yabuta, T.; Yoshio, T.; Nakamura, T.; Komori, M.; Kawai, N.; et al. Scheduled endoscopic surveillance controls secondary cancer after curative endoscopic resection for early gastric cancer: A multicentre retrospective cohort study by Osaka University ESD study group. *Gut* **2013**, *62*, 1425–1432. [CrossRef]
102. Li, L.; Yu, C. *Helicobacter pylori* Infection following Endoscopic Resection of Early Gastric Cancer. *Biomed. Res. Int.* **2019**, *2019*, 9824964. [CrossRef]
103. Mladenova, I. Clinical Relevance of Helicobacter pylori Infection. *J. Clin. Med.* **2021**, *10*, 3473. [CrossRef] [PubMed]

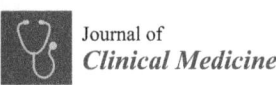

Article

Experience with Rifabutin-Containing Therapy in 500 Patients from the European Registry on *Helicobacter pylori* Management (Hp-EuReg)

Olga P. Nyssen [1], Dino Vaira [2], Ilaria Maria Saracino [2], Giulia Fiorini [2], María Caldas [1], Luis Bujanda [3], Rinaldo Pellicano [4], Alma Keco-Huerga [5], Manuel Pabón-Carrasco [5], Elida Oblitas Susanibar [6], Alfredo Di Leo [7], Giuseppe Losurdo [7], Ángeles Pérez-Aísa [8], Antonio Gasbarrini [9], Doron Boltin [10], Sinead Smith [11], Perminder Phull [12], Theodore Rokkas [13], Dominique Lamarque [14], Anna Cano-Català [15,16], Ignasi Puig [15,16], Francis Mégraud [17], Colm O'Morain [11] and Javier P. Gisbert [1,*]

1. Centro de Investigación Biomédica en Red de Enfermedades Hepáticas y Digestivas (CIBERehd), Hospital Universitario de La Princesa, Instituto de Investigación Sanitaria Princesa (IIS-IP), Universidad Autónoma de Madrid (UAM), 28006 Madrid, Spain; opn.aegredcap@aegastro.es (O.P.N.); m.caldas.a@gmail.com (M.C.)
2. Department of Surgical and Medical Sciences, IRCCS S. Orsola, University of Bologna, 40138 Bologna, Italy; berardino.vaira@unibo.it (D.V.); saracinoilariamaria@gmail.com (I.M.S.); giulia.fiorini@aosp.bo.it (G.F.)
3. Hospital Donostia, Instituto Biodonostia, Centro de Investigación Biomédica en Red de Enfermedades Hepáticas y Digestivas (CIBERehd), Universidad del País Vasco (UPV/EHU), 20014 San Sebastián, Spain; medik@telefonica.net
4. Unit of Gastroenterology, Molinette Hospital, 10126 Turin, Italy; rpellicano@cittadellasalute.to.it
5. Servicio de Gastroenterolgía, Hospital de Valme, 41014 Sevilla, Spain; almakh94@hotmail.com (A.K.-H.); mpabon@cruzroja.es (M.P.-C.)
6. Unit of Gastroenterology, Consorci Sanitari de Terrassa, 08221 Terrassa, Spain; eosusanibar@gmail.com
7. Section of Gastroenterology, Department of Emergency and Organ Transplantation, University Hospital Policlinico Consorziale, 70124 Bari, Italy; alfredo.dileo@uniba.it (A.D.L.); giuseppelos@alice.it (G.L.)
8. Agencia Sanitaria Costa del Sol, Red de Investigación en Servicios de Salud en Enfermedades Crónicas (REDISSEC), 29651 Marbella, Spain; drapereza@hotmail.com
9. Medicina Interna, Fondazione Policlinico Universitario A, Gemelli IRCCS, Università Cattolica del Sacro Cuore, 00168 Roma, Italy; antonio.gasbarrini@unicatt.it
10. Division of Gastroenterology, Rabin Medical Center, Sackler School of Medicine, Tel Aviv University, Tel Aviv 49100, Israel; dboltin@gmail.com
11. Faculty of Health Sciences, Trinity College Dublin, D02PN40 Dublin, Ireland; smithsi@tcd.ie (S.S.); colmomorain@gmail.com (C.O.)
12. Department of Digestive Disorders, Aberdeen Royal Infirmary, Foresterhill Health Campus, Aberdeen AB25 2ZN, UK; p.s.phull@abdn.ac.uk
13. Gastroenterology Clinic, Henry Dunant Hospital, 11526 Athens, Greece; sakkor@otenet.gr
14. Hôpital Ambroise Paré, Université de Versailles St-Quentin en Yvelines, Boulogne Billancourt, 92100 Paris, France; lamarquedominique@gmail.com
15. Gastroenterology Service, Althaia Xarxa Assistencial Universitària de Manresa, 08243 Manresa, Spain; acano@aegastro.es (A.C.-C.); ignasi.puig@aegastro.es (I.P.)
16. Medicine Department, Universitat de Vic-Universitat Central de Catalunya (UVicUCC), 08500 Manresa, Spain
17. INSERM U1312, Université de Bordeaux, 33076 Bordeaux, France; francis.megraud@u-bordeaux.fr
* Correspondence: javier.p.gisbert@gmail.com; Tel.: +349-1309-3911; Fax: +349-1520-4013

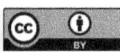

Abstract: Background: First-line *Helicobacter pylori* (*H. pylori*) treatments have been relatively well evaluated; however, it remains necessary to identify the most effective rescue treatments. Our aim was to assess the effectiveness and safety of *H. pylori* regimens containing rifabutin. METHODS: International multicentre prospective non-interventional European Registry on *H. pylori* Management (Hp-EuReg). Patients treated with rifabutin were registered in AEG-REDCap e-CRF from 2013 to 2021. Modified intention-to-treat and per-protocol analyses were performed. Data were subject to quality control. Results: Overall, 500 patients included in the Hp-EuReg were treated with rifabutin (mean age 52 years, 72% female, 63% with dyspepsia, 4% with peptic ulcer). Culture was performed in 63% of cases: dual resistance (to both clarithromycin and metronidazole) was reported in 46% of the cases, and triple resistance (to clarithromycin, metronidazole, and levofloxacin) in 39%. In 87% of cases rifabutin was utilised as part of a triple therapy together with amoxicillin and a proton-pump-inhibitor, and in an additional 6% of the patients, bismuth was added to this triple regimen. Rifabutin was mainly used in second-line (32%), third-line (25%), and fourth-line (27%) regimens, achieving overall 78%, 80% and 66% effectiveness by modified intention-to-treat, respectively. Compliance with treatment was 89%. At least one adverse event was registered in 26% of the patients (most frequently nausea), and one serious adverse event (0.2%) was reported in one patient with leukopenia and thrombocytopenia with fever requiring hospitalisation. Conclusion: Rifabutin-containing therapy represents an effective and safe strategy after one or even several failures of *H. pylori* eradication treatment.

Keywords: *Helicobacter pylori*; *H. pylori*; rifabutin; treatment; eradication failure; culture; bismuth; rescue; Hp-EuReg

1. Introduction

Helicobacter pylori (*H. pylori*) is a worldwide spread bacterium that causes mainly gastritis, as well as peptic ulcer disease and gastric cancer [1]. Currently, the most used first-line therapies fail in more than 20% of cases [2]. One of the major factors affecting our ability to cure *H. pylori* infection is antibiotic resistance, mainly to the macrolide clarithromycin, which is growing dramatically in many geographic areas [3,4].

A rescue regimen including a quadruple combination of a proton pump inhibitor (PPI), bismuth, tetracycline, and metronidazole has been introduced as the optimal rescue therapy after experiencing *H. pylori* eradication failure [5]. However, this treatment results in eradication failure in at least 20% of cases [2,6–8]. In addition, administration of this regimen is relatively complex, is associated with a high incidence of adverse events (AEs), and many countries are currently experiencing a general unavailability of tetracycline and/or bismuth. Furthermore, mainly levofloxacin-containing rescue regimens, produce a mean eradication rate of only approximately 80%, probably due to the rising *H. pylori* resistance to quinolones [9].

And thus, even after two or more eradication treatments, *H. pylori* infection persists in several cases, and these patients constitute a therapeutic dilemma. Currently, the international guidelines recommend performing culture in the aforementioned patients to select a rescue treatment according to microbial sensitivity to antibiotics, as a standard third/fourth-line therapy is lacking, although this approach is not always practical [10]. Therefore, it seems worthwhile to perform an evaluation of drugs without cross-resistance to macrolides, nitroimidazole or quinolones as components of retreatment combination therapies [11].

Rifabutin, also known as ansamycin (LM 427), is a well-established antimicrobial agent that belongs to the S-rifamycin derivative group and has been previously successfully utilised, among others, for the treatment of atypical *Mycobacterium* infections such as *Mycobacterium avium-intracellulare* complex [12]. Rifabutin may be useful against *H. pylori* because this pathogen has high in vitro sensitivity to this drug, which does not share resistance mechanisms with clarithromycin, metronidazole, or levofloxacin [11,13,14]. Furthermore, the selection of resistant *H. pylori* strains has been low in experimental conditions [15]. Consequently, rifabutin-based rescue therapies could represent a potential and attractive strategy for *H. pylori* eradication failures [12].

The "European Registry on *H. pylori* Management" (Hp-EuReg) is an international multicentre prospective non-interventional registry starting in 2013 aimed to evaluate the decisions and outcomes in *H. pylori* management, in real-world clinical practice, by European gastroenterologists from more than 30 countries [2,16]. Therefore, the Hp-EuReg represents a valued long-lasting overview of current *H. pylori* management enabling continuous evaluation of treatment for enhancement. The present study is a sub-analysis of this large-scale international multicentre registry, which aimed to assess the effectiveness and safety of rifabutin-containing regimens used in the management of *H. pylori* in Europe.

2. Methods

2.1. European Registry on H. pylori Management (Hp-EuReg)

Hp-EuReg is an international, multicentre, prospective, non-interventional registry that has been recording information on the management of *H. pylori* infection since 2013. Hp-EuReg has a Scientific Committee that ensures coherence, continued quality and scientific integrity of the analyses performed and manuscripts produced. Additionally, the Hp-EuReg protocol [16] selected national coordinators in the 30 participating countries, where gastroenterologists are currently recruited at approximately 300 centres to provide their contribution to the study. The investigators assemble and upload a series of variables and outcomes into the registry's database (REDCap) using an Electronic Case Report Form (e-CRF). The variables include: the patient's demographic information; any previous attempts for eradication and the treatments employed; the outcomes of any treatment, recording details such as compliance, cure rate, follow-up, and any reported AE. The REDCap database [17] is managed and hosted by the "Asociación Española de Gastroenterología" (AEG, Madrid, Spain, www.aegastro.es, last accessed 10 March 2022), a non-profit Scientific and Medical Society that focuses on Gastroenterology research. The study was conducted according to the guidelines of the 1975 Declaration of Helsinki and was approved in 2012 by the Ethics Committee of La Princesa University Hospital (Madrid, Spain), that acted as reference Institutional Review Board, was classified by the Spanish Drug and Health Product Agency, and was prospectively registered at ClinicalTrials.gov (NCT02328131).

2.2. Data Analysis

Data from June 2013 to November 2021 were extracted, and a quality review was performed on all the records included for each country and centre. The PPI dose used for *H. pylori* eradication treatment was grouped into three categories as reported by Graham [18] and Kirchheiner [19]: Low dose, if the potency of PPI was between 4.5 and 27 mg omeprazole equivalents when given twice daily; standard dose, for PPI between 32 and 40 mg omeprazole equivalents when given twice daily; and high dose, for PPI between 54 and 128 mg omeprazole equivalents when given twice daily. Treatment duration was evaluated according to three categories: 10, 12 and 14 days, based on the most frequent treatment durations.

2.3. Effectiveness Analysis

The main outcome used to evaluate the effectiveness was the eradication rate achieved with the treatment. *H. pylori* eradication was confirmed at least one month after completing eradication treatment with at least one of the following diagnostic methods: Urea breath test, stool antigen test and/or histology.

Effectiveness was analysed in three sub-groups of patients: (1) an intention-to-treat (ITT) group that included all patients registered up to November 2021 who had at least a six-month follow-up, in this group lost to follow-up cases were deemed treatment failures; (2) a per-protocol (PP) group which included all cases that had a complete follow-up and had achieved at least 90% treatment compliance, as defined in the protocol; and (3) a modified ITT (mITT) group that aimed to reflect the closest result to that obtained in clinical practice; this group included all cases that had completed the follow-up (i.e., that had undertaken a confirmatory test after the eradication treatment), regardless of compliance.

All different treatments prescribed with rifabutin were examined *a priori* for effectiveness according to the rifabutin dose, the PPI dose, the duration of therapy and, whenever possible, to the line of treatment.

2.4. Statistical Analysis

Continuous variables were expressed as the mean and standard deviation, whereas qualitative variables were presented as the absolute and relative frequencies, displayed as percentages (%) and corresponding 95% confidence intervals.

A multivariate analysis (using a backward modelling strategy, and comparing models using the log-likelihood ratio) was performed to study in the mITT population the relation between the eradication rate of rifabutin-containing regimens and the following variables: age, sex (female [ref.] vs. male), indication (dyspepsia and others [ref] vs. ulcer disease), compliance (no [ref] vs. yes, defined as taking >90% of the total drug prescribed), PPI dose (low [ref.] vs. standard, and low vs. high); treatment length (10 [ref.], 12, and 14 days); treatment line (first-line [ref] vs. second-line vs. all remaining rescue therapies).

3. Results

3.1. Baseline Characteristics

Until November 2021, 500 patients from seven countries had been treated with a rifabutin-containing regimen and were registered in Hp-EuReg. Three countries accounted for the majority of cases (90% of the data): Italy (333 patients) and Spain (117 patients) followed by Israel (33 patients). The remaining participating countries registered less than 10 patients each: France (7 cases), United Kingdom (5 cases), Ireland (3 cases) and Greece (2 cases).

Mean age was 52 years (±13), 72% of them were female, 63% suffered from dyspepsia, and 4% from peptic ulcer.

The ^{13}C-urea breath test represented the most frequently (86%) used non-invasive diagnostic method, while culture and antibiogram was performed in 63% of the patients. Resistance to at least one of the following antibiotics: clarithromycin, metronidazole and levofloxacin was reported in 52%, 49% and 47% of the patients, respectively. Dual resistance (to both clarithromycin and metronidazole) was reported in 46% of the cases, and triple resistance (to clarithromycin, metronidazole, and levofloxacin) in 39%. No resistance was reported in 2.2% of those patients with culture testing.

Confirmation of the eradication was at least performed by means of one of the following methods: ^{13}C-urea breath test (81%), monoclonal stool antigen test (3%), histology (1.4%), polyclonal stool antigen test (0.6%), rapid urease test (0.6%), and culture (0.6%).

3.2. Prescriptions

In total, 18 different rifabutin-containing treatments including two or three other antibiotics in the scheme were registered. However, in 87% of the cases, rifabutin was used as part of a triple therapy together with amoxicillin and a PPI, and in an additional 6% of the patients, bismuth was added to this triple regimen, while the others correspond to different drug combinations (Table 1).

Table 1. Rifabutin-containing regimens registered in Hp-EuReg between 2013 and 2021.

Prescriptions	n (%)
Triple-PPI + A+R	434 (86.8)
Quadruple-PPI + A+R + B	32 (6.4)
Triple-PPI + R+Tc	5 (1.0)
Triple-PPI + L+R	4 (0.8)
Quadruple-PPI + R+D + B	4 (0.8)
Triple-PPI + M+R	3 (0.6)
Quadruple-PPI + L+R + Tc	3 (0.6)

Table 1. Cont.

Prescriptions	n (%)
Quadruple-PPI + R+B + minocycline	3 (0.6)
Triple-PPI + R+minocycline	2 (0.4)
Quadruple-PPI + A+R + Tc	2 (0.4)
Quadruple-PPI + A+R	1 (0.2)
Triple-PPI + R+D	1 (0.2)
Dual-PPI + R	1 (0.2)
Triple-PPI + C+R	1 (0.2)
Quadruple-PPI + L+R + B	1 (0.2)
Quadruple-PPI + C+R + B	1 (0.2)
Quadruple-PPI + A+L + R+Tc	1 (0.2)
Sequential-PPI + C+A + R	1 (0.2)
Total	500 (100)

A: amoxicillin; B: bismuth; C: clarithromycin; D: doxycycline; L: levofloxacin; M: metronidazole; R: rifabutin; Tc: tetracycline; PPI: proton pump inhibitor; N: Number of patients with prescribed treatment.

Rifabutin was mainly used in second-line (32%), third-line (25%), and fourth-line (27%) regimens; in addition, rifabutin was also used to a lesser extent as part of a first-line (9%), fifth-line (6%) or sixth-line (2%) therapy (Table 2).

Table 2. Rifabutin-containing prescriptions and overall effectiveness according to treatment line.

	Use, n (%)	mITT, n (%)	95%CI	PP, n (%)	95%CI
Total	500 (100)	426 (73.5)	69–77	415 (74)	70–78
1st line	43 (9)	41 (73)	58–88	41 (73)	58–88
2nd line	160 (32)	139 (78)	70–85	136 (78)	71–85
3rd line	124 (25)	100 (80)	72–88	97 (81)	73–90
4th line	134 (27)	114 (66)	57–75	109 (67)	58–76
5th line	29 (5)	24 (58)	36–79	24 (58)	36–80
6th line	10 (2)	8 (75)	35–97	8 (75)	35–97

mITT: modified intention-to-treat; PP: per protocol, CI: confidence interval, n: total number of patients analysed.

Overall, the antibiotic treatments were mostly combined with low (46%) or high-dose PPIs (46%), and administered most frequently for 12 days (58%), and in lower proportion for 10 (25%) or 14 days (17.5%).

Rifabutin was prescribed at two main dosages: 150 mg once a day (56%) or 150 mg every 12 h, i.e., 300 mg daily (41%).

Triple therapy together with a PPI, amoxicillin and rifabutin was mainly prescribed in second- (35%), third- (25%) or fourth-line (24%); and in most of the cases (66%) for 12 days and with low-dose PPIs (51%).

Finally, quadruple therapy with a PPI, amoxicillin, rifabutin and bismuth was prescribed mainly in fourth-line treatment (66%), in 10-day regimens (84%) and with high-dose PPIs (78%).

3.3. Effectiveness

Overall mITT effectiveness in first-, second-, third, fourth-, fifth- and six-line regimens was 73% ($n = 30/41$), 78% ($n = 108/139$), 80% ($n = 80/100$), 66% ($n = 75/114$), 58% ($n = 14/24$) and 75% ($n = 6/8$), respectively, as further detailed in Table 2.

Although the overall eradication with 12 days therapy was numerically higher (78%: $n = 188/241$) than when prescribed for 10 or 14 days (69% in both cases: $n = 79/115$ and $n = 42/61$, respectively), these differences were not statistically significant ($p = 0.78$).

Similarly, the overall effectiveness of rifabutin regimens was higher when high-dose PPIs were used (85%, 152/179) as compared to low- or standard-dose PPIs (66%, 138/208 and 58%, 22/38, respectively), however these differences were not statistically significant ($p = 0.86$).

Overall effectiveness with a daily rifabutin dosage of 150 mg was higher (78%, $n = 187/239$) when compared to the 300 mg daily dosage (67%, $n = 110/166$), although the difference was not statistically significant ($p = 0.53$). On the other hand, when only naïve patients were assessed, the eradication rate was higher (100%, $n = 4/4$) in the 300 mg group than in the 150 mg one (69%, $n = 25/36$), although such difference did not reach a statistical significance ($p = 0.73$).

Figure 1 shows data on the mITT effectiveness of the two most frequent prescriptions of rifabutin-containing regimens (triple therapy with a PPI, amoxicillin and rifabutin and quadruple therapy with a PPI, amoxicillin, rifabutin and bismuth) according to treatment length, PPI dose and treatment line (from second- to fourth-line). These data are further detailed in Supplementary Table S1 and compared below independently for treatment length and PPI dose.

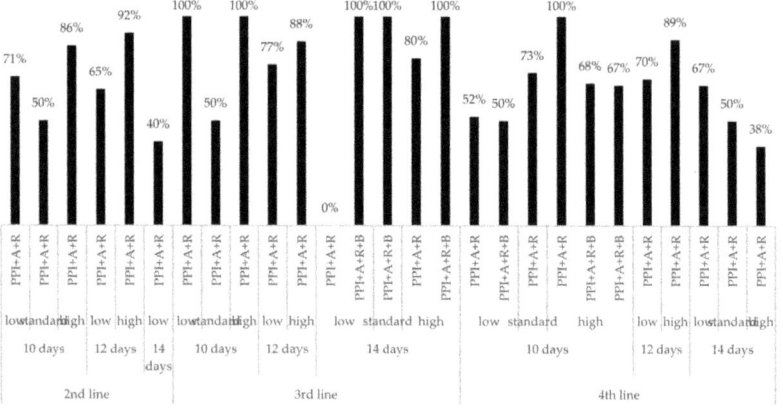

Figure 1. Effectiveness by modified intention-to-treat analysis of both triple therapy with amoxicillin and rifabutin and quadruple therapy with amoxicillin, rifabutin and bismuth, according to duration, potency of acid inhibition and treatment line. A: amoxicillin; B: bismuth; R: rifabutin; PPI: proton pump inhibitor (low-dose PPI: 4.5–27 mg omeprazole equivalents (OE) twice daily (bid) (i.e., 20 mg OE bid), standard-dose PPI: 32–40 mg omeprazole equivalents bid (i.e., 40 mg OE bid), high-dose PPI: 54–128 mg omeprazole equivalents bid (i.e., 60 mg OE bid).

The overall eradication rate achieved with the triple therapy with amoxicillin and rifabutin was 73% ($n = 265/363$); however, in second- and third-line (77%, $n = 103/133$ and 79%, $n = 66/84$, respectively) cure rate was higher than in fourth-line (64%, $n = 53/83$), with no statistical differences in the eradication rate between treatment lines ($p = 0.51$). Effectiveness was numerically higher (78%, $n = 187/240$) for 12-day treatment than that of 10-day (70%, $n = 53/76$) or 14-day (54%, $n = 21/39$) treatment, but these differences were not statistically significant ($p = 0.30$). Additionally, higher PPI doses provided better outcomes with this same regimen (87.5%, $n = 119/136$) than when combined with either low (66%,

$n = 129/196$) or standard PPI doses (53%, $n = 16/30$), with statistically significant differences in the eradication rate ($p = 0.000$). Further details are presented in Supplementary Table S1.

The overall eradication rate achieved with the quadruple therapy with amoxicillin, rifabutin and bismuth in fourth-line was 68% ($n = 21/31$), and was similar when prescribed for a duration of 10 days (68%, $n = 18/27$) or when combined with high-dose PPIs (68%, $n = 16/24$). Likewise, no statistically significant difference ($p = 0.20$) was reported in the eradication rate with quadruple therapy with amoxicillin, rifabutin and bismuth according to treatment duration, nor PPI dose. Further details are presented in Supplementary Table S1.

3.4. Safety and Compliance

At least one AE was registered in 26% ($n = 126/480$) of the patients: the most common AEs were nausea (7.6%, $n = 38$)—lasting in over 80% of cases between 4 and 5 days—, and asthenia (6.2%, $n = 31$)—lasting in 79% of cases between 5 and 7 days. Intensity of both AEs was mild or moderate in all patients. One serious AE (0.2%) was reported in one patient (treated with the triple therapy with amoxicillin and rifabutin), with leukopenia, thrombocytopenia and accompanying fever that required hospitalisation; but this patient recovered spontaneously and was discharged from hospital without further complications.

Triple therapy with amoxicillin and rifabutin exhibited significantly ($p = 0.001$) lower overall AE incidence (23%, $n = 97/417$) than the quadruple rifabutin regimen with bismuth (52%, $n = 16/31$); however, the latter provided better results in terms of treatment compliance (97%, $n = 30/31$) than the triple therapy (86%, $n = 369/416$), with no significant differences ($p = 0.13$).

Overall compliance with treatment was 89% ($n = 428$), although 25% ($n = 13$, where nine were treated with the triple therapy with amoxicillin and rifabutin, and one with the quadruple with rifabutin and bismuth) of patients interrupted the treatment due to AEs.

3.5. Univariate Analysis

In order to equate conditions, the effectiveness of triple therapy with amoxicillin and rifabutin versus quadruple therapy with amoxicillin, rifabutin and bismuth was compared when both were prescribed for 10 days and in fourth-line treatment (that is, in those subgroups where more data were available). In this context, no statistically significant difference in mITT eradication rate was found between triple therapy and the bismuth-rifabutin quadruple regimen (66% [$n = 27/41$] vs. 67% [$n = 14/21$], $p = 0.59$).

The analysis was also stratified by PPI dose with both regimens, and a comparison could be performed when both were combined with high-dose PPIs (during 10 days and in fourth-line treatment): triple therapy reported a numerically higher mITT eradication rate (100%, $n = 5/5$) than quadruple therapy (68%, $n = 13/19$); but these differences were not statistically significant ($p = 0.28$).

Additionally, no subgroup analysis was performed by dosage schedule as a whole; however, it is noteworthy that one patient was prescribed 150 mg of rifabutin every 12 h (i.e., 300 mg rifabutin per day).

3.6. Multivariate Analysis

Stepwise multivariate logistic regression analysis was further performed to determine those variables influencing the most the mITT eradication rate of triple therapy with amoxicillin and rifabutin (as it was the only regimen with a sufficient sample size for multivariate analysis).

The analysis revealed that among all the covariates being analysed (age, sex, indication, compliance, PPI dose; treatment length; treatment line), compliance (OR = 13.1, 95%CI = 2.1–81.4), a high-dose PPI (OR = 4.4, 95%CI = 2.3–8.3), as well as the age (OR = 1.03, 95%CI = 1.01–1.05) were significantly associated with higher therapy success. Additionally, 14-day treatment duration was associated with a tendency (although not significant) towards lower effectiveness, as compared to 10-day therapy.

4. Discussion

A relevant proportion of patients still fail to eradicate *H. pylori* infection, even with the current most effective treatment regimens. Nowadays, clinicians have to take into account treatment failures apart from substantiating first-line eradication regimens. In this context, rifabutin presents potential utility against *H. pylori*.

Hp-EuReg, an international multicentre prospective non-interventional European Registry on *H. pylori* management [16], has allowed us to recruit the largest series of patients treated with rifabutin, with 500 patients included from 2013 to 2021. Our results, with approximately 80% *H. pylori* cure rate—in agreement with previous reviews [12,20,21]—could be considered relatively encouraging, especially taking into account that rifabutin regimens were prescribed mainly after two-to-four eradication failures with key antibiotics such as clarithromycin, metronidazole, tetracycline and levofloxacin. In fact, resistance to clarithromycin, metronidazole and levofloxacin was reported in 52%, 49% and 47% of our patients, respectively. Furthermore, dual resistance (to both clarithromycin and metronidazole) was reported in almost half of the cases, and triple resistance (to clarithromycin, metronidazole, and levofloxacin) in more than a third.

The encouraging results obtained with rifabutin-containing regimens are probably due to the low *H. pylori* resistance rate to this antibiotic [13,22,23]. Thus, in a previous systematic review including 39 studies and almost 10,000 patients, rifabutin resistance was reported in only 0.13% of the cases; furthermore, when only naïve *H. pylori* participants were considered, this rate was even lower (0.07%) [12]. In our study, no prevalence data on the rifabutin resistance were available, and therefore the reduced effect of the resistance to this antibiotic on the high effectiveness of treatments could not be confirmed. Resistance to rifabutin is due to mutations in the *rpoB* gene and there is no cross-reaction with the resistance mechanisms to the other antibiotics; accordingly, in cases with *H. pylori* infection with primary resistance to clarithromycin or metronidazole (or both), rifabutin therapy has been reported highly effective [24–31], and even in patients with triple resistance to these two antibiotics plus quinolones [14], which is the usual real-life scenario after several treatment eradication attempts.

When prescribed as a second-line regimen, a rifabutin-containing regimen was effective in 78% of the patients in our study; even when used as a sixth-line therapy this regimen was able to cure the infection in 75% of our cases. These results are consistent with those summarised in a previous relevant review [12]. Accordingly, a recent study found that the efficacy of rifabutin treatment was not significantly influenced by the number of previous treatment failures: eradication rates in patients with one, two, three, and four or more previous failures were 78.3%, 89.6%, 68.6%, and 88.9%, respectively (non-statistically significant differences) [32].

Regarding the specific regimen prescribed in Hp-EuReg, rifabutin was used as part of a triple therapy together with amoxicillin and a PPI in most ($\approx$90%) of the cases, which achieved cure rates of 77% in second-line, 79% in third-line, and 64% in fourth-line treatments. Liu et al. conducted a meta-analysis of clinical trials for eradication of *H. pylori* that included a treatment arm with a PPI, rifabutin, and amoxicillin; twenty-one studies were included, and the overall reported eradication rate was 70% [20]. More recently, Gingold-Belfer et al. performed another meta-analysis of randomised controlled trials with a treatment arm consisting of PPI, amoxicillin, and rifabutin, and the pooled cure rate in the 33 studies selected was 71.8% [21].

With respect to rifabutin dose and frequency in *H. pylori* eradication regimens, the majority of studies prescribe rifabutin 300 mg/day [12]. However, in our study, approximately 50% of the patients received only 150 mg/day. The *H. pylori* cure rate in published small number of previous studies using rifabutin 150 mg/day was about 40–70% only [33,34], although other studies have reported higher eradication rates [14,29,35]. There is only one study directly comparing both doses: Perri et al. [33] performed a randomised study where patients persistently infected after one or more courses of standard regimens were treated for 10 days with pantoprazole, amoxicillin, and rifabutin 150 mg once daily or

300 mg once daily. In intention-to-treat analysis, eradication rates were 67% in the rifabutin 150 mg group and significantly higher (87%) in the rifabutin 300 mg group. As opposed to these results, our study showed a similar effectiveness with a daily rifabutin dosage of 150 mg (78%) to that of the 300 mg daily dosage (67%); however, when only naïve patients were assessed, the eradication rate was higher (100%) in the 300 mg group than in the 150 mg one (69%), although such difference remained not statistically significant. This may probably due to the small sample size ($n=4$ patients) in our 300 mg group, which may not be very representative and therefore the lack of statistical significance may not imply the real effect.

The ideal length of rifabutin treatment remains unclear, but 10 to 12-day regimens are generally recommended [12], as it was the case in Hp-EuReg, where ≈80% of the patients received this regimen. In some reports, a 7-day course was as efficacious as 10 to 14-day regimens, while this shorter duration dramatically reduced the efficacy, with eradication rates of only 44%, as reported elsewhere [36]. Although rifabutin treatment could be more likely to be successful when treatment duration is 14 days, as suggested in some studies [21], many other exposed that therapy between 12 and 14 days achieves similar results to the 10-day course and is likely to rise the incidence of AEs [37]. A recent randomised controlled trial compared 10-day vs. 14-day eradication therapy with PPI, amoxicillin and rifabutin and determined that over 90% of patients resulted in successful eradication with 14-day therapy, but stated that considering the tolerability of therapy, 10-day treatment may be enough to obtain a successful eradication rate [38]. In line with these results, in our study, therapy with amoxicillin and rifabutin was prescribed mostly for 12 days, achieving higher effectiveness (78%) than when prescribed for 10 (70%) or even 14 days (54%), although these differences were not statistically significant.

Bismuth is one of the few antimicrobials to which resistance is not developed [39]. In addition, bismuth has an additive effect with antibiotics, overcomes levofloxacin and clarithromycin resistance and its efficacy is not affected by metronidazole resistance [39,40]. Therefore, combining bismuth and rifabutin in the same regimen may be a promising option. Some authors have evaluated a combination of a triple therapy with a PPI, amoxicillin and rifabutin, with bismuth—and thus converting this triple regimen into a quadruple one—, with encouraging results [41–43]. Ciccaglione et al. reported, in a small sample size population, that the addition of bismuth to a triple therapy that included PPI, amoxicillin, and rifabutin in patients treated for the third time for *H. pylori* infection resulted in 30% therapeutic gain compared to rifabutin-based triple therapy alone [42]. In our study, the addition of bismuth did not seem to increase the effectiveness of the rifabutin-triple regimen 68% vs. 73%, respectively), although the number of patients receiving the quadruple regimen was considerably low ($n = 32$) and in most of them was utilised as a fourth-line rescue regimen. And so, as previously stated this lack of statistical differences between the triple and the bismuth quadruple therapies, may be due to the differences in sample sizes between groups or potentially that the finding could reliably exclude several covariates that may introduce some bias.

In Hp-EuReg, compliance with treatment was quite satisfactory (89%) and the safety profile was acceptable. At least one AE was registered in 28% of the patients (most frequently nausea and asthenia), but most of them (>95%) were of mild-to-moderate intensity. This seems to be a favourable safety profile, mainly when compared to other well stablished eradication regimens, such as the bismuth and non-bismuth quadruple therapies [44,45]. In a recent meta-analysis of all studies including rifabutin for *H. pylori* eradication, mean rate of AEs was 15% [12]. In our study, only one serious AE (0.2%) was reported in a single patient with leukopenia and thrombocytopenia with fever requiring hospitalisation. Accordingly, a recent review on the use of rifabutin for *H. pylori* infection [21], only found one severe AE reported in the literature [31].

Myelotoxicity is the most significant AE of rifabutin [46,47]. Overall, this complication is rare and is far more likely when high dose (600 mg/day) and prolonged duration therapy is used [46,47]. Several cases of myelotoxicity during *H. pylori* therapy have been mentioned in the literature [27,28,35,37,48–52]. However, myelotoxicity was not reported in most of the studies evaluating rifabutin for *H. pylori* infection. In the studies describing this complication, myelotoxicity was observed in 1.5% to 3% of the patients [27,28,37,50,52], although some studies reported higher incidence [49,51]. In the meta-analysis conducted by Gingold-Belfer et al., neutropenia was addressed in 27 studies, where 19 of them reported no cases of neutropenia and eight studies reported at least one case; and so, in total, only 17 patients developed neutropenia across all studies [21]. All patients reported in the literature recovered from myelotoxicity uneventfully within few days, with spontaneous recovery from leukopenia. In several cases, the leukopenia was clinically apparent with fever [37,49]. Infections or other adverse outcomes related to reduced white cell count have not been reported in the setting of *H. pylori* treatment [27,28,37,48–52].

Only few studies have compared a triple combination of a PPI, amoxicillin and rifabutin with the widely used "classic" bismuth quadruple regimen [27,30,33,36]. As an example, in the randomised study by Perri et al., side effects were less frequent in rifabutin-treated patients than in those on bismuth quadruple therapy; additionally, the eradication rates were reported the same in both groups (67%) when rifabutin was prescribed at 150 mg, and even higher (87%) when prescribed at 300 mg [33]. Miehlke et al. [30] compared, also in a randomised study, rifabutin-based triple therapy for 7 days vs. high-dose dual therapy for 14 days, for rescue treatment of *H. pylori*; premature discontinuation of treatment occurred in 2% and 5% of patients respectively. Finally, one study directly compared rifabutin to levofloxacin as third-line therapy for *H. pylori*, and AEs were reported in 60% and 50% of the cases, respectively. However, in this study, the intention-to-treat eradication rate was reported lower (45%) in the rifabutin group as compared to the levofloxacin one (85%) [51].

The major limitation of our study was that the rifabutin regimens in the studied cohort were heterogeneous, including several schemes, doses, and durations. Nonetheless, most of the regimens included a triple combination of rifabutin together with a PPI and amoxicillin administered for 10-to-12 days. Heterogeneity was inherent to the study design of Hp-EuReg (i.e., observational, non-interventional) and therefore difficult to avoid, as wide selection criteria were initially established to reflect as much as possible real clinical practice. Most of patients came from only three countries, and this might introduce selection bias. Another point to highlight is that culture was performed in only 63% of the cases; however, this reflects real routine gastroenterology practice in Europe, where antibiograms are not performed on a routine basis and treatments are mainly empirically prescribed [10]; furthermore, as previously noted, resistance to rifabutin is exceptional, occurring in less than 1% of the cases [12].

In summary, from the analysis of Hp-EuReg, it can be deduced that rifabutin-containing therapy represents a relatively effective and safe strategy after one or even several failures of *H. pylori* eradication treatment, although still insufficient as not reaching the desired 90% threshold of eradication [7]. Since resistance to rifabutin is practically non-existent, and rifabutin therapy is highly effective even in patients with primary resistance to clarithromycin, metronidazole, and levofloxacin, rifabutin usage in an empirical manner may be suggested as "rescue" therapy without culture in those patients in whom these antibiotics have failed. Recent studies have also evaluated the role of rifabutin in *H. pylori* treatment in naïve patients, with encouraging results [31,53]. Nevertheless, the consideration of rifabutin as a novel first-line treatment option for *H. pylori* infection should be carefully weighed against concerns regarding microbial resistance, treatment cost (rifabutin is quite expensive), and the availability and effectiveness of alternative drugs.

Supplementary Materials: The following supporting information can be downloaded at: https://www.mdpi.com/article/10.3390/jcm11061658/s1, Table S1: Effectiveness of both triple therapy with amoxicillin and rifabutin and quadruple therapy with amoxicillin, rifabutin and bismuth, according to duration, potency of acid inhibition and treatment line.

Author Contributions: Conceptualization, J.P.G.; Data curation, O.P.N. and J.P.G.; Formal analysis, O.P.N. and J.P.G.; Investigation, O.P.N.; Methodology, O.P.N. and J.P.G.; Project administration, A.C.-C.; Software, O.P.N. and A.C.-C.; Supervision, O.P.N. and J.P.G.; Validation, O.P.N., D.V., I.M.S., G.F., M.C., L.B., R.P., A.K.-H., E.O.S., A.D.L., G.L., Á.P.-A., A.G., D.B., S.S., P.P., T.R., D.L., I.P., F.M., C.O. and J.P.G.; Visualization, O.P.N. and M.P.-C.; Writing—original draft, O.P.N. and J.P.G.; Writing—review & editing, O.P.N., D.V., I.M.S., G.F., M.C., L.B., R.P., A.K.-H., M.P.-C., E.O.S., A.D.L., Á.P.-A., A.G., D.B., S.S., P.P., T.R., D.L., I.P., F.M., C.O. and J.P.G. All authors have read and agreed to the published version of the manuscript.

Funding: This project was promoted and funded by the European Helicobacter and Microbiota Study Group (EHMSG), the Spanish Association of Gastroenterology (AEG) and the Centro de Investigación Biomédica en Red de Enfermedades Hepáticas y Digestivas (CIBERehd).

Institutional Review Board Statement: The study was conducted according to the guidelines of the 1975 Declaration of Helsinki and was approved in 2012 by the Ethics Committee of La Princesa University Hospital (Madrid, Spain), that acted as reference Institutional Review Board, was classified by the Spanish Drug and Health Product Agency, and was prospectively registered at ClinicalTrials.gov (NCT02328131).

Informed Consent Statement: Informed consent was obtained from all subjects involved in the study.

Data Availability Statement: The data that support the findings of this study are not publicly available given that containing information could compromise the privacy of research participants. However, previous published data on the Hp-EuReg study, or de-identified raw data referring to current study, as well as further information on the methods used to explore the data could be shared, with no particular time constraint. Individual participant data will not be shared.

Conflicts of Interest: Gisbert has served as speaker, consultant, and advisory member for or has received research funding from Mayoly, Allergan, Diasorin, Gebro Pharma, and Richen. Nyssen has received research funding from Mayoly and Allergan. Pérez-Aisa has received compensation from Allergan and Mylan for formative actions. A. Di Leo served as consultant for T.H.D. spa. The remaining authors declare no conflict of interest.

Abbreviations

Adverse event	AE
Helicobacter pylori	*H. pylori*
proton pump inhibitor	PPI

References

1. Crowe, S.E. *Helicobacter pylori* Infection. *N. Engl. J. Med.* **2019**, *380*, 1158–1165. [CrossRef] [PubMed]
2. Nyssen, O.P.; Bordin, D.; Tepes, B.; Perez-Aisa, A.; Vaira, D.; Caldas, M.; Bujanda, L.; Castro-Fernandez, M.; Lerang, F.; Leja, M.; et al. European Registry on *Helicobacter pylori* management (Hp-EuReg): Patterns and trends in first-line empirical eradication prescription and outcomes of 5 years and 21 533 patients. *Gut* **2021**, *70*, 40–54. [CrossRef] [PubMed]
3. Megraud, F.; Bruyndonckx, R.; Coenen, S.; Wittkop, L.; Huang, T.-D.; Hoebeke, M.; Bénéjat, L.; Lehours, P.; Goossens, H.; Glupczynski, Y. *Helicobacter pylori* resistance to antibiotics in Europe in 2018 and its relationship to antibiotic consumption in the community. *Gut* **2021**, *70*, 1815–1822. [CrossRef] [PubMed]
4. Savoldi, A.; Carrara, E.; Graham, D.Y.; Conti, M.; Tacconelli, E. Prevalence of Antibiotic Resistance in *Helicobacter pylori*: A Systematic Review and Meta-analysis in World Health Organization Regions. *Gastroenterology* **2018**, *155*, 1372.e17–1382.e17. [CrossRef] [PubMed]
5. Gisbert, J.P.; Alcedo, J.; Amador, J.; Bujanda, L.; Calvet, X.; Castro-Fernandez, M.; Gené, E.; Lanas, Á.; Lucendo, A.; Molina-Infante, J. V Spanish Consensus Conference on *Helicobacter pylori* infection treatment. *Gastroenterol. Hepatol.* **2021**. [CrossRef] [PubMed]
6. Fallone, C.A.; Chiba, N.; Van Zanten, S.V.; Fischbach, L.; Gisbert, J.P.; Hunt, R.H.; Jones, N.L.; Render, C.; Leontiadis, G.I.; Moayyedi, P.; et al. The Toronto Consensus for the Treatment of *Helicobacter pylori* Infection in Adults. *Gastroenterology* **2016**, *151*, 51.e14–69.e14. [CrossRef] [PubMed]
7. Malfertheiner, P.; Megraud, F.; O'Morain, C.A.; Gisbert, J.P.; Kuipers, E.J.; Axon, A.T.; Bazzoli, F.; Gasbarrini, A.; Atherton, J.; Graham, D.Y.; et al. Management of *Helicobacter pylori* infection—The Maastricht V/Florence Consensus Report. *Gut* **2017**, *66*, 6–30. [CrossRef] [PubMed]
8. Chey, W.D.; Leontiadis, G.I.; Howden, C.W.; Moss, S.F. ACG Clinical Guideline: Treatment of *Helicobacter pylori* Infection. *Am. J. Gastroenterol.* **2017**, *112*, 212–239. [CrossRef]

9. Gisbert, J.P.; Morena, F. Systematic review and meta-analysis: Levofloxacin-based rescue regimens after *Helicobacter pylori* treatment failure. *Aliment. Pharmacol. Ther.* **2006**, *23*, 35–44. [PubMed]
10. Gisbert, J.P. Empirical or susceptibility-guided treatment for *Helicobacter pylori* infection? A comprehensive review. *Ther. Adv. Gastroenterol.* **2020**, *13*, 1–16. [CrossRef] [PubMed]
11. Megraud, F. Basis for the management of drug-resistant *Helicobacter pylori* infection. *Drugs* **2004**, *64*, 1893–1904. [CrossRef]
12. Gisbert, J.P. Rifabutin for the Treatment of *Helicobacter pylori* Infection: A Review. *Pathogens* **2020**, *10*, 15. [CrossRef] [PubMed]
13. Heep, M.; Beck, D.; Bayerdörffer, E.; Lehn, N. Rifampin and Rifabutin Resistance Mechanism in *Helicobacter pylori*. *Antimicrob. Agents Chemother.* **1999**, *43*, 1497–1499. [CrossRef] [PubMed]
14. Fiorini, G.; Zullo, A.; Vakil, N.; Saracino, I.M.; Ricci, C.; Castelli, V.; Gatta, L.; Vaira, D. Rifabutin Triple Therapy is Effective in Patients with Multidrug-resistant Strains of *Helicobacter pylori*. *J. Clin. Gastroenterol.* **2018**, *52*, 137–140. [CrossRef] [PubMed]
15. Gisbert, J.P.; Calvet, X. Review article: Rifabutin in the treatment of refractory *Helicobacter pylori* infection. *Aliment. Pharmacol. Ther.* **2011**, *35*, 209–221. [CrossRef] [PubMed]
16. McNicholl, A.G.; O'Morain, C.A.; Megraud, F.; Gisbert, J.P. As Scientific Committee of the Hp-Eureg on Behalf of the National, C. Protocol of the European Registry on the management of *Helicobacter pylori* infection (Hp-EuReg). *Helicobacter* **2019**, *24*, e12630. [CrossRef]
17. Harris, P.A.; Taylor, R.; Thielke, R.; Payne, J.; Gonzalez, N.; Conde, J.G. Research electronic data capture (REDCap)—A metadata-driven methodology and workflow process for providing translational research informatics support. *J. Biomed. Inform.* **2009**, *42*, 377–381. [CrossRef]
18. Graham, D.Y.; Lu, H.; Dore, M.P. Relative potency of proton-pump inhibitors, *Helicobacter pylori* therapy cure rates, and meaning of double-dose PPI. *Helicobacter* **2019**, *24*, e12554. [CrossRef] [PubMed]
19. Kirchheiner, J.; Glatt, S.; Fuhr, U.; Klotz, U.; Meineke, I.; Seufferlein, T.; Brockmöller, J. Relative potency of proton-pump inhibitors—Comparison of effects on intragastric pH. *Eur. J. Clin. Pharmacol.* **2009**, *65*, 19–31. [CrossRef] [PubMed]
20. Liu, X.; Wang, H.; Lv, Z.; Wang, Y.; Wang, B.; Xie, Y.; Zhou, X.; Lv, N. Rescue Therapy with a Proton Pump Inhibitor Plus Amoxicillin and Rifabutin for *Helicobacter pylori* Infection: A Systematic Review and Meta-Analysis. *Gastroenterol. Res. Pract.* **2015**, *2015*, 415648. [CrossRef] [PubMed]
21. Gingold-Belfer, R.; Niv, Y.; Levi, Z.; Boltin, D. Rifabutin triple therapy for first-line and rescue treatment of *Helicobacter pylori* infection: A systematic review and meta-analysis. *J. Gastroenterol. Hepatol.* **2021**, *36*, 1392–1402. [CrossRef] [PubMed]
22. De Francesco, V.; Giorgio, F.; Hassan, C.; Manes, G.; Vannella, L.; Panella, C.; Ierardi, E.; Zullo, A. Worldwide *H. pylori* antibiotic resistance: A systematic review. *J. Gastrointestin. Liver Dis.* **2010**, *19*, 409–414.
23. Megraud, F.; Coenen, S.; Versporten, A.; Kist, M.; Lopez-Brea, M.; Hirschl, A.M.; Andersen, L.P.; Goossens, H.; Glupczynski, Y.; Study Group participants. Helicobacter pylori resistance to antibiotics in Europe and its relationship to antibiotic consumption. *Gut* **2013**, *62*, 34–42.
24. Bock, H.; Koop, H.; Lehn, N.; Heep, M. Rifabutin-based triple therapy after failure of *Helicobacter pylori* eradication treatment: Preliminary experience. *J. Clin. Gastroenterol.* **2000**, *31*, 222–225. [CrossRef] [PubMed]
25. Pilotto, A.; Franceschi, M.; Rassu, M.; Furlan, F.; Scagnelli, M. In vitro activity of rifabutin against strains of *Helicobacter pylori* resistant to metronidazole and clarithromycin. *Am. J. Gastroenterol.* **2000**, *95*, 833–834. [CrossRef] [PubMed]
26. Beales, I.L. Efficacy of *Helicobacter pylori* eradication therapies: A single centre observational study. *BMC Gastroenterol.* **2001**, *1*, 7. [CrossRef]
27. Wong, W.M.; Gu, Q.; Lam, S.K.; Fung, F.M.Y.; Lai, K.C.; Hu, W.H.C.; Yee, Y.K.; Chan, C.K.; Xia, H.H.X.; Yuen, M.F.; et al. Randomized controlled study of rabeprazole, levofloxacin and rifabutin triple therapy vs. quadruple therapy as second-line treatment for *Helicobacter pylori* infection. *Aliment. Pharmacol. Ther.* **2003**, *17*, 553–560. [CrossRef] [PubMed]
28. Toracchio, S.; Capodicasa, S.; Soraja, D.; Cellini, L.; Marzio, L. Rifabutin based triple therapy for eradication of *H. pylori* primary and secondary resistant to tinidazole and clarithromycin. *Dig. Liver Dis.* **2005**, *37*, 33–38. [CrossRef]
29. Borody, T.J.; Pang, G.; Wettstein, A.R.; Clancy, R.; Herdman, K.; Surace, R.; Llorente, R.; Ng, C. Efficacy and safety of rifabutin-containing 'rescue therapy' for resistant *Helicobacter pylori* infection. *Aliment. Pharmacol. Ther.* **2006**, *23*, 481–488. [CrossRef] [PubMed]
30. Miehlke, S.; Hansky, K.; Schneider-Brachert, W.; Kirsch, C.; Morgner, A.; Madisch, A.; Kuhlisch, E.; Bästlein, E.; Jacobs, E.; Bayerdörffer, E.; et al. Randomized trial of rifabutin-based triple therapy and high-dose dual therapy for rescue treatment of *Helicobacter pylori* resistant to both metronidazole and clarithromycin. *Aliment. Pharmacol. Ther.* **2006**, *24*, 395–403. [CrossRef]
31. Graham, D.Y.; Canaan, Y.; Maher, J.; Wiener, G.; Hulten, K.G.; Kalfus, I.N. Rifabutin-Based Triple Therapy (RHB-105) for *Helicobacter pylori* Eradication: A Double-Blind, Randomized, Controlled Trial. *Ann. Intern. Med.* **2020**, *172*, 795–802. [CrossRef] [PubMed]
32. Miehlke, S.; Schneider-Brachert, W.; Kirsch, C.; Morgner, A.; Madisch, A.; Kuhlisch, E.; Haferland, C.; Bästlein, E.; Jebens, C.; Zekorn, C.; et al. One-Week Once-Daily Triple Therapy with Esomeprazole, Moxifloxacin, and Rifabutin for Eradication of Persistent *Helicobacter pylori* Resistant to Both Metronidazole and Clarithromycin. *Helicobacter* **2008**, *13*, 69–74. [CrossRef] [PubMed]
33. Perri, F.; Festa, V.; Clemente, R.; Villani, M.R.; Quitadamo, M.; Caruso, N.; Bergoli, M.L.; Andriulli, A. Randomized study of two "rescue" therapies for helicobacter pylori-infected patients after failure of standard triple therapies. *Am. J. Gastroenterol.* **2001**, *96*, 58–62.

34. Saracino, I.M.; Pavoni, M.; Zullo, A.; Fiorini, G.; Saccomanno, L.; Lazzarotto, T.; Antonelli, G.; Cavallo, R.; Borghi, C.; Vaira, D. Rifabutin-Based Triple Therapy or Bismuth-Based Quadruple Regimen as Rescue Therapies for *Helicobacter pylori* Infection. *Eur. J. Intern. Med.* **2020**, *81*, 50–53. [CrossRef]
35. Fiorini, G.; Vakil, N.; Zullo, A.; Saracino, I.M.; Castelli, V.; Ricci, C.; Zaccaro, C.; Gatta, L.; Vaira, D. Culture-based Selection Therapy for Patients Who Did Not Respond to Previous Treatment for *Helicobacter pylori* Infection. *Clin. Gastroenterol. Hepatol.* **2013**, *11*, 507–551. [CrossRef] [PubMed]
36. Navarro-Jarabo, J.M.; Fernández, N.; Sousa, F.L.; Cabrera, M.; Castro, M.; Ramírez, L.M.; Rivera, R.; Ubiña, E.; Vera, F.; Méndez, I.; et al. Efficacy of rifabutin-based triple therapy as second-line treatment to eradicate *Helicobacter pylori* infection. *BMC Gastroenterol.* **2007**, *7*, 31. [CrossRef]
37. Van der Poorten, D.; Katelaris, P.H. The effectiveness of rifabutin triple therapy for patients with difficult-to-eradicate *Helicobacter pylori* in clinical practice. *Aliment. Pharmacol Ther.* **2007**, *26*, 1537–1542. [CrossRef] [PubMed]
38. Mori, H.; Suzuki, H.; Matsuzaki, J.; Tsugawa, H.; Fukuhara, S.; Miyoshi, S.; Hirata, K.; Seino, T.; Matsushita, M.; Nishizawa, T.; et al. Rifabutin-based 10-day and 14-day triple therapy as a third-line and fourth-line regimen for *Helicobacter pylori* eradication: A pilot study. *United Eur. Gastroenterol. J.* **2016**, *4*, 380–387. [CrossRef]
39. Malfertheiner, P. Infection: Bismuth improves PPI-based triple therapy for *H. pylori* eradication. *Nat. Rev. Gastroenterol. Hepatol.* **2010**, *7*, 538–539. [CrossRef]
40. Liao, J.; Zheng, Q.; Liang, X.; Zhang, W.; Sun, Q.; Liu, W.; Xiao, S.; Graham, D.Y.; Lu, H. Effect of Fluoroquinolone Resistance on 14-day Levofloxacin Triple and Triple Plus Bismuth Quadruple Therapy. *Helicobacter* **2013**, *18*, 373–377. [CrossRef]
41. Tay, C.Y.; Windsor, H.M.; Thirriot, F.; Lu, W.; Conway, C.; Perkins, T.T.; Marshall, B.J. *Helicobacter pylori* eradication in Western Australia using novel quadruple therapy combinations. *Aliment. Pharmacol. Ther.* **2012**, *36*, 1076–1083. [CrossRef] [PubMed]
42. Ciccaglione, A.F.; Tavani, R.; Grossi, L.; Cellini, L.; Manzoli, L.; Marzio, L. Rifabutin Containing Triple Therapy and Rifabutin with Bismuth Containing Quadruple Therapy for Third-Line Treatment of *Helicobacter pylori* Infection: Two Pilot Studies. *Helicobacter* **2016**, *21*, 375–381. [CrossRef]
43. Ierardi, E.; Giangaspero, A.; Losurdo, G.; Giorgio, F.; Amoruso, A.; De Francesco, V. Quadruple rescue therapy after first and second line failure for *Helicobacter pylori* treatment: Comparison between two tetracycline-based regimens. *J. Gastrointestin. Liver Dis.* **2014**, *23*, 36–70. [CrossRef]
44. Gisbert, J.P.; Calvet, X. Review article: Non-bismuth quadruple (concomitant) therapy for eradication of *Helicobater pylori*. *Aliment. Pharmacol. Ther.* **2011**, *34*, 604–617. [CrossRef] [PubMed]
45. Nyssen, O.P.; Perez-Aisa, A.; Tepes, B.; Castro-Fernandez, M.; Kupcinskas, J.; Jonaitis, L.; Bujanda, L.; Lucendo, A.; Jurecic, N.B.; Perez-Lasala, J.; et al. Adverse Event Profile During the Treatment of *Helicobacter pylori*: A Real-World Experience of 22,000 Patients from the European Registry on *H. pylori* Management (Hp-EuReg). *Am. J. Gastroenterol.* **2021**, *116*, 1220–1229. [CrossRef] [PubMed]
46. Griffith, D.E.; Brown, B.A.; Girard, W.M.; Wallace, J.R.J. Adverse Events Associated with High-Dose Rifabutin in Macrolide-Containing Regimens for the Treatment of *Mycobacterium avium* Complex Lung Disease. *Clin. Infect. Dis.* **1995**, *21*, 594–598. [CrossRef]
47. Apseloff, G.; Foulds, G.; LaBoy-Goral, L.; Kraut, E.; Vincent, J. Severe neutropenia caused by recommended prophylactic doses of rifabutin. *Lancet* **1996**, *348*, 685. [CrossRef]
48. Perri, F.; Festa, V.; Clemente, R.; Quitadamo, M.; Andriulli, A. Rifabutin-based 'rescue therapy' for *Helicobacter pylori* infected patients after failure of standard regimens. *Aliment. Pharmacol. Ther.* **2000**, *14*, 311–316. [CrossRef]
49. Canducci, F.; Ojetti, V.; Pola, P.; Gasbarrini, G.; Gasbarrini, A. Rifabutin-based *Helicobacter pylori* eradication 'rescue therapy'. *Aliment. Pharmacol Ther.* **2001**, *15*, 143. [CrossRef]
50. Qasim, A.; Sebastian, S.; Thornton, O.; Dobson, M.; McLoughlin, R.; Buckley, M.; O'Connor, H.; O'Morain, C. Rifabutin- and furazolidone-based *Helicobacter pylori* eradication therapies after failure of standard first- and second-line eradication attempts in dyspepsia patients. *Aliment. Pharmacol. Ther.* **2005**, *21*, 91–96. [CrossRef]
51. Gisbert, J.P.; Marcos, S.; Moreno-Otero, R.; Pajares, J.M. Third-line rescue therapy with levofloxacin is more effective than rifabutin rescue regimen after two *Helicobacter pylori* treatment failures. *Aliment. Pharmacol. Ther.* **2006**, *24*, 1469–1474. [CrossRef] [PubMed]
52. Gisbert, J.P.; Castro-Fernandez, M.; Perez-Aisa, A.; Cosme, A.; Molina-Infante, J.; Rodrigo, L.; Modolell, I.; Cabriada, J.L.; Lamas, E.; Marcos, E.; et al. Fourth-line rescue therapy with rifabutin in patients with three *Helicobacter pylori* eradication failures. *Aliment. Pharmacol. Ther.* **2012**, *35*, 941–947. [CrossRef] [PubMed]
53. Kalfus, I.N.; Graham, D.Y.; Riff, D.S.; Panas, R.M. Rifabutin-Containing Triple Therapy (RHB-105) for Eradication of *Helicobacter pylori*: Randomized ERADICATE Hp Trial. *Antibiotics* **2020**, *9*, 685. [CrossRef] [PubMed]

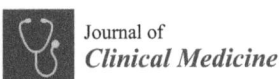

Article

Efficacy of a Third-Generation High-Vision Ultrathin Endoscope for Evaluating Gastric Atrophy and Intestinal Metaplasia in *Helicobacter pylori*-Eradicated Patients

Junichi Uematsu [1], Mitsushige Sugimoto [1,*], Mariko Hamada [1], Eri Iwata [1], Ryota Niikura [1], Naoyoshi Nagata [1], Masakatsu Fukuzawa [2], Takao Itoi [2] and Takashi Kawai [1]

[1] Department of Gastroenterological Endoscopy, Tokyo Medical University Hospital, Shinjuku, Tokyo 160-0023, Japan; juju1113u@yahoo.co.jp (J.U.); mahamada0820@gmail.com (M.H.); eiwata@tokyo-med.ac.jp (E.I.); rniikuratritonocn@gmail.com (R.N.); nnagata_ncgm@yahoo.co.jp (N.N.); t-kawai@tokyo-med.ac.jp (T.K.)

[2] Department of Gastroenterology and Hepatology, Tokyo Medical University Hospital, Shinjuku, Tokyo 160-0023, Japan; masakatu8055@yahoo.co.jp (M.F.); itoitakao@gmail.com (T.I.)

* Correspondence: sugimo@tokyo-med.ac.jp; Tel.: +81-3-3342-6111; Fax: +81-3-3345-5359

Abstract: Background: Image-enhanced endoscopy methods such as narrow-band imaging (NBI) are advantageous over white-light imaging (WLI) for detecting gastric atrophy, intestinal metaplasia, and cancer. Although new third-generation high-vision ultrathin endoscopes improve image quality and resolution over second-generation endoscopes, it is unclear whether the former also enhances color differences surrounding atrophy and intestinal metaplasia for endoscopic detection. We compared the efficacy of a new third-generation ultrathin endoscope and an older second-generation endoscope. Methods: We enrolled 50 *Helicobacter pylori*-eradicated patients who underwent transnasal endoscopy with a second-generation and third-generation endoscope (GIF-290N and GIF-1200N, respectively) in our retrospective study. Color differences based on the International Commission on Illumination 1976 (L*, a*, b*) color space were compared between second-generation and third-generation high-vision endoscopes. Results: Color differences surrounding atrophy produced by NBI on the GIF-1200N endoscope were significantly greater than those on GIF-290N (19.2 ± 8.5 vs. 14.4 ± 6.2, p = 0.001). In contrast, color differences surrounding intestinal metaplasia using both WLI and NBI were similar on GIF-1200N and GIF-290N endoscopes. NBI was advantageous over WLI for detecting intestinal metaplasia on both endoscopes. Conclusions: NBI using a third-generation ultrathin endoscope produced significantly greater color differences surrounding atrophy and intestinal metaplasia in *H. pylori*-eradicated patients compared with WLI.

Keywords: third-generation ultrathin endoscope; transnasal endoscopy; narrow-band imaging; Kyoto classification of gastritis; gastric atrophy and intestinal metaplasia

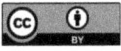

1. Introduction

In Japan, the Kyoto classification of gastritis was developed to identify patients at high risk of developing gastric cancer using a grading system for endoscopic risk that is based on endoscopic characteristics of gastritis related to *Helicobacter pylori* infection [1,2]. This system assesses patients for gastric cancer risk by scoring five endoscopic parameters, namely atrophy, intestinal metaplasia, enlarged folds, nodularity, and diffuse redness [1,2]. Given that gastric cancer arising from long-term *H. pylori* infection is a major concern around the world, and *H. pylori*-positive patients develop gastric cancer at a rate of 0.4% annually [3], it is important to accurately evaluate the endoscopic risk of gastric cancer, especially in terms of gastric atrophy and intestinal metaplasia, in *H. pylori*-positive and previously eradicated patients at high risk of gastric cancer [2,4,5].

Recent developments in endoscopic instrumentation and image-enhancement techniques, known together as image-enhanced endoscopy (IEE), including narrow-band imaging (NBI), blue laser imaging, linked color imaging, and texture and color enhancement imaging with or without magnification, have improved the detection rate of gastric atrophy, intestinal metaplasia, and cancer [6–10]. Although transnasal and oral endoscopes differ in their detection rates for gastrointestinal diseases and the assessment of the severity of gastritis [11,12], in 2020, Olympus Co. developed a third-generation high-vision ultrathin endoscope called GIF-1200N with a new high-quality complementary metal-oxide semiconductor sensor that could improve resolution, noise, and graduation over older second-generation endoscopes such as GIF-290N. In addition, the development of a new processor called EVIS X-1 has improved image quality over older processors such as EXERA III and LUCERA ELITE. Therefore, combining the new third-generation ultrathin endoscope with the new processor is expected to increase the detection rate of endoscopic atrophy, intestinal metaplasia, and cancer over a combination of the older second-generation endoscope and older processor [13]. Although determining color differences according to the International Commission on Illumination (CIE) 1976 (L*a*b*) color space is a typical objective endoscopic analysis method [10,14,15], it is unclear whether third-generation endoscopes produce significantly greater color differences surrounding atrophy and intestinal metaplasia for endoscopic detection.

In Japan, transnasal endoscopy using an ultrathin endoscope has become a popular medical screening test because it is relatively pain-free for patients. Given their widespread use, it is prudent to evaluate the usefulness of these tests. Here, we investigated whether a new high-vision third-generation ultrathin endoscope using white-light imaging (WLI) and NBI improves the detection of gastric cancer risk assessed based on the Kyoto classification of gastritis compared with an older second-generation endoscope in *H. pylori*-eradicated patients.

2. Materials and Methods

2.1. Study Design and Patients

This study was a retrospective trial conducted at Tokyo Medical University Hospital to investigate the efficacy of transnasal endoscopy for evaluating the severity of gastritis in patients who had received eradication therapy for *H. pylori* infection. Of patients who had a history of transnasal endoscopy with a second-generation endoscope (GIF-290N, Olympus Co., Tokyo, Japan), we enrolled 50 patients aged $\geq$ 20 years who had subsequently undergone endoscopy with a high-vision third-generation ultrathin endoscope as part of a health check-up (GIF-1200N, Olympus Co., Tokyo, Japan). Exclusion criteria were patients with a history of gastric surgery, a lack of clear images to evaluate endoscopic gastritis, atrophy and intestinal metaplasia, and no history of eradication therapy for *H. pylori* infection.

The study protocol adhered to the ethical principles of the Declaration of Helsinki and was approved by the institutional review board of Tokyo Medical University (T2020-0059). Because this study was conducted under a retrospective design, and written informed consent was not obtained from each enrolled patient, a document describing an opt-out policy through which potential patients and/or relatives could refuse inclusion was uploaded on the Tokyo Medical University Hospital website.

2.2. Endoscopy and Severity of Gastritis

Endoscopy was performed using the older second-generation GIF-290N (from March 2015 to June 2020) and new third-generation ultrathin GIF-1200N endoscopes (from April 2021 to January 2022) (Figure 1). The severity of gastritis was retrospectively scored according to the Kyoto classification of gastritis and the Kimura–Takemoto classification [1,16]. In the Kyoto classification, the total score is calculated by summing the scores for five parameters, namely atrophy, intestinal metaplasia, hypertrophy of gastric folds, nodularity, and diffuse redness [2,17–19]. The 1st and 2nd endoscopies were performed by an expert endoscopist (KT). Two expert endoscopists independently evaluated the severity of gastritis using

WBI. When scores assigned by the two endoscopists differed, a consensus was reached by reviewing patient images.

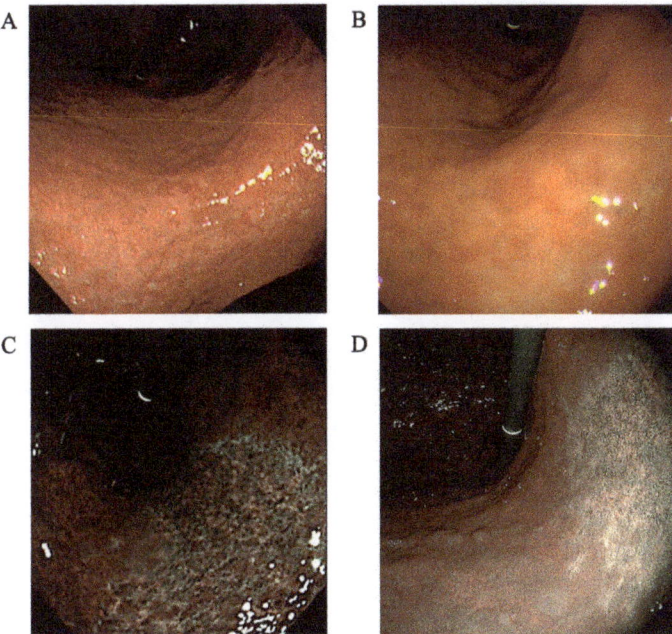

Figure 1. Images taken using a second-generation GIF-290N ultrathin endoscope by white-light imaging (**A**), third-generation GIF-1200N ultrathin endoscope by white-light imaging (**B**), second-generation endoscope by narrow-band imaging (**C**), and third-generation endoscope by narrow-band imaging (**D**). The endoscopic features of mucosal atrophy are characterized by a discolored mucosa and visible capillary network in the atrophic area (**A**–**D**). Intestinal metaplasia is defined as multiple ashen nodular or cobblestone-like lesions on atrophic mucosa observed (**A,B**). Villous appearance, whitish mucosa, and rough mucosal surface are helpful indicators for the endoscopic diagnosis of intestinal metaplasia. Map-like redness is defined as reddish depressed areas of various shape and sizes in the atrophic area (**A**).

2.3. Measurement of Colors

Color differences surrounding atrophic borders and intestinal metaplasia were measured and compared between GIF-290N and GIF-1200N endoscopes [10]. We randomly set three pairs (with and without) of regions (atrophy or intestinal metaplasia) of interest and calculated the color difference in each patient using pictures of similar anatomical location (i.e., antrum and lesser curve of lower body) at both GIF-290N and GIF-1200N endoscopes. Color differences were calculated using the CIE 1976 (L*, a*, b*) color space [20,21], a three-dimensional model composed of a black-white axis (L*, brightness), a red-green axis (a*, red-green component), and a yellow-blue axis (b*, yellow-blue component). The color difference was defined as ΔE, which expresses the distance between two points in the color space. ΔE was calculated using the following formula: $\{(\Delta L^*)^2 + (\Delta a^*)^2 + (\Delta b^*)^2\}^{1/2}$, where ΔL^*, Δa^*, and Δb^* are differences in the L*, a*, and b* values, respectively, between regions with and without atrophy and intestinal metaplasia. Each ΔL^*, Δa^*, and Δb^* value was determined by a computer operator who was blinded to clinical information using Adobe Photoshop, version 22.5.1 (Adobe KK, Tokyo, Japan).

2.4. Statistical Analysis

Parameters including age, height, body weight, and Kyoto classification score are expressed as mean ± standard deviation (SD). Categorical variables for GIF-290N and GIF-1200N endoscopes are summarized as n (%) and were compared using χ^2 tests. Statistically significant differences in mean Kyoto classification scores and mean ΔE between GIF-290N and GIF-1200N endoscopes were determined using Student's t-test. A p-value < 0.05 was considered statistically significant, and all p-values were two-sided. All statistical analyses were performed using the statistical analysis software SPSS, version 27.0 (IBM Japan, Tokyo, Japan).

3. Results

3.1. Patient Characteristics

Of patients who had a history of endoscopy using GIF-290N, we randomly enrolled 50 H. pylori-eradicated patients, who had subsequently undergone transnasal endoscopy using the GIF-1200N endoscope as part of a health check-up. The mean age was 74.3 ± 6.6 years and 54.0% of patients were male (Table 1). Baseline diseases included peptic ulcers in 10.0% of patients (n = 5), gastric cancer in 6.0% (n = 3), and other cancers in 24.0% (n = 12). Drugs taken included proton pump inhibitors in 32.0% of patients (n = 16), antiplatelet drugs in 32.0% (n = 16), and anticoagulants in 8.0% (n = 4) (Table 1). The mean duration from 1st to 2nd endoscopies was 35.5 ± 19.8 (months ± SD).

Table 1. Characteristics of patients enrolled in this study.

	All Patients (n = 50)
Age (years ± SD)	74.3 ± 6.6
Sex [male, n (%)]	27 (54.0%)
Height (cm ± SD)	160.8 ± 8.7
Body weight (kg ± SD)	58.8 ± 9.7
H. pylori infection, Negative/Current/Eradicated [n/n/n]	0/0/50
Smoking, Never/Current/Past [n/n/n]	32/1/17
Alcohol [n (%)]	32 (64.0%)
Diseases	
Peptic ulcer [n (%)]	5 (10.0%)
Gastric cancer [n (%)]	3 (6.0%)
Cancer (others) [n (%)]	12 (24.0%)
Hyperlipidemia [n (%)]	17 (34.0%)
Hypertension [n (%)]	28 (56.0%)
Diabetes mellitus [n (%)]	7 (14.0%)
Drugs	
Proton pump inhibitor [n (%)]	16 (32.0%)
NSAID [n (%)]	0 (0%)
Antihypertensive drug [n (%)]	32 (64.0%)
Antihyperlipidemic drug [n (%)]	20 (40.0%)
Antiplatelet drug [n (%)]	16 (32.0%)
Anticoagulant [n (%)]	4 (8.0%)
Antidiabetic drug [n (%)]	9 (18.0%)
Bisphosphonate [n (%)]	2 (4.0%)
Mean duration from 1st to 2nd endoscopies (months ± SD)	35.5 ± 19.8

Abbreviations: H. pylori: Helicobacter pylori, NSAID: non-steroidal anti-inflammatory drug, SD: standard deviation.

3.2. Severity of Gastritis Assessed Using WLI on GIF-290N and GIF-1200N Endoscopes

On WLI, the severity of gastritis based on the degree of atrophy scored according to the Kimura–Takemoto classification, and the degree of atrophy, intestinal metaplasia, enlarged folds, nodular gastritis, and diffuse redness scored according to the Kyoto classification of gastritis were similar between GIF-290N and GIF-1200N endoscopes (Table 2). The rates of detection of xanthoma, multiple white and flat elevated lesions and map-like redness were also similar between GIF-290N and GIF-1200N endoscopes (data not shown).

Table 2. Severity of gastritis by white-light imaging according to the Kimura–Takemoto classification and Kyoto classification of gastritis.

Category/Characteristic		GIF-1200N Endoscope (WLI)	GIF-290N Endoscope (WLI)	p-Value
Kimura–Takemoto classification				
Atrophy	C-0–C-II	9 (18.0%)	8 (16.0%)	0.240
	C-III–O-I	29 (58.0%)	36 (72.0%)	
	O-II–O-III	12 (24.0%)	6 (12.0%)	
Kyoto classification of gastritis				
Atrophy	A0	2 (4.0%)	0 (0%)	0.420
	A1	13 (26.0%)	16 (16.7%)	
	A2	35 (70.0%)	34 (66.7%)	
Intestinal metaplasia	IM0	15 (30.0%)	11 (22.0%)	0.662
	IM1	12 (24.0%)	15 (30.0%)	
	IM2	23 (46.0%)	24 (48.0%)	
Enlarged folds	H0	49 (98.0%)	50 (100%)	1
	H1	1 (2.0%)	0 (0%)	
Nodular gastritis	N0	50 (100%)	50 (100%)	1
	N1	0 (0%)	0 (0%)	
Diffuse redness	DR0	46 (92.0%)	46 (92.0%)	1
	DR1	4 (8.0%)	4 (8.0%)	
	DR2	0 (0%)	0 (0%)	

Similarly, mean endoscopic scores of gastritis evaluated using WLI according to the Kyoto classification of gastritis were not significantly different between GIF-290N and GIF-1200N endoscopes (Table 3).

Table 3. Endoscopic severity of gastritis by white-light imaging according to the Kyoto classification of gastritis.

Endoscopic Characteristic	GIF-1200N Endoscope	GIF-290N Endoscope	p-Value
Atrophy	1.66 ± 0.56	1.68 ± 0.47	0.709
Intestinal metaplasia	1.16 ± 0.87	1.26 ± 0.80	0.168
Enlarged folds	0.02 ± 0.14	0.00 ± 0.00	0.322
Nodular gastritis	0.00 ± 0.00	0.00 ± 0.00	
Diffuse redness	0.08 ± 0.27	0.08 ± 0.33	1.000
Total score	2.94 ± 1.641	3.12 ± 1.29	0.060

Data show mean ± standard deviation.

3.3. Color Differences in Endoscopic Atrophy and Intestinal Metaplasia on GIF-290N and GIF-1200N Endoscopes

The color difference surrounding atrophic borders evaluated using NBI was 14.4 ± 6.2 on the GIF-290N endoscope and 19.2 ± 8.5 on the GIF-1200N endoscope; the difference was significantly greater on the GIF-1200N than the GIF-290N endoscope ($p = 0.001$, Table 4). Significant differences evaluated using NBI were also observed along the black–white (ΔL^*) and the red–green axis (Δa^*) surrounding atrophy between GIF-290N and GIF-1200N endoscopes. In contrast, there was no significant color difference surrounding atrophic borders observed using WLI between the two endoscopes (Table 4).

Table 4. Color differences between areas with and without atrophy and between regions with and without intestinal metaplasia.

Finding		GIF-1200N Endoscope WLI	GIF-290N Endoscope WLI	p-Value	GIF-1200N Endoscope NBI	GIF-290N Endoscope NBI	p-Value
Atrophy	ΔL*	5.8 ± 11.0	5.7 ± 7.9	0.954	12.3 ± 13.0	5.6 ± 11.5	**0.030**
	Δa*	−6.0 ± 4.7	−8.8 ± 7.3	**0.015**	−1.6 ± 10.3	5.5 ± 6.5	**0.002**
	Δb*	−0.6 ± 3.0	−2.4 ± 4.1	**0.012**	2.0 ± 3.7	2.3 ± 2.9	0.733
	ΔE*	13.4 ± 6.4	15.0 ± 4.8	0.133	19.2 ± 8.5	14.4 ± 6.2	**0.001**
Intestinal metaplasia	ΔL*	2.2 ± 4.7	3.3 ± 4.9	0.034	5.0 ± 6.7	3.0 ± 8.5	0.388
	Δa*	−0.6 ± 5.3	−2.5 ± 6.0	0.076	−9.3 ± 5.8	−9.0 ± 5.0	0.819
	Δb*	−0.5 ± 2.7	−1.7 ± 3.3	**0.043**	−2.3 ± 3.6	−2.9 ± 2.0	0.415
	ΔE*	7.1 ± 3.3	6.9 ± 3.1	0.738	13.7 ± 4.2	13.3 ± 4.4	0.760

Abbreviations: WLI: white-light imaging, ΔL*: change in brightness, Δa*: change in red-green component, Δb*: change in yellow-blue component, ΔE: color difference; * $p < 0.05$. Bold meant data with $p < 0.05$ with significant different.

Likewise, there were no significant differences in ΔE surrounding intestinal metaplasia using either WLI (7.1 ± 3.3 and 6.9 ± 3.1) or NBI (13.7 ± 4.23 and 13.3 ± 4.4) on the GIF-290N compared to the GIF-1200N endoscope (Table 4).

When color differences surrounding atrophic borders were compared between WLI and NBI on the GIF-1200N endoscope, the difference in NBI (19.2 ± 8.5) was significantly greater than that in WLI (13.4 ± 6.4, $p < 0.001$, Figure 2). In contrast, no significant differences were observed in ΔE surrounding atrophic borders between WLI and NBI on the GIF-290N endoscope. The color differences surrounding intestinal metaplasia using NBI on the GIF-290N and GIF-1200N endoscopes were 13.3 ± 4.4 and 13.7 ± 4.2, which were significantly greater than those observed using WLI (6.9 ± 3.1 and 7.1 ± 3.3, both $p < 0.001$, respectively) (Figure 2).

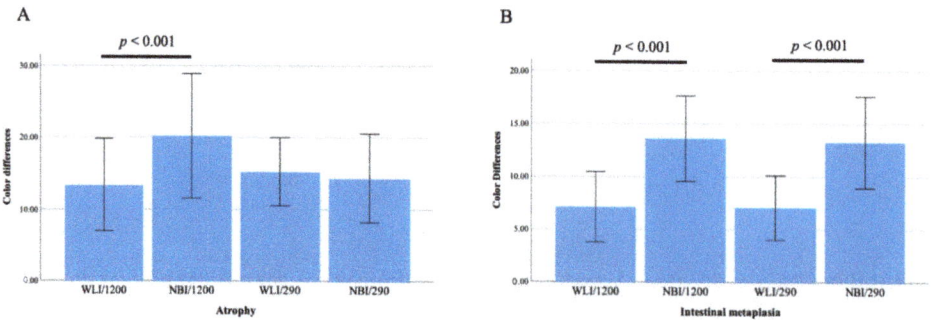

Figure 2. Color differences surrounding atrophic borders (A) and intestinal metaplasia (B) between WLI and NBI using third-generation GIF-1200N and second-generation GIF-290N ultrathin endoscopes.

4. Discussion

We demonstrated that NBI with a third-generation ultrathin endoscope produced significantly greater color differences based on the CIE 1976 (L*, a*, b*) color space surrounding atrophic borders than a second-generation endoscope in *H. pylori*-eradicated patients. In addition, NBI using a third-generation endoscope produced significantly greater color differences surrounding atrophy and intestinal metaplasia compared with WLI. Therefore, combining third-generation endoscopes with IEE methods such as NBI may be useful for identifying patients at a high risk of gastric cancer at health check-ups through not only improved image quality, resolution, noise, and graduation, but also increased color differences.

4.1. Efficacy of Third-Generation High-Vision Ultrathin Endoscope for Detecting Gastric Cancer Risk

Given that advances in endoscopic technology have markedly enhanced the diagnostic capability of endoscopy, it is important to determine the best method for identifying patients with a higher risk of gastric cancer and the best endoscopic method for diagnosing early-stage gastric cancer in *H. pylori*-positive and *H. pylori*-eradicated patients. The detection rate of gastric cancer and diagnostic efficiency for gastritis among those at a high risk of developing gastric cancer is affected by the skill of the endoscopist (e.g., experience and knowledge concerning endoscopy and gastric cancer), gastric environment (e.g., *H. pylori* infection, mucus, mucosal redness, and the severity of atrophy and intestinal metaplasia), tumor-related factors (e.g., location, size, form, number of tumors, and pathological types), and endoscope image-related factors (e.g., image quality, resolution, noise, graduation, type of IEE, field of view and ease of passage).

Because transnasal endoscopy performed using an ultrathin endoscope is safe and can be performed without any sedation, endoscopic examination is often performed transnasally to reduce invasiveness and distress to the patient [22–24]. However, major disadvantages of transnasal endoscopy include the need for complex considerations (e.g., anesthesia of the nasal cavity, use of vasoconstrictors, limited manipulations, and lower power aspiration and air supply), poor image quality, lower detection rate of gastrointestinal diseases, and different evaluation methods for the severity of gastritis compared with oral endoscopy [12,25]. In fact, when we investigated the capability of a second-generation endoscope for diagnosing gastric cancer in 255 consecutive patients who underwent gastrointestinal screening, the sensitivity, specificity, and diagnostic accuracy for gastric cancer diagnosis using WLI were as low as 50.0%, 63.6%, and 61.5%, respectively [11]. Likewise, Toyoizumi et al. [12] reported that the sensitivity and specificity of a second-generation ultrathin endoscope for diagnosing gastric cancer were significantly lower than that of a high-resolution oral endoscope (sensitivity 58.5% vs 78%, $p = 0.021$; specificity 91.8% vs 100%, $p = 0.014$). However, the introduction of a third-generation ultrathin endoscope (GIF-1200N; Olympus Co., Tokyo, Japan) with improved resolution in 2020 has made it possible to obtain high-definition images of the microsurface of the mucosa. Although few studies have reported the usefulness of this third-generation ultrathin endoscope with high image quality for detecting gastric cancer, our previous preliminary study showed that the sensitivity of WLI with the third-generation GIF-1200N endoscope was 85.7% for gastric cancer diagnosis, which is a significant improvement on the second-generation GIF-XP290N endoscope (31.8%) [13]. Clearly, distinguishable colors at the border of a tumor, atrophy and intestinal metaplasia can enhance an endoscopist's ability to determine the extent of the tumor, atrophy, and intestinal metaplasia. Therefore, in addition to endoscope image-related factors such as image quality, resolution, noise, and graduation, assessing color differences according to the CIE 1976 (L*a*b*) color space is also an objective endoscopic analysis method (e.g., detection of intestinal metaplasia and atrophic border between WLI and IEE) [10,14,15]. In this study, we demonstrated for the first time that NBI using a third-generation ultrathin endoscope produces significantly greater color differences surrounding atrophic borders than a second-generation endoscope. The high image quality, high resolution, and low noise of the third-generation ultrathin endoscope are expected to improve the detection rate of gastric cancer, and screening for gastric cancer using third-generation ultrathin endoscopes will become increasingly important as the number of patients who have received *H. pylori* eradication therapy increases.

4.2. NBI Using Ultrathin Endoscopy for Identifying Patients at High Risk of Gastric Cancer

Gastric cancer is relatively common worldwide, with over 1,000,000 new cases reported in 2018, and an estimated 783,000 reported deaths [26]. A recent meta-analysis showed that eradication therapy reduces the risk of gastric cancer, with a relative risk of 0.51–0.67 [27], although it cannot prevent gastric cancer development in all patients. Therefore, the surveillance of all *H. pylori*-eradicated patients is important for the early diagnosis of gastric cancer. In fact, regular endoscopic surveillance increases the survival rate of gastric cancer, with a Japanese cohort study showing that >95% of cases with gastric cancer identified by annual endoscopy surveillance can be cured by endoscopic resection [28].

The current *H. pylori* infection rate in Japan is about 35%, and most Japanese patients with atrophy undergoing a health check-up by endoscopy have previously received eradication therapy for *H. pylori* infection. Because endoscopic characteristics differ between *H. pylori*-positive and eradicated patients, we focused on strategies for detecting atrophy and intestinal metaplasia in *H. pylori*-eradicated patients in this study. Although WLI is currently the most common endoscopic technique for the stomach, a diagnosis by WLI is based on the size and color of the lesion, and the characteristics of the lesion surface, surrounding mucosa, and gastric rugae. This makes the experience of the endoscopist immensely important and causes great variability in diagnostic findings. Despite sufficient illumination by a new processor for endoscopy, abnormalities in mucosal discoloration and morphological changes to the mucosal surface go undetected using WLI or a combination of WLI and indigocarmine chromoendoscopy in 18.9–21.6% of early-stage gastric cancer cases [29,30]. A recent multicenter randomized controlled trial also failed to show the efficacy of second-generation NBI for early-stage gastric cancer detection in high-risk patients (1.9% in WLI and 2.3% in second-generation NBI, $p = 0.412$) [31]. However, recent studies have reported that the vessel plus surface (VS) classification system, which uses innovative optical image-enhancing technology in magnifying NBI endoscopy to enable the better visualization of surface structures and blood vessels than WLI, has high diagnostic capability for determining the extent of invasion of early-stage gastric cancer and superficial squamous cell carcinoma of the head and neck and the esophagus [29,30,32,33]. In fact, the MAPS II guideline, an official statement from the European Society of Gastrointestinal Endoscopy, states that using a high-definition endoscope with IEE is more effective for detecting atrophy and intestinal metaplasia than high-definition WLI alone [34]. Similarly, guidelines for the endoscopic diagnosis of early gastric cancer from the Japan Gastroenterological Endoscopy Society Guideline Committee [5] recommend using conventional WLI for determining the depth of invasion of early gastric cancer (Strength of recommendation: 2, Level of evidence: C) and IEE for diagnosing the extent of invasion (Strength of recommendation: 1, Level of evidence: B). A randomized controlled trial by Asada-Hirayama et al. reported that magnifying NBI endoscopy produced significantly better results than indigocarmine chromoendoscopy in endoscopic submucosal dissection (ESD) cases (89.4% vs. 75.9%, $p = 0.007$) [29]. Additionally, we previously reported that the diagnostic accuracy of a second-generation ultrathin endoscope using WLI is as low as 61.5% but can be increased to 92.3% by adding observation with NBI [11]. In this study, color differences surrounding atrophic borders and intestinal metaplasia were significantly greater on a third-generation ultrathin endoscope using NBI (19.2 ± 8.5 and 13.7 ± 4.2, $p < 0.001$) than WLI (13.4 ± 6.4 and 7.1 ± 3.3, both $p < 0.001$). Our findings provide the first evidence of the efficacy of NBI with a third-generation ultrathin endoscope for detecting gastric atrophy and intestinal metaplasia as indicators of precancerous lesions over WLI. Large-scale multi-center prospective studies are needed to investigate the efficacy of NBI with a third-generation endoscopy for detecting atrophy, intestinal metaplasia, and gastric cancer, and for identifying those at high risk among not only *H. pylori*-eradicated patients, but also *H. pylori*-positive and naive patients.

4.3. Limitations

This study has a few limitations. First, it was a retrospective single-center study and the sample size was small. Second, endoscopic evaluations of gastritis using GIF-290N and GIF-1200N were performed at different times. In general, gastric atrophy and intestinal metaplasia after eradication therapy in any patients are gradually recovered depended on age, severity of atrophy, and intestinal metaplasia at eradication, and environmental and genetic factors [35,36]. In this study, because the mean duration from first to second endoscopies was 35.5 ± 19.8 months, the severity of gastritis may differ between GIF-290N and GIF-1200N endoscopes. Because two endoscopies should be carried out at the same time to compare ability, this study may have potential biases. However, mean endoscopic scores of gastritis evaluated using WLI according to the Kyoto classification of gastritis were not significantly different between GIF-290N and GIF-1200N endoscopes, of which the difference in gastric mucosal situation by the duration from first to second endoscopies may ignore. However, we will plan to clarify the clinical endoscopic significance between GIF-290N and GIF-1200N at the same time, as part of further study. Third, we evaluated the severity of gastritis by combining GIF-1200N with the EVIS X-1 processor and GIF-290N with the LUCERA ELITE processor; therefore, differences in processor functionality may have affected the results. Fourth, although pathological examination is considered the gold standard for the evaluation of gastric atrophy and intestinal metaplasia, we did not evaluate pathological gastritis in this study. Therefore, we cannot completely deny a hypothesis that the apparently better image quality of a particular imaging technique for an evaluation of atrophy and intestinal metaplasia may actually be an artifact during the image management process.

5. Conclusions

We showed that NBI with a third-generation high-vision ultrathin endoscope enhanced color differences surrounding atrophy and intestinal metaplasia according to the CIE 1976 (L*a*b*) color space compared to a second-generation endoscope in *H. pylori*-eradicated patients. Thus, third-generation ultrathin endoscopes may possess greater diagnostic efficiency for screening and improve risk stratification for gastric cancer.

Author Contributions: Conceptualization, M.S. and T.K.; methodology, M.S. and T.K.; software, J.U. and M.S.; formal analysis, J.U. and M.S.; investigation, M.S. and T.K.; Writing—Original draft preparation, J.U. and M.S.; Writing—Review and editing, J.U., M.S., M.H., N.N., E.I., R.N., M.F., T.I. and T.K.; supervision, T.I. and T.K.; project administration, M.S. All authors have read and agreed to the published version of the manuscript.

Funding: This research received no external funding.

Institutional Review Board Statement: The study was conducted in accordance with the Declaration of Helsinki, and approved by the Institutional Review Board of Tokyo Medical University (protocol code T2020-0265 and date of approval: 4 November 2020).

Informed Consent Statement: Because this study was conducted under a retrospective design and written informed consent was not obtained from each enrolled patient, a document describing an opt-out policy through which potential patients and/or relatives could refuse inclusion was uploaded on the Tokyo Medical University Hospital website.

Data Availability Statement: The data presented in this study are available on request from the corresponding author.

Acknowledgments: We thank Heidi Tran and Guy Harris from DMC Corp. (http://www.dmed.co.jp/, accessed on 14 April 2022) for editing a draft of this manuscript.

Conflicts of Interest: The authors declare no conflict of interest.

References

1. Kamada, T.; Haruma, K.; Inoue, K.; Shiotani, A. Helicobacter pylori infection and endoscopic gastritis-Kyoto classification of gastritis. *Nihon Shokakibyo Gakkai Zasshi* **2015**, *112*, 982–993. [CrossRef] [PubMed]
2. Sugimoto, M.; Ban, H.; Ichikawa, H.; Sahara, S.; Otsuka, T.; Inatomi, O.; Bamba, S.; Furuta, T.; Andoh, A. Efficacy of the Kyoto Classification of Gastritis in Identifying Patients at High Risk for Gastric Cancer. *Intern. Med.* **2017**, *56*, 579–586. [CrossRef] [PubMed]
3. Uemura, N.; Okamoto, S.; Yamamoto, S.; Matsumura, N.; Yamaguchi, S.; Yamakido, M.; Taniyama, K.; Sasaki, N.; Schlemper, R.J. Helicobacter pylori infection and the development of gastric cancer. *N. Engl. J. Med.* **2001**, *345*, 784–789. [CrossRef] [PubMed]

4. Graham, D.Y. Helicobacter pylori infection in the pathogenesis of duodenal ulcer and gastric cancer: A model. *Gastroenterology* **1997**, *113*, 1983–1991. [CrossRef]
5. Yao, K.; Uedo, N.; Kamada, T.; Hirasawa, T.; Nagahama, T.; Yoshinaga, S.; Oka, M.; Inoue, K.; Mabe, K.; Yao, T.; et al. Guidelines for endoscopic diagnosis of early gastric cancer. *Dig. Endosc.* **2020**, *32*, 663–698. [CrossRef]
6. Dohi, O.; Yagi, N.; Naito, Y.; Fukui, A.; Gen, Y.; Iwai, N.; Ueda, T.; Yoshida, N.; Kamada, K.; Uchiyama, K.; et al. Blue laser imaging-bright improves the real-time detection rate of early gastric cancer: A randomized controlled study. *Gastrointest. Endosc.* **2019**, *89*, 47–57. [CrossRef]
7. Majima, A.; Dohi, O.; Takayama, S.; Hirose, R.; Inoue, K.; Yoshida, N.; Kamada, K.; Uchiyama, K.; Ishikawa, T.; Takagi, T.; et al. Linked color imaging identifies important risk factors associated with gastric cancer after successful eradication of Helicobacter pylori. *Gastrointest. Endosc.* **2019**, *90*, 763–769. [CrossRef]
8. Ono, S.; Kato, M.; Tsuda, M.; Miyamoto, S.; Abiko, S.; Shimizu, Y.; Sakamoto, N. Lavender Color in Linked Color Imaging Enables Noninvasive Detection of Gastric Intestinal Metaplasia. *Digestion* **2018**, *98*, 222–230. [CrossRef]
9. Ono, S.; Kawada, K.; Dohi, O.; Kitamura, S.; Koike, T.; Hori, S.; Kanzaki, H.; Murao, T.; Yagi, N.; Sasaki, F.; et al. Linked Color Imaging Focused on Neoplasm Detection in the Upper Gastrointestinal Tract: A Randomized Trial. *Ann. Intern. Med.* **2021**, *174*, 18–24. [CrossRef]
10. Mizukami, K.; Ogawa, R.; Okamoto, K.; Shuto, M.; Fukuda, K.; Sonoda, A.; Matsunari, O.; Hirashita, Y.; Okimoto, T.; Kodama, M.; et al. Objective Endoscopic Analysis with Linked Color Imaging regarding Gastric Mucosal Atrophy: A Pilot Study. *Gastroenterol. Res. Pract.* **2017**, *2017*, 5054237. [CrossRef]
11. Kawai, T.; Yanagizawa, K.; Naito, S.; Sugimoto, H.; Fukuzawa, M.; Gotoda, T.; Matsubayashi, J.; Nagao, T.; Hoshino, S.; Tsuchida, A.; et al. Evaluation of gastric cancer diagnosis using new ultrathin transnasal endoscopy with narrow-band imaging: Preliminary study. *J. Gastroenterol. Hepatol.* **2014**, *29* (Suppl. 4), 33–36. [CrossRef]
12. Toyoizumi, H.; Kaise, M.; Arakawa, H.; Yonezawa, J.; Yoshida, Y.; Kato, M.; Yoshimura, N.; Goda, K.; Tajiri, H. Ultrathin endoscopy versus high-resolution endoscopy for diagnosing superficial gastric neoplasia. *Gastrointest. Endosc.* **2009**, *70*, 240–245. [CrossRef]
13. Kawai, Y.; Kawai, T.; Hamada, M.; Iwata, E.; Niikura, R.; Nagata, N.; Yanagisawa, K.; Sugimoto, M.; Yamagishi, T. Examination of endoscopic findings in the diagnosis of early gastric cancer associated with the evolution of transnasal endoscope. Japanese association for cancer detection and diagnosis. *Jpn. Assoc. Cancer Detect. Diagn.* **2022**, *29*, 178–184. (In Japanese)
14. Ono, S.; Shimoda, Y.; Tanaka, I.; Kinowaki, S.; Inoue, M.; Ono, M.; Yamamoto, K.; Shimizu, Y.; Sakamoto, N. Optical effect of spraying l-menthol on gastric intestinal metaplasia visualized by linked color imaging. *Eur. J. Gastroenterol. Hepatol.* **2021**, *33*, 358–363. [CrossRef]
15. Kawai, Y.; Sugimoto, M.; Hamada, M.; Iwata, E.; Niikura, R.; Nagata, N.; Fukuzawa, M.; Itoi, T.; Kawai, T. Linked color imaging effectively detects the endoscopic atrophic border in transnasal endoscopy. *J. Clin. Biochem. Nutr.* **2022**, in press. [CrossRef]
16. Kimura, K.; Takemoto, T. An Endoscopic Recognition of the Atrophic Border and its Significance in Chronic Gastritis. *Endoscopy* **1969**, *1*, 87–97. [CrossRef]
17. Dixon, M.F.; Genta, R.M.; Yardley, J.H.; Correa, P. Classification and grading of gastritis. The updated Sydney System. International Workshop on the Histopathology of Gastritis, Houston 1994. *Am. J. Surg. Pathol.* **1996**, *20*, 1161–1181. [CrossRef]
18. Rugge, M.; Correa, P.; Di Mario, F.; El-Omar, E.; Fiocca, R.; Geboes, K.; Genta, R.M.; Graham, D.Y.; Hattori, T.; Malfertheiner, P.; et al. OLGA staging for gastritis: A tutorial. *Dig. Liver. Dis.* **2008**, *40*, 650–658. [CrossRef]
19. Rugge, M.; Meggio, A.; Pennelli, G.; Piscioli, F.; Giacomelli, L.; De Pretis, G.; Graham, D.Y. Gastritis staging in clinical practice: The OLGA staging system. *Gut* **2007**, *56*, 631–636. [CrossRef]
20. Kuehni, R.G. Color-tolerance data and the tentative CIE 1976 L a b formula. *J. Opt. Soc. Am.* **1976**, *66*, 497–500. [CrossRef]
21. Sato, Y.; Sagawa, T.; Hirakawa, M.; Ohnuma, H.; Osuga, T.; Okagawa, Y.; Tamura, F.; Horiguchi, H.; Takada, K.; Hayashi, T.; et al. Clinical utility of capsule endoscopy with flexible spectral imaging color enhancement for diagnosis of small bowel lesions. *Endosc. Int. Open* **2014**, *2*, E80–E87. [CrossRef] [PubMed]
22. Garcia, R.T.; Cello, J.P.; Nguyen, M.H.; Rogers, S.J.; Rodas, A.; Trinh, H.N.; Stollman, N.H.; Schlueck, G.; McQuaid, K.R. Unsedated ultrathin EGD is well accepted when compared with conventional sedated EGD: A multicenter randomized trial. *Gastroenterology* **2003**, *125*, 1606–1612. [CrossRef] [PubMed]
23. Tatsumi, Y.; Harada, A.; Matsumoto, T.; Tani, T.; Nishida, H. Feasibility and tolerance of 2-way and 4-way angulation videoscopes for unsedated patients undergoing transnasal EGD in GI cancer screening. *Gastrointest. Endosc.* **2008**, *67*, 1021–1027. [CrossRef] [PubMed]
24. Dumortier, J.; Josso, C.; Roman, S.; Fumex, F.; Lepilliez, V.; Prost, B.; Lot, M.; Guillaud, O.; Petit-Laurent, F.; Lapalus, M.G.; et al. Prospective evaluation of a new ultrathin one-plane bending videoendoscope for transnasal EGD: A comparative study on performance and tolerance. *Gastrointest. Endosc.* **2007**, *66*, 13–19. [CrossRef]
25. Parker, C.; Alexandridis, E.; Plevris, J.; O'Hara, J.; Panter, S. Transnasal endoscopy: No gagging no panic! *Frontline Gastroenterol.* **2016**, *7*, 246–256. [CrossRef]
26. Bray, F.; Ferlay, J.; Soerjomataram, I.; Siegel, R.L.; Torre, L.A.; Jemal, A. Global cancer statistics 2018: GLOBOCAN estimates of incidence and mortality worldwide for 36 cancers in 185 countries. *CA Cancer J. Clin.* **2018**, *68*, 394–424. [CrossRef]
27. Sugimoto, M.; Murata, M.; Yamaoka, Y. Chemoprevention of gastric cancer development after Helicobacter pylori eradication therapy in an East Asian population: Meta-analysis. *World J. Gastroenterol.* **2020**, *26*, 1820–1840. [CrossRef]

28. Nakajima, T.; Oda, I.; Gotoda, T.; Hamanaka, H.; Eguchi, T.; Yokoi, C.; Saito, D. Metachronous gastric cancers after endoscopic resection: How effective is annual endoscopic surveillance? *Gastric Cancer* **2006**, *9*, 93–98. [CrossRef]
29. Asada-Hirayama, I.; Kodashima, S.; Sakaguchi, Y.; Ono, S.; Niimi, K.; Mochizuki, S.; Tsuji, Y.; Minatsuki, C.; Shichijo, S.; Matsuzaka, K.; et al. Magnifying endoscopy with narrow-band imaging is more accurate for determination of horizontal extent of early gastric cancers than chromoendoscopy. *Endosc. Int. Open* **2016**, *4*, E690–E698. [CrossRef]
30. Nagahama, T.; Yao, K.; Maki, S.; Yasaka, M.; Takaki, Y.; Matsui, T.; Tanabe, H.; Iwashita, A.; Ota, A. Usefulness of magnifying endoscopy with narrow-band imaging for determining the horizontal extent of early gastric cancer when there is an unclear margin by chromoendoscopy (with video). *Gastrointest. Endosc.* **2011**, *74*, 1259–1267. [CrossRef]
31. Yoshida, N.; Doyama, H.; Yano, T.; Horimatsu, T.; Uedo, N.; Yamamoto, Y.; Kakushima, N.; Kanzaki, H.; Hori, S.; Yao, K.; et al. Early gastric cancer detection in high-risk patients: A multicentre randomised controlled trial on the effect of second-generation narrow band imaging. *Gut* **2021**, *70*, 67–75. [CrossRef]
32. Muto, M.; Minashi, K.; Yano, T.; Saito, Y.; Oda, I.; Nonaka, S.; Omori, T.; Sugiura, H.; Goda, K.; Kaise, M.; et al. Early detection of superficial squamous cell carcinoma in the head and neck region and esophagus by narrow band imaging: A multicenter randomized controlled trial. *J. Clin. Oncol.* **2010**, *28*, 1566–1572. [CrossRef]
33. Yao, K.; Anagnostopoulos, G.K.; Ragunath, K. Magnifying endoscopy for diagnosing and delineating early gastric cancer. *Endoscopy* **2009**, *41*, 462–467. [CrossRef]
34. Pimentel-Nunes, P.; Libanio, D.; Marcos-Pinto, R.; Areia, M.; Leja, M.; Esposito, G.; Garrido, M.; Kikuste, I.; Megraud, F.; Matysiak-Budnik, T.; et al. Management of epithelial precancerous conditions and lesions in the stomach (MAPS II): European Society of Gastrointestinal Endoscopy (ESGE), European Helicobacter and Microbiota Study Group (EHMSG), European Society of Pathology (ESP), and Sociedade Portuguesa de Endoscopia Digestiva (SPED) guideline update 2019. *Endoscopy* **2019**, *51*, 365–388. [CrossRef]
35. Kodama, M.; Murakami, K.; Okimoto, T.; Sato, R.; Uchida, M.; Abe, T.; Shiota, S.; Nakagawa, Y.; Mizukami, K.; Fujioka, T. Ten-year prospective follow-up of histological changes at five points on the gastric mucosa as recommended by the updated Sydney system after Helicobacter pylori eradication. *J. Gastroenterol.* **2012**, *47*, 394–403. [CrossRef]
36. Kodama, M.; Okimoto, T.; Mizukami, K.; Hirashita, Y.; Wada, Y.; Fukuda, M.; Matsunari, O.; Okamoto, K.; Ogawa, R.; Fukuda, K.; et al. Gastric mucosal changes, and sex differences therein, after Helicobacter pylori eradication: A long-term prospective follow-up study. *J. Gastroenterol. Hepatol.* **2021**, *36*, 2210–2216. [CrossRef]

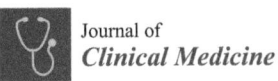

Article

Evaluation of a New Monoclonal Chemiluminescent Immunoassay Stool Antigen Test for the Diagnosis of *Helicobacter pylori* Infection: A Spanish Multicentre Study

Elena Resina [1], María G. Donday [1], Samuel J. Martínez-Domínguez [2], Emilio José Laserna-Mendieta [3,4,5,6], Ángel Lanas [2], Alfredo J. Lucendo [4,5,6,7], Marta Sánchez-Luengo [2], Noelia Alcaide [8], Luis Fernández-Salazar [8], Luisa De La Peña-Negro [9], Luis Bujanda [10], Marta Gómez-Ruiz de Arbulo [11], Javier Alcedo [12], Ángeles Pérez-Aísa [13], Raúl Rodríguez [14], Sandra Hermida [1], Yanire Brenes [1], Olga P. Nyssen [1,†] and Javier P. Gisbert [1,*,†]

1. Gastroenterology Unit, Hospital Universitario de La Princesa, Instituto de Investigación Sanitaria Princesa (IIS-Princesa), Universidad Autónoma de Madrid (UAM), and Centro de Investigación Biomédica en Red de Enfermedades Hepáticas y Digestivas (CIBERehd), 28006 Madrid, Spain
2. Hospital Clínico Universitario Lozano Blesa de Zaragoza, Instituto de Investigación Sanitaria de Aragón (IIS Aragón) and Universidad de Zaragoza, 50009 Zaragoza, Spain
3. Laboratory Medicine Department, Hospital Universitario de La Princesa, 28006 Madrid, Spain
4. Department of Gastroenterology, Hospital General de Tomelloso, 13700 Tomelloso, Spain
5. Instituto de Investigación Sanitaria La Princesa (IIS-Princesa), 28006 Madrid, Spain
6. Instituto de Investigación Sanitaria de Castilla-La Mancha (IDISCAM), 28006 Madrid, Spain
7. Centro de Investigación Biomédica en Red Enfermedades Hepáticas y Digestivas (CIBERehd), 28006 Madrid, Spain
8. Gastroenterology Unit, Hospital Clínico Universitario de Valladolid, Gerencia Regional de Salud (SACYL) and Universidad de Valladolid, 47003 Valladolid, Spain
9. Gastroenterology Unit, Hospital de Viladecans, 08840 Barcelona, Spain
10. Gastroenterology Unit, Hospital Donostia/Instituto Biodonostia, Universidad del País Vasco (UPV/EHU), Centro de Investigación Biomédica en Red de Enfermedades Hepáticas y Digestivas (CIBERehd), 20014 San Sebastián, Spain
11. Microbiology Department, Hospital Donostia/Instituto Biodonostia, Centro de Investigación Biomédica en Red de Enfermedades Respiratorias (CIBERES), 20014 San Sebastián, Spain
12. Gastroenterology Unit, Hospital Universitario Miguel Servet, 50009 Zaragoza, Spain
13. Gastroenterology Unit, Agencia Sanitaria Costa del Sol, 29651 Marbella, Spain
14. Hospital General Universitario de Castellón, 20014 Castellón de la Plana, Spain
* Correspondence: javier.p.gisbert@gmail.com; Tel.: +34-913-093-911; Fax: +34-915-204-013
† These authors contributed equally to this work.

Abstract: The stool antigen test (SAT) represents an attractive alternative for detection of *Helicobacter pylori*. The aim of this study was to assess the accuracy of a new SAT, the automated LIAISON® Meridian *H. pylori* SA based on monoclonal antibodies, compared to the defined gold standard ^{13}C-urea breath test (UBT). This prospective multicentre study (nine Spanish centres) enrolled patients ≥18 years of age with clinical indication to perform UBT for the initial diagnosis and for confirmation of bacterial eradication. Two UBT methods were used: mass spectrometry (MS) including citric acid (CA) or infrared spectrophotometry (IRS) without CA. Overall, 307 patients (145 naïve, 162 with confirmation of eradication) were analysed. Using recommended cut-off values (negative SAT < 0.90, positive ≥ 1.10) the sensitivity, specificity, positive predictive value, negative predictive value and accuracy were 67%, 97%, 86%, 92% and 91%, respectively, obtaining an area under the receiver operating characteristic (ROC) curve (AUC) of 0.85. Twenty-eight patients, including seven false positives and 21 false negatives, presented a discordant result between SAT and UBT. Among the 21 false negatives, four of six tested with MS and 11 of 15 tested with IRS presented a borderline UBT delta value. In 25 discordant samples, PCR targeting *H. pylori* DNA was performed to re-assess positivity and SAT accuracy was re-analysed: sensitivity, specificity, positive predictive value, negative predictive value, accuracy and AUC were 94%, 97%, 86%, 99%, 97% and 0.96, respectively. The new LIAISON® Meridian *H. pylori* SA SAT showed a good accuracy for diagnosis of *H. pylori* infection.

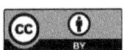

Keywords: diagnosis; *Helicobacter pylori*; stool antigen test; urea breath test

1. Introduction

Helicobacter pylori (*H. pylori*) is a highly prevalent worldwide infection and is the main cause not only of gastritis, but also of peptic ulcer and gastric cancer. Therefore, an accurate diagnosis remains crucial [1]. *H. pylori* screening and eradication is indicated in several clinical contexts including gastric cancer precursor lesions, peptic ulcer disease and gastric mucosa-associated lymphoid tissue lymphoma, among others [2,3]. However, more recently, consensus has been reached on eradicating *H. pylori* regardless of the associated clinical condition [4].

Although different methods have been established to detect *H. pylori* infection, identifying *H. pylori*-infected patients is a challenge. *H. pylori* infection diagnostic methods are classically divided into invasive and non-invasive. Invasive methods are based on the detection of the organism in the stomach by means of gastric biopsy samples (histology, rapid urease test (RUT), culture and molecular diagnostic methods), which require an endoscopy. This strategy should be considered in patients with alarm symptoms or in older (i.e., >50–55 years) patients. On the other hand, non-invasive methods do not require an endoscopic examination and are currently the most widely used diagnostic techniques [5–7].

Uninvestigated dyspepsia represents one-quarter of primary care referrals to the gastroenterologist in Spain [8]. In the absence of alarm symptoms, and in those younger than 50–55, a "test-and-treat" strategy would be appropriate for diagnosis, preferring non-invasive tests such as urea breath test (UBT) or stool antigen test (SAT) rather than prescribing proton pump inhibitors (PPIs) or endoscopy [9–11].

The UBT has been classically considered the preferred non-invasive technique due to its excellent sensitivity and specificity (>95–100%) demonstrated in countless studies and meta-analyses. Moreover, UBT has been the most widely used diagnostic method in recent years, making it an optimal gold standard [12,13]. Although UBT is safe, some disadvantages have been described: point-of-care testing, significant consumption of patient time (30–60 min), fasting requirement, the high cost of qualified personnel or sending the collected samples to an analytical laboratory [14]. In addition, there are physical difficulties for certain populations (e.g., children and disabled) in performing the test [15].

The SAT is a low-cost diagnostic method, without the previously described disadvantages, suitable for at-risk populations [16]. Indeed, some studies have suggested its better cost-effectiveness compared to other techniques [17,18].

Two types of SATs have been described: the enzyme immunoassays, such as enzyme-linked immunosorbent assay (ELISA) or the more recently developed, chemiluminescence-based immunoassays (CLIA), and "rapid" or "in-office" tests (immunochromatography assay or ICA). These methods can be based either on polyclonal or monoclonal antibodies [6,16]. With regard to "rapid" or "in-office" tests, controversial results have been reported [19] and they are not recommended in clinical practice guidelines due to their limited accuracy [20].

The diagnostic performance of different SATs is heterogeneous, although there is no doubt that the use of monoclonal antibodies has resulted in a higher accuracy compared to polyclonal antibodies, both in adults and children [15,19,21].

The high accuracy of SAT has been widely demonstrated in most reviews and meta-analyses, providing a sensitivity above 80–90%. Additionally, a sensitivity of 83% has been reported in a very recent Cochrane meta-analysis, with no discrimination between monoclonal and polyclonal antibodies [12], while other studies evaluating the monoclonal technique showed a higher sensitivity and specificity (96.2% and 94.7%, respectively), in the paediatric population [21].

Another study, also in children, showed a sensitivity and specificity of 97% [15]. A meta-analysis by Gisbert et al. reported sensitivity and specificity data >93% both before and after *H. pylori* treatment [19]. Additionally, a clinical review by the Canadian Drug Agency described a sensitivity and specificity of 90.0–92.4% and 91.0–100%, respectively, with monoclonal SAT [22]. Therefore, SAT is currently recommended by the main international guidelines as a valid and reliable diagnostic method [2,20,23].

As previously mentioned, the CLIA technique for the identification of *H. pylori* in faeces has proven similar accuracy to that reported for both ELISA and the best performing lateral flow immunoassays, with additional advantages [24].

In the current study, we evaluated the accuracy of the LIAISON® Meridian *H. pylori* SA test for the diagnosis and confirmation of eradication of *H. pylori* infection. This new test is a fully automated, time saving, objective and traceable CLIA, which detects the presence of *H. pylori* antigen in human stools using unique monoclonal antibodies.

2. Materials and Methods

2.1. Patients and Design

This is a prospective, comparative, multicentre study that aimed to evaluate the accuracy of the new LIAISON® Meridian *H. pylori* SA stool antigen test. Nine Spanish centres participated in the study. Consecutive adult patients with indication of *H. pylori* infection primary diagnosis or confirmation of the bacterial eradication according to standard clinical practice were enrolled between November 2019 and May 2021. Patients were included for both pre- and post-treatment tests, and the signing of an informed consent for each test was required.

Inclusion criteria were indication to perform an *H. pylori* infection diagnosis; capacity and willingness to give written informed consent; prior prescribed ^{13}C-UBT; and, for confirmation of eradication (if the patient was included for post-eradication treatment diagnosis), performance of the test at least four weeks after the treatment was discontinued. Exclusion criteria were age below 18 years; advanced chronic disease that would not allow the patient to complete follow-up or attend follow-up visits; previous gastric surgery; alcohol or drug abuse; antibiotic or bismuth salts consumption four weeks prior to testing; and PPI intake two weeks prior to testing.

The study protocol was approved by the Ethics Committee of all participant hospitals.

2.2. Stool Antigen Test

Patients were instructed to obtain a faecal sample within 24–36 h either before or after the UBT was performed.

H. pylori was detected using a new automated LIAISON® Meridian *H. pylori* SA assay (REF 318200, DiaSorin, Stillwater, MN, USA) (Supplementary File S1). The test is a CLIA in sandwich format that uses novel monoclonal antibodies for capture and detection of *H. pylori* stool antigen. Testing was performed following the manufacturer's instructions at the laboratory of Hospital de La Princesa (Madrid, Spain). Specimens had to be stored at least at -20 °C.

The process was performed automatically by the LIAISON® XL analyser (DiaSorin SpA, Saluggia, Italy). Two hundred microlitres of the diluted sample (mixture of sample diluent and stool) was incubated with paramagnetic particles coated with capture antibodies. Isoluminol conjugated antibodies for *H. pylori* antigen were subsequently added and incubated and the unbound material was washed. Then the flash chemiluminescent reaction was initiated and chemiluminescent light was measured by a photomultiplier. Relative light units (RLU) were recorded. RLU were proportional to the concentration of the *H. pylori* stool antigen present.

Specimens were classified as negative, equivocal or positive based on their index (<0.9, 0.9–1.1 and >1.1, respectively). The trained operator was unaware of the results of the reference tests.

Equivocal LIAISON® results (CLIA values of 0.9–1.1) were solved by immediately repeating SAT on another sample from the same specimen using a kit from a different batch. This latter result was the one valid for analysis.

2.3. Urea Breath Test

The gold standard was defined by the ^{13}C-UBT. Two UBT methods were used according to the available and standard clinical practice from the participating centres. The professionals analysing the UBT test were unaware of the SAT results.

2.3.1. Isotope Ratio Mass Spectrometry (IRMS)

The commercial test TAU-KIT® (Isomed, S.L., Madrid, Spain) was used. The patient had to fast at least six hours before the test was performed. Initially, a citric acid solution (4.2 g, Citral pylori®) dissolved in 200 mL of water was administered. After 10 min, samples were collected to determine the reference value of the test. The urea solution was prepared by dissolving a 100 mg tablet of this substrate in 125 mL of water. After 30 min following the administration of the urea solution, samples of exhaled breath were again collected. Samples were classified as either negative, unclear or positive based on delta values (<4‰, 4–5‰ and 5‰, respectively).

Patients with unclear UBT results (delta values between 4‰ and 5‰ measured by mass spectrometer) were asked to repeat both the UBT and the stool sample at least four weeks after testing. These latter results were used for the analysis.

2.3.2. Non-Dispersive Isotope-Selective Infrared Spectrometry (NDIRS)

The UBT was performed using UBTest 100 mg (Ferrer Internacional, Barcelona, Spain). Determinations were performed in accordance with the manufacturer's specifications. The patient had to fast at least eight hours before the test performance. A basal breath sample was collected by blowing into a specially designed bag. After this, patient swallowed a pill of 100 mg of ^{13}C-labelled urea in 100 mL of water, and 20 min later filled a second breath bag. Samples were immediately processed by NDIRS (POCone^{TM} or POConePlus, Infrared Spectrophotometer, Otsuka Pharmaceutical, Tokyo, Japan). In accordance with the manufacturer's specifications, an increase in the proportion ^{13}C/^{12}C ($\Delta^{13}CO_2$ (‰)) of 2.5‰ or more after urea intake was considered as indicative of *H. pylori* infection. No unclear values are described by the manufacturer.

2.4. H. pylori Detection by PCR

Faecal samples with discrepant results between UBT and SAT data were subjected to two different polymerase chain reactions (PCR) in an external laboratory for confirmation of *H. pylori* presence. Samples were transported at a temperature of at least −20 °C. First, DNA was extracted in an automated extractor device (KingFisher, Thermo Scientific, Waltham, MA, USA) employing magnetic particles (MagMax CORE Nucleic Acid Purification Kit, Applied Biosystems, Foster City, CA, USA) and following the instructions from the manufacturers. PCR amplification was performed in 100 ng of DNA (final volume 50 µL) by using primer oligonucleotides for the glmM gene and the 16S rRNA region of *H. pylori* (SYNLAB Diagnósticos Globales S.A.U., Barcelona, Spain). The threshold detection limit of the aforementioned techniques is 200–300 copies per gram of faeces. For the amplification of the *H. pylori* 16S rRNA region, a nested PCR assay was performed with 30 cycles in each amplification and hybridisation temperatures of 34 °C and 41 °C in the first and second amplifications, respectively. For the amplification of the glmM gene, a PCR assay was performed with 40 cycles at a hybridisation temperature of 48 °C. Detection of the specific amplified bands (398 bp for 16S rRNA and 294 bp for glmM gene) was performed in 3% agarose gels. All tests were performed by experienced laboratory professionals, blinded to the *H. pylori* status of the samples and to the results of the other tests. To confirm the presence or absence of *H. pylori* in faecal samples, the results of both PCRs must be positive or negative, respectively.

2.5. Statistical Analysis

Quantitative variables are provided as the mean and the standard deviation (SD). Categorical variables are expressed as percentages and 95% confidence intervals (CIs). The statistical significance threshold was set at a p-value < 0.05.

Sensitivity, specificity, positive predictive value (PPV) and negative predictive value (NPV) and their 95% CIs were calculated by standard methods, and positive and negative likelihood ratios (LR+ and LR−, respectively), using the UBT results as study gold standard. The study was reported in compliance with the Standards for the Reporting of Diagnostic Accuracy Studies (STARD) recommendations [25].

The sample size was calculated based on the formula by Jones et al. [26]. Two different sample size calculations were performed: one each for the pre-treatment and post-treatment analyses.

Calculations were performed using an expected (desired) sensitivity and specificity of 97%, a precision of 5% and a CI of 95%. Based on published data and previous experience in our country, the expected pre-treatment prevalence was 45% (of dyspeptic patients attending a gastroenterology outpatient clinic) and post-treatment prevalence would range from 20 to 30% depending on the administered treatment (as the effectiveness in clinical practice ranges from 70 to 80%).

Under these conditions, the estimated required sample size was 100 and 166 patients for pre-treatment and post-treatment, respectively. It should be taken into consideration that some doctors are prescribing optimized treatments (four drugs, 14 days), which may reduce the post-treatment prevalence down to 10–15%. In the worst case scenario (with only a 10% post-treatment prevalence), given this sample size, and maintaining a 95% CI and an expected accuracy at 97%, the precision would be 8%.

3. Results

A total of 321 patients were screened in nine centres; of these, 14 were excluded, leaving 307 patients for enrolment in the study (Figure 1). The baseline characteristics of the included subjects are shown in Table 1.

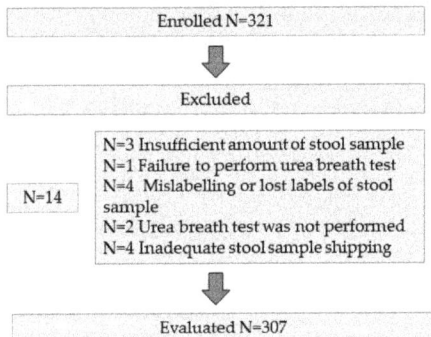

Figure 1. Flow diagram of the enrolled patients.

A STARD flow diagram of the study is shown in Figure 2, including the overall pool of patients evaluated, the pre-treatment group (i.e., treatment-naïve patients) and the post-treatment group (i.e., those where a confirmation of eradication was requested).

In two patients, delta values were unclear (between 4‰ and 5‰, measured by IRMS). In these two patients, the UBT was repeated, and a new stool sample was collected at least four weeks after the baseline test. Another two faecal samples provided equivocal LIAISON® results (CLIA values of 0.9–1.1). This problem was solved by immediately repeating the SAT on another sample from the same specimen, obtaining valid results.

Table 1. Characteristics of the included patients.

Variables	
Age (mean ± SD)	47.1 ± 14.4
	N (%)
Gender (female)	207 (67)
Clinical indication	
○ Pre-treatment/naïve	145 (47)
○ Post-treatment/confirmation	162 (53)
UBT method	
○ IRMS	118 (38)
○ NDIRS	189 (62)
History of peptic ulcer	14 (5)
H. pylori infection prevalence (by UBT)	% (95% CI)
○ Overall	21 (16–26%)
○ Pre-treatment/naïve	29 (21–37%)
○ Post-treatment/confirmation	14 (8–19%)
	N = 307

N: number of patients included; CI: confidence intervals; UBT: urea breath test; IRMS: isotope ratio mass spectrometry; NDIRS: non-dispersive isotope-selective infrared spectrometry.

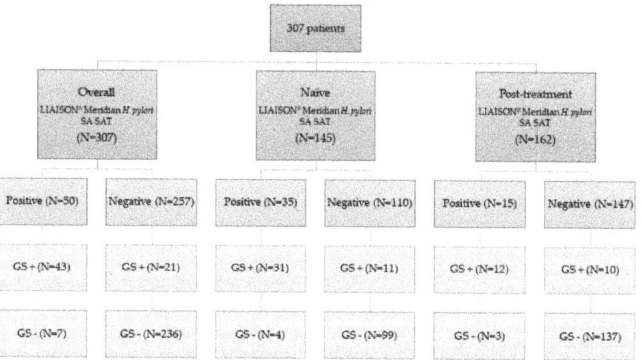

Figure 2. Standards for the Reporting of Diagnostic Accuracy Studies (STARD) flow diagram of the study. N: number of patients included; SAT: stool antigen test; GS+: gold standard positive; GS−: gold standard negative.

The LIAISON® Meridian *H. pylori* SA test had an overall sensitivity of 67% (95% CI 55–79%) and a specificity of 97% (95–99%). PPV and NPV were 86% (75–97%) and 92% (88–95%), respectively. The LR+ and LR− were 23 (11–49) and 0.34 (0.24–0.48), respectively. Global accuracy was 91% (88–94%) with an area under the ROC curve (AUC) of 0.85 (0.78–0.92).

Sensitivity, specificity, PPV, NPV, accuracy, LR+, LR−, and AUC were calculated separately for treatment-naïve patients and in the post-treatment group. Results are shown in Tables 2 and 3, respectively.

In total, 28/307 patients (including seven false positives and 21 false negatives) presented a discordant result between SAT and UBT. Among the 21 false negatives, four of six tested with IRMS had a UBT delta value very close to the cut-off point (values between 5.2 and 5.8 being the cut-off point with IRMS 5‰). In addition, 11/15 tested with NDIRS had a UBT delta value near the cut-off point (with values below 10), and 10/15 had values equal to or lower than 8.5 (the cut-off point with NDIRS 2.5‰).

Twenty-five of these samples were subjected to a confirmatory PCR. In three discordant samples, all of them classified as false negatives, the remaining sample was insufficient for PCR analysis. All stool PCRs were negative for *H. pylori* DNA detection. The accuracy of the LIAISON® Meridian *H. pylori* SA assay was re-analysed, considering these patients as non-infected. Results are shown in Table 4.

Table 2. Accuracy of the LIAISON® Meridian *H. pylori* SA test in treatment-naïve patients.

Comparison SAT vs. UBT	Sensitivity (95% CI)	Specificity (95% CI)	PPV (95% CI)	NPV (95% CI)	LR+ (95% CI)	LR− (95% CI)	Global Accuracy (95% CI)	AUC (95% CI)
Naïve	74% (59–88)	96% (92–100)	89% (77–100)	90% (84–96)	19 (7–51)	0.27 (0.16–0.45)	90% (84–95)	0.88 (0.80–0.96)
NDIRS naïve	73% (54–92)	93% (86–100)	83% (65–100)	89% (80–97)	11 (4–29)	0.29 (0.15–0.55)	87% (80–95)	0.86 (0.75–0.96)
IRMS naïve	75% (51–99)	100% (99–100)	100% (96–100)	92% (82–100)	-	0.25 (0.11–0.58)	93% (86–100)	0.91 (0.79–1.0)

SAT: stool antigen test; UBT: urea breath test; PPV: positive predictive value; NPV: negative predictive value; LR+: positive likelihood ratio; LR−: negative likelihood ratio; AUC: area under the ROC curve; IRMS: isotope ratio mass spectrometry, cut-off value 5‰; NDIRS: non-dispersive isotope-selective infrared spectrometry, cut-off value 2.5‰.

Table 3. Accuracy of the LIAISON® Meridian *H. pylori* SA test in post-treatment patients.

Comparison SAT vs. UBT	Sensitivity (95% CI)	Specificity (95% CI)	PPV (95% CI)	NPV (95% CI)	LR+ (95% CI)	LR− (95% CI)	Global Accuracy (95% CI)	AUC (95% CI)
Post-treatment	55% (31–78)	98% (95–100)	80% (56–100)	93% (89–98)	25 (8–82)	0.46 (0.29–0.73)	92% (87–96)	0.79 (0.65–0.93)
NDIRS post-treatment	53% (26–80)	99% (96–100)	90% (66–100)	91% (85–98)	46 (6–336)	0.48 (0.29–0.79)	91% (85–97)	0.81 (0.67–0.95)
IRMS post-treatment	60% (7–100)	96% (90–100)	60% (7–100)	96% (90–100)	16 (3–75)	0.42 (0.14–1.22)	93% (86–100)	0.78 (0.44–1.0)

SAT: stool antigen test; UBT: urea breath test; PPV: positive predictive value; NPV: negative predictive value; LR+: positive likelihood ratio; LR−: negative likelihood ratio; AUC: area under the ROC curve; IRMS: isotope ratio mass spectrometry, cut-off value 5‰; NDIRS: non-dispersive isotope-selective infrared spectrometry, cut-off value 2.5‰.

Table 4. Accuracy of the LIAISON® Meridian *H. pylori* SA test after performing PCR in stool of discordant samples.

Comparison SAT vs. UBT	Sensitivity (95% CI)	Specificity (95% CI)	PPV (95% CI)	NPV (95% CI)	LR+ (95% CI)	LR− (95% CI)	Global Accuracy (95% CI)	AUC (95% CI)
Overall	94% (85–100)	97% (95–99)	86% (75–97)	99% (97–100)	35 (17–73)	0.07 (0.02–0.20)	97% (95–99)	0.96 (0.91–1.0)
Naïve	91% (80–100)	96% (93–100)	89% (77–100)	97% (94–100)	25 (10–67)	0.09 (0.03–0.27)	95% (91–99)	0.996 (0.99–1.0)
Post-treatment	100% (96–100)	98% (95–100)	80% (56–100)	100% (99–100)	50 (16–153)	0.00	98% (96–100)	0.94 (0.88–1.0)

SAT: stool antigen test; UBT: urea breath test; PPV: positive predictive value; NPV: negative predictive value; LR+: positive likelihood ratio; LR−: negative likelihood ratio; AUC: area under the ROC curve.

Mean UBT value (±SD) in treatment-naïve positive patients was 43.3 ± 28.4 and 18.4 ± 15.2 measured by IRMS and NDIRS, respectively. Mean UBT value (±SD) in post-treatment negative patients was 0.96 ± 0.98 and 0.54 ± 0.52 measured by IRMS and NDIRS, respectively.

4. Discussion

The present study evaluated the accuracy of an *H. pylori* diagnostic method, a chemiluminescent immunoassay of the LIAISON® Meridian *H. pylori* SA versus the performance of the ^{13}C-UBT, defined as the gold standard.

Although high levels of global accuracy (91%) and specificity (97%) were shown with this novel strategy, the sensitivity was sub-optimal (67%) both in naïve diagnostic testing (74%) and in post-treatment eradication confirmatory testing (55%). Even though the results were lower than expected, they were within the range of variability found in a recent meta-analysis of SATs, which described a high heterogeneity of performance depending on the brand, or even for the same brand in different populations [22]. Several methodological aspects should be taken into consideration when extracting conclusions from our results.

First, the choice of ^{13}C-UBT as the unique gold standard method might represent a limitation in the correct classification of patients as positive or negative for *H. pylori* infection. The concern arises because no invasive diagnostic method, such as histological evaluation, RUT or culture was used as the gold standard, neither a combination of two or more diagnostic tests. Therefore, using ^{13}C-UBT only as the reference method, misdiagnosis by the UBT may hide the existence of correct stool classifications by SAT.

Second, and regarding the two different UBT technologies used, multiple studies and meta-analyses support the high accuracy of NDIRS and its high correlation with IRMS, with sensitivity and specificity for *H. pylori* infection diagnosis > 90–95% for both techniques [27,28]. Conversely, recent studies [29–31] have suggested that NDIRS tests offer a low specificity, between 47 and 88%, and a low PPV (with Otsuka equipment, including the POCone spectrophotometer used in our study), with a relatively high false-positive rate. This could be a consequence of the NDIRS cut-off point set by the manufacturer, as there is evidence of an increase in specificity from 60 to 90% [30], or from 47.1% to 95.7% [31] by raising the currently recommended cut-off point from 2.5‰ to 8.5‰. In fact, other studies [29,31] suggest an even larger "grey or borderline area" of 2–10‰ where the positive UBT results obtained with NDIRS may be less reliable and could possibly be classified as false positive.

Kwon et al., basing their results on a post-treatment group of 223 UBT-positive patients with values ranging from 2.5‰ to 10.0‰, found that 34% were false positives as determined by endoscopic biopsy [31]. Furthermore, there is evidence that when the UBT is positive, delta figures are usually much higher than the cut-off point [32], in line with our study, where results showed mean positive UBT values of 43 and 18 measured by IRMS and NDIRS, respectively.

In this respect, it should be highlighted in our study that the majority of "false negatives" of the SAT (11/15 analysed with NDIRS) were within these borderline values (2.5‰ to 10.0‰). In addition, very recent guidelines recommended the use of IRMS technology as a first choice UBT reference method, leaving NDIRS as an alternative [33]. Furthermore, it is remarkable that citric acid is not included in the NDIRS protocol, in contrast to that of IRMS, as citric acid has proven to make the UBT more robust and is an essential component of the protocol [2,13].

All the above-mentioned considerations might explain the lower sensitivity of the LIAISON® Meridian *H. pylori* SA assay (65%) in the present study when compared to NDIRS, which raised (to 71%) when compared to IRMS. These data suggest a slightly lower PPV and specificity of the NDIRS UBT than would be expected. Moreover, it can be assumed that the higher accuracy of the IRMS UBT is probably due, at least in part, to the use of citric acid in its protocol.

Focusing on the benefits of using SAT as a non-invasive method, several advantages such as rapidity are to be highlighted, since the sample can be delivered with no need to remain in the hospital or medical centre, thereby reducing work absenteeism, tending to simplicity in the procedure and subsequently lowering the costs. In addition, some studies suggested that SAT has the same diagnostic value in patients with distal gastrectomy as in patients without surgery [14,34] and regardless of treatment with PPIs [35]. However, these statements are not widely accepted, and further studies are needed. Hence, we excluded these patients from our protocol. On the other hand, the SAT also has some disadvantages, including that negative SAT results may not indicate the absence of *H. pylori* infection but rather low density of *H. pylori* in the stomach and a low antigen load in the stool [16]. However, this disadvantage is common for most non-invasive methods, for instance, with UBT it has even been suggested to select a lower cut-off value (compared to the pre-treatment setting) in order to maintain the diagnostic accuracy for the monitoring of *H. pylori* eradication [32].

Concerning the SAT methodology, as mentioned in Section 1, SATs can be either based on ELISA, CLIA or ICA [7]. The former has been the most widely studied and recommended by international guidelines due to its high diagnostic accuracy [2]. Laboratory-based CLIAs are widely used in clinical laboratories. This technique has elevated sensitivity due to the broad contact surface area provided by the particles of the reagent for antigen–antibody interaction, as well as the increased intra- and inter-assay accuracy inherent to CLIA versus ELISA methodology. Luminescent transitions of excited molecules or atoms to a state of lower energy are characterised by electromagnetic radiation dissipated as photons in the ultraviolet (UV), visible or near-infrared region. These luminescent reactions are classified according to the energy source involved during the excitation step; thus, most classical light-emission reactions are referred to as bioluminescence (from in vivo systems), chemiluminescence (from a chemical reaction, as is the case of this study protocol), electroluminescence (from electrochemical reaction) and photoluminescence (from UV, visible or near-infrared radiations). Chemiluminescence reactions are generally oxidoreduction processes and the excited compound, which is the reaction product, has a different chemical structure from the initial reactant [36,37]. The technology has the ability to detect minimal quantities of antigen in stool samples (4 ng/mL), and by using a photomultiplier, the luminescence signal can be measured down to a few photons [24]. Additionally, automation enables processing a large number of samples in a short period of time, thereby saving time, providing objective results, minimising mishandling and ensuring proper traceability. Altogether these characteristics warrant validation studies of this technique in our setting.

Technological advances allow the use of techniques such as chemiluminescence for the diagnosis of *H. pylori* infection, and technological developments also enable progress in the treatment or control of infection through the use of sensors capable of detecting anti-biofilm drugs or urease inhibitors [38,39].

The accuracy of the automated LIAISON® Meridian *H. pylori* SA assay has been previously evaluated in a limited number of publications. Opekun et al. [40] included 277 patients and combined different methods including histology, culture and RUT as gold standard, obtaining a high sensitivity and specificity (95.5% and 97.6%, respectively). However, only eight patients were included in the post-treatment group. Ramírez-Lázaro et al. [24] included 252 untreated patients. Compared to the gold standard (concordance of the RUT, histopathology and UBT), the test had a sensitivity of 90.1% and a specificity of 92.4%, with PPV and NPV > 90%. Another evaluation of the test in 103 untreated patients with dyspepsia was performed in Spain [41] using the same gold standard (UBT) as in the present study and reporting results similar to ours, with a sensitivity of 72% and a specificity of 96.2%. However, this latter study was reported only as a conference abstract. Thus, to the best of our knowledge, our study included the largest number of post-treatment patients in which confirmation of *H. pylori* eradication was assessed.

It has been suggested that in the post-treatment setting the SAT may have a suboptimal performance given the low prevalence of infection, with PPV around 50% [42]. In this regard, the present study is in accordance with current literature as the LIAISON® Meridian *H. pylori* SA assay accuracy was inferior in the post-treatment setting (sensitivity 55%, specificity 98%, AUC 0.79) than in naïve patients (sensitivity 74%, specificity 96%, AUC 0.88) while maintaining an acceptable post-treatment PPV of 80% despite a prevalence of *H. pylori* of only 14% (consequence of an eradication rate of 86%). Therefore, despite the fact that meta-analyses claim that *H. pylori* monoclonal SAT can also be used in the post-treatment setting with high sensitivity and specificity [19], it may have worse diagnostic performance than in the naïve setting. Nevertheless, considering the data after performing PCR on stool from discordant samples, excellent accuracy values were also obtained in the post-treatment setting (sensitivity 100%, specificity 98%, AUC 0.94).

The use of molecular techniques, such as stool PCR, is increasing not only for diagnosis but also for non-invasive detection of bacterial antibiotic resistance [43]. The overall sensitivity of stool PCR as a diagnostic test, depending on target gene, ranges between 40 and 100%, being the highest for the 23s RNA and 16s RNA genes, the latter with sensitivity and specificity close to 100% in some studies [44]. The two most consistent meta-analyses, one including twenty-six studies and the other one including seven studies in children, calculated a sensitivity range of 70–80% [15,45].

The genes used in our study, glmM and 16s rRNA, have a sensitivity of 56% and 74%, and a high specificity of 99% and 87%, respectively, with an excellent AUC (≥ 0.95), placing them as two of the first-choice genes for stool PCR testing [45]. In addition, we used a nested PCR for the amplification of the 16s rRNA gene, a front-line technique due to its higher sensitivity and the ability to amplify the target sequence at a lower concentration, as it involves two rounds of amplification [15,16,45]. Furthermore, combination of several target genes might help to improve the diagnostic performance by reducing the possibility of missed detection [16]. The combination of these two genes in gastric biopsies of 387 patients provided a sensitivity and specificity of 92.9% and 92.4%, respectively, which is superior to histopathology and RUT [46].

Therefore, we re-analysed the data by considering our 25 discordant patients as "true negatives", with both negative genes in stool samples, especially in view of the borderline positive value of the UBT in most of them. This improved the accuracy of the LIAISON® *H. pylori* SA up to a sensitivity of 94%, a specificity of 97%, and an AUC of 0.96.

Our study has some limitations, such as not having an invasive method or a combination of several diagnostic methods as the gold standard or using two different UBT technologies. On the other hand, our study has several strengths: the inclusion of prospectively evaluated patients, the multicentre study design, its large sample size, the inclusion not only of pre-treatment but also post-treatment patients, and the performance of stool PCR analysis of discordant samples.

5. Conclusions

In conclusion, the LIAISON® *H. pylori* SA chemiluminescent diagnostic assay showed a good accuracy for diagnosis of *H. pylori* infection, both pre- and post-treatment.

Supplementary Materials: The following are available online at https://www.mdpi.com/article/10.3390/jcm11175077/s1, File S1: Stool antigen test protocol [47–54].

Author Contributions: Writing—original draft, E.R.; project administration, M.G.D., S.H., Y.B., J.P.G., E.R., S.J.M.-D., E.J.L.-M., Á.L., A.J.L., M.S.-L., N.A., L.F.-S., L.D.L.P.-N., L.B., M.G.-R.d.A., J.A., Á.P.-A. and R.R. acted as recruiters, collected or helped to interpret data, critically reviewed the manuscript drafts, and approved the submitted manuscript; methodology and study design, E.R., J.P.G. and O.P.N.; writing—review & editing, J.P.G. and O.P.N. All authors have read and agreed to the published version of the manuscript.

Funding: This is an independent study financed by a DIASORIN IBERIA S.A. (Grant number: 3800). DIASORIN had no access to clinical data and was not involved in study design, statistical analysis and manuscript writing.

Institutional Review Board Statement: Protocol was approved by the Ethics Committee of the participant hospitals and the ethics committee of La Princesa University Hospital (Madrid, Spain), which acted as the reference institution. Date of approval: 20 June 2019. The study protocol conforms to the ethical guidelines of the 1975 Declaration of Helsinki as reflected in a prior approval by the institution's human research committee.

Informed Consent Statement: Written informed consent has been obtained from all the patients involved in the study.

Data Availability Statement: The data presented in this study are available on request from the corresponding author.

Conflicts of Interest: Javier P. Gisbert served as a speaker, a consultant and advisory member for or has received research funding from Mayoly, Allergan, Diasorin, Gebro Pharma, and Richen. Olga P. Nyssen received research funding from Allergan and Mayoly Spindler. Luis Bujanda served as consultant or has received research funding from Ikan Biotech. Javier Alcedo served as a speaker, an advisory member for, or has received research funding from Allergan and Isomed Pharma. The remaining authors have no potential conflict of interest. The funders had no role in the design of the study; in the collection, analyses, or interpretation of data; in the writing of the manuscript, or in the decision to publish the results.

References

1. Crowe, S.E. *Helicobacter pylori* Infection. *N. Engl. J. Med.* **2019**, *380*, 1158–1165. [CrossRef]
2. Malfertheiner, P.; Megraud, F.; O'Morain, C.A.; Gisbert, J.P.; Kuipers, E.J.; Axon, A.T.; Bazzoli, F.; Gasbarrini, A.; Atherton, J.; Graham, D.Y.; et al. Management of *Helicobacter pylori* infection-the Maastricht V/Florence Consensus Report. *Gut* **2017**, *66*, 6–30. [CrossRef]
3. Pimentel-Nunes, P.; Libânio, D.; Marcos-Pinto, R.; Areia, M.; Leja, M.; Esposito, G.; Garrido, M.; Kikuste, I.; Megraud, F.; Matysiak-Budnik, T.; et al. Management of epithelial precancerous conditions and lesions in the stomach (MAPS II): European Society of Gastrointestinal Endoscopy (ESGE), European Helicobacter and Microbiota Study Group (EHMSG), European Society of Pathology (ESP), and Sociedade Portuguesa de Endoscopia Digestiva (SPED) guideline update 2019. *Endoscopy* **2019**, *51*, 365–388. [CrossRef] [PubMed]
4. Cubiella, J.; Pérez Aisa, Á.; Cuatrecasas, M.; Díez Redondo, P.; Fernández Esparrach, G.; Marín-Gabriel, J.C.; Moreira, L.; Núñez, H.; Pardo López, M.L.; Rodríguez de Santiago, E.; et al. Gastric cancer screening in low incidence populations: Position statement of AEG, SEED and SEAP. *Gastroenterol. Hepatol.* **2021**, *44*, 67–86. [CrossRef] [PubMed]
5. Godbole, G.; Mégraud, F.; Bessède, E. Review: Diagnosis of *Helicobacter pylori* infection. *Helicobacter* **2020**, *25* (Suppl. S1), e12735. [CrossRef] [PubMed]
6. Sabbagh, P.; Mohammadnia-Afrouzi, M.; Javanian, M.; Babazadeh, A.; Koppolu, V.; Vasigala, V.R.; Nouri, H.R.; Ebrahimpour, S. Diagnostic methods for *Helicobacter pylori* infection: Ideals, options, and limitations. *Eur. J. Clin. Microbiol. Infect Dis.* **2019**, *38*, 55–66. [CrossRef] [PubMed]
7. Dore, M.P.; Pes, G.M. What Is New in *Helicobacter pylori* Diagnosis. An Overview. *J. Clin. Med.* **2021**, *10*, 2091. [CrossRef]
8. McNicholl, A.G.; Amador, J.; Ricote, M.; Cañones-Garzón, P.J.; Gene, E.; Calvet, X.; Gisbert, J.P. Spanish primary care survey on the management of *Helicobacter pylori* infection and dyspepsia: Information, attitudes, and decisions. *Helicobacter* **2019**, *24*, e12593. [CrossRef]
9. Ford, A.C.; Qume, M.; Moayyedi, P.; Arents, N.L.; Lassen, A.T.; Logan, R.F.; McColl, K.E.; Myres, P.; Delaney, B.C. *Helicobacter pylori* "test and treat" or endoscopy for managing dyspepsia: An individual patient data meta-analysis. *Gastroenterology* **2005**, *128*, 1838–1844. [CrossRef]
10. Beresniak, A.; Malfertheiner, P.; Franceschi, F.; Liebaert, F.; Salhi, H.; Gisbert, J.P. *Helicobacter pylori* "Test-and-Treat" strategy with urea breath test: A cost-effective strategy for the management of dyspepsia and the prevention of ulcer and gastric cancer in Spain-Results of the Hp-Breath initiative. *Helicobacter* **2020**, *25*, e12693. [CrossRef]
11. Gisbert, J.P.; Calvet, X. *Helicobacter pylori* "Test-and-Treat" Strategy for Management of Dyspepsia: A Comprehensive Review. *Clin. Transl. Gastroenterol.* **2013**, *4*, e32. [CrossRef]
12. Best, L.M.; Takwoingi, Y.; Siddique, S.; Selladurai, A.; Gandhi, A.; Low, B.; Yaghoobi, M.; Gurusamy, K.S. Non-invasive diagnostic tests for *Helicobacter pylori* infection. *Cochrane Database Syst. Rev.* **2018**, *3*, Cd012080. [CrossRef]
13. Gisbert, J.P.; Pajares, J.M. Review article: 13C-urea breath test in the diagnosis of *Helicobacter pylori* infection—A critical review. *Aliment. Pharmacol. Ther.* **2004**, *20*, 1001–1017. [CrossRef]

14. Shimoyama, T. Stool antigen tests for the management of *Helicobacter pylori* infection. *World J Gastroenterol* **2013**, *19*, 8188–8191. [CrossRef]
15. Leal, Y.A.; Cedillo-Rivera, R.; Simón, J.A.; Velázquez, J.R.; Flores, L.L.; Torres, J. Utility of stool sample-based tests for the diagnosis of *Helicobacter pylori* infection in children. *J. Pediatr. Gastroenterol. Nutr.* **2011**, *52*, 718–728. [CrossRef]
16. Qiu, E.; Li, Z.; Han, S. Methods for detection of *Helicobacter pylori* from stool sample: Current options and developments. *Braz. J. Microbiol.* **2021**, *52*, 2057–2062. [CrossRef]
17. Elwyn, G.; Taubert, M.; Davies, S.; Brown, G.; Allison, M.; Phillips, C. Which test is best for *Helicobacter pylori*? A cost-effectiveness model using decision analysis. *Br. J. Gen. Pract.* **2007**, *57*, 401–403.
18. Schulz, T.R.; McBryde, E.S.; Leder, K.; Biggs, B.A. Using stool antigen to screen for *Helicobacter pylori* in immigrants and refugees from high prevalence countries is relatively cost effective in reducing the burden of gastric cancer and peptic ulceration. *PLoS ONE* **2014**, *9*, e108610. [CrossRef]
19. Gisbert, J.P.; de la Morena, F.; Abraira, V. Accuracy of monoclonal stool antigen test for the diagnosis of *H. pylori* infection: A systematic review and meta-analysis. *Am. J. Gastroenterol.* **2006**, *101*, 1921–1930. [CrossRef]
20. Gisbert, J.P.; Calvet, X.; Bermejo, F.; Boixeda, D.; Bory, F.; Bujanda, L.; Castro-Fernández, M.; Dominguez-Muñoz, E.; Elizalde, J.I.; Forné, M.; et al. III Spanish Consensus Conference on *Helicobacter pylori* infection. *Gastroenterol. Hepatol.* **2013**, *36*, 340–374. [CrossRef]
21. Zhou, X.; Su, J.; Xu, G.; Zhang, G. Accuracy of stool antigen test for the diagnosis of *Helicobacter pylori* infection in children: A meta-analysis. *Clin. Res. Hepatol. Gastroenterol.* **2014**, *38*, 629–638. [CrossRef] [PubMed]
22. CADTH. Stool Antigen Tests for Helicobacter pylori Infection: A Review of Clinical and Cost-Effectiveness and Guidelines. In *Rapid Response Reports: Summary with Critical Appraisal*; Canadian Agency for Drugs and Technologies in Health (CADTH): Ottawa, ON, Canada, 2015.
23. Chey, W.D.; Leontiadis, G.I.; Howden, C.W.; Moss, S.F. ACG Clinical Guideline: Treatment of *Helicobacter pylori* Infection. *Am. J. Gastroenterol.* **2017**, *112*, 212–239. [CrossRef]
24. Ramírez-Lázaro, M.J.; Lite, J.; Lario, S.; Pérez-Jové, P.; Montserrat, A.; Quílez, M.E.; Martínez-Bauer, E.; Calvet, X. Good diagnostic accuracy of a chemiluminescent immunoassay in stool samples for diagnosis of *Helicobacter pylori* infection in patients with dyspepsia. *J. Investig. Med.* **2016**, *64*, 388–391. [CrossRef] [PubMed]
25. Bossuyt, P.M.; Reitsma, J.B.; Bruns, D.E.; Gatsonis, C.A.; Glasziou, P.P.; Irwig, L.M.; Lijmer, J.G.; Moher, D.; Rennie, D.; de Vet, H.C. Towards complete and accurate reporting of studies of diagnostic accuracy: The STARD initiative. Standards for Reporting of Diagnostic Accuracy. *Clin. Chem.* **2003**, *49*, 1–6. [CrossRef] [PubMed]
26. Jones, S.R.; Carley, S.; Harrison, M. An introduction to power and sample size estimation. *Emerg. Med. J.* **2003**, *20*, 453–458. [CrossRef] [PubMed]
27. Gisbert, J.P.; Gomollón, F.; Domínguez-Muñoz, J.E.; Borda, F.; Jiménez, I.; Vázquez, M.A.; Gallego, S.; Iglesias, J.; Pastor, G.; Pajares, J.M. Comparison between two 13C-urea breath tests for the diagnosis of *Helicobacter pylori* infection: Isotope ratio mass spectrometer versus infrared spectrometer. *Gastroenterol. Hepatol.* **2003**, *26*, 141–146. [CrossRef] [PubMed]
28. Kato, M.; Saito, M.; Fukuda, S.; Kato, C.; Ohara, S.; Hamada, S.; Nagashima, R.; Obara, K.; Suzuki, M.; Honda, H.; et al. 13C-Urea breath test, using a new compact nondispersive isotope-selective infrared spectrophotometer: Comparison with mass spectrometry. *J. Gastroenterol.* **2004**, *39*, 629–634. [CrossRef]
29. Kwon, Y.H.; Kim, N.; Yoon, H.; Shin, C.M.; Park, Y.S.; Lee, D.H. Effect of Citric Acid on Accuracy of (13)C-Urea Breath Test after *Helicobacter pylori* Eradication Therapy in a Region with a High Prevalence of Atrophic Gastritis. *Gut Liver* **2019**, *13*, 506–514. [CrossRef]
30. Calvet, X.; Sánchez-Delgado, J.; Montserrat, A.; Lario, S.; Ramírez-Lázaro, M.J.; Quesada, M.; Casalots, A.; Suárez, D.; Campo, R.; Brullet, E.; et al. Accuracy of diagnostic tests for *Helicobacter pylori*: A reappraisal. *Clin. Infect Dis.* **2009**, *48*, 1385–1391. [CrossRef]
31. Kwon, Y.H.; Kim, N.; Lee, J.Y.; Choi, Y.J.; Yoon, K.; Hwang, J.J.; Lee, H.J.; Lee, A.; Jeong, Y.S.; Oh, S.; et al. The Diagnostic Validity of Citric Acid-Free, High Dose (13)C-Urea Breath Test After *Helicobacter pylori* Eradication in Korea. *Helicobacter* **2015**, *20*, 159–168. [CrossRef]
32. Gisbert, J.P.; Olivares, D.; Jimenez, I.; Pajares, J.M. Long-term follow-up of 13C-urea breath test results after *Helicobacter pylori* eradication: Frequency and significance of borderline delta13CO2 values. *Aliment. Pharmacol. Ther.* **2006**, *23*, 275–280. [CrossRef]
33. Keller, J.; Hammer, H.F.; Afolabi, P.R.; Benninga, M.; Borrelli, O.; Dominguez-Munoz, E.; Dumitrascu, D.; Goetze, O.; Haas, S.L.; Hauser, B.; et al. European guideline on indications, performance and clinical impact of (13) C-breath tests in adult and pediatric patients: An EAGEN, ESNM, and ESPGHAN consensus, supported by EPC. *United Eur. Gastroenterol. J.* **2021**, *9*, 598–625. [CrossRef]
34. Yan, J.; Yamaguchi, T.; Odaka, T.; Suzuki, T.; Ohyama, N.; Hara, T.; Sudo, K.; Nakamura, K.; Denda, T.; Takiguchi, N.; et al. Stool antigen test is a reliable method to detect Helicobacter pylori in the gastric remnant after distal gastrectomy for gastric cancer. *J. Clin. Gastroenterol.* **2010**, *44*, 73–74. [CrossRef]
35. Kodama, M.; Murakami, K.; Okimoto, T.; Fukuda, Y.; Shimoyama, T.; Okuda, M.; Kato, C.; Kobayashi, I.; Fujioka, T. Influence of proton pump inhibitor treatment on *Helicobacter pylori* stool antigen test. *World J. Gastroenterol.* **2012**, *18*, 44–48. [CrossRef]
36. Roda, A.; Pasini, P.; Mirasoli, M.; Michelini, E.; Guardigli, M. Biotechnological applications of bioluminescence and chemiluminescence. *Trends Biotechnol.* **2004**, *22*, 295–303. [CrossRef]

37. Marquette, C.A.; Blum, L.J. Chemiluminescent enzyme immunoassays: A review of bioanalytical applications. *Bioanalysis* **2009**, *1*, 1259–1269. [CrossRef]
38. Xiao, S.; Shang, K.; Zhang, L.; Li, W.; Wang, X. A rapid anti-*Helicobacter pylori* biofilm drug screening biosensor based on AlpB outer membrane protein and colloidal gold/nanoporous gold framework. *Biosens. Bioelectron.* **2022**, *215*, 114599. [CrossRef]
39. Xiao, S.; Shang, K.; Li, W.; Wang, X. An efficient biosensor based on the synergistic catalysis of *Helicobacter pylori* urease b subunit and nanoplatinum for urease inhibitors screening and antagonistic mechanism analyzing. *Sens. Actuators B Chem.* **2022**, *355*, 131284. [CrossRef]
40. Opekun, A.R.; Zierold, C.; Rode, A.; Blocki, F.A.; Fiorini, G.; Saracino, I.M.; Vaira, D.; Sutton, F.M. Clinical Performance of the Automated LIAISON® Meridian *H. pylori* SA Stool Antigen Test. *Biomed. Res. Int.* **2020**, *2020*, 7189519. [CrossRef]
41. Vargas, J.; López-Sánchez, M.; Pabón, M.; Lamas, E.; Parra, M.; CastroFernández, M. Evaluation of a novel chemiluminiscent inmunoassay for the detection of *Helicobacter pylori* antigen and their correlation with immunochromatographic rapid test in stools samples from adults patients. *Helicobacter* **2013**, *18*, 121. [CrossRef]
42. Sánchez Delgado, J.; García-Iglesias, P.; Titó, L.; Puig, I.; Planella, M.; Gené, E.; Saló, J.; Martínez-Cerezo, F.; Molina-Infante, J.; Gisbert, J.P.; et al. Update on the management of *Helicobacter pylori* infection. Position paper from the Catalan Society of Digestology. *Gastroenterol. Hepatol.* **2018**, *41*, 272–280. [CrossRef] [PubMed]
43. Yang, H.; Hu, B. Diagnosis of *Helicobacter pylori* Infection and Recent Advances. *Diagnostics* **2021**, *11*, 1305. [CrossRef]
44. Shuber, A.P.; Ascaño, J.J.; Boynton, K.A.; Mitchell, A.; Frierson, H.F., Jr.; El-Rifai, W.; Powell, S.M. Accurate, noninvasive detection of *Helicobacter pylori* DNA from stool samples: Potential usefulness for monitoring treatment. *J. Clin. Microbiol.* **2002**, *40*, 262–264. [CrossRef] [PubMed]
45. Khadangi, F.; Yassi, M.; Kerachian, M.A. Review: Diagnostic accuracy of PCR-based detection tests for *Helicobacter Pylori* in stool samples. *Helicobacter* **2017**, *22*, e12444. [CrossRef]
46. Zhou, L.; Zhao, F.; Hu, B.; Fang, Y.; Miao, Y.; Huang, Y.; Ji, D.; Zhang, J.; Xu, L.; Zhang, Y.; et al. A Creative *Helicobacter pylori* Diagnosis Scheme Based on Multiple Genetic Analysis System: Qualification and Quantitation. *Helicobacter* **2015**, *20*, 343–352. [CrossRef] [PubMed]
47. Kusters, J.G.; van Vliet, A.H.; Kuipers, E.J. Pathogenesis of *Helicobacter pylor* infection. *Clin. Microbiol. Rev.* **2006**, *19*, 449–490. [PubMed]
48. Brown, L.M. *Helicobacter pylor*: Epidemiology and routes of transmission. *Epidemiol. Rev.* **2000**, *22*, 283–297.
49. Megraud, F. Transmission of *Helicobacter pylor*: Faecal-oral versus oral-oral route. *Aliment. Pharmacol. Ther.* **1995**, *9* (Suppl. S2), 85–91.
50. Amieva, M.R.; El-Omar, E.M. Host-bacterial interactions in *Helicobacter pylor* infection. *Gastroenterology* **2008**, *134*, 306–323.
51. Clinical and Laboratory Standards Institute (CLSI). *Statistical Quality Control for Quantitiative Measurements: Priciples and Definition: Approved Guideline*, 3rd ed.; CLSI Document C24-A3; Clinical and Laboratory Standards Institute (CLSI): Wayne, PA, USA, 2006; Volume 26, ISBN 1-56238-613-1.
52. Clinical and Laboratory Standards Institute (CLSI). *Evaluation of Precision Performance of Quantitative Measure Methods; Approved Guideline*, 3rd ed.; EP5-A3; Clinical and Laboratory Standards Institute (CLSI): Wayne, PA, USA, 2014; Volume 34.
53. Clinical and Laboratory Standards Institute (CLSI). *User Verification of Precision and Estimation of Bias; Approved Guideline*, 3rd ed.; EP15-A3; Clinical and Laboratory Standards Institute (CLSI): Wayne, PA, USA, 2014; Volume 28.
54. Clinical and Laboratory Standards Institute (CLSI). *Interference Testing in Clinical Chemistry; Approved Guideline*, 2nd ed.; EP7-A2; Clinical and Laboratory Standards Institute (CLSI): Wayne, PA, USA, 2005; Volume 28.

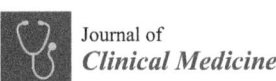

Review

Current and Future Perspectives in the Diagnosis and Management of *Helicobacter pylori* Infection

Malek Shatila and Anusha Shirwaikar Thomas *

Department of Gastroenterology, Hepatology and Nutrition, The University of Texas MD Anderson Cancer Center, Houston, TX 77030, USA
* Correspondence: asthomas1@mdanderson.org; Tel.: +1-832-7859155

Abstract: *Helicobacter pylori* (*Hp*) is a prevalent organism infecting almost half the global population. It is a significant concern, given its associated risk of gastric cancer, which is the third leading cause of cancer death globally. Infection can be asymptomatic or present with dyspeptic symptoms. It may also present with alarm symptoms in the case of progression to cancer. Diagnosis can be achieved non-invasively (breath tests, stool studies, or serology) or invasively (rapid urease test, biopsy, or culture). Treatment involves acid suppression and regimens containing several antibiotics and is guided by resistance rates. Eradication is essential, as it lowers the risk of complications and progression to cancer. Follow-up after eradication is similarly important, as the risk of cancer progression remains. There have been many recent advances in both diagnosis and treatment of *Hp*. In particular, biosensors may be effective diagnostic tools, and nanotechnology, vaccines, and potassium-competitive acid blockers may prove effective in enhancing eradication rates.

Keywords: *Helicobacter pylori*; gastric cancer; peptic ulcer disease; triple therapy; bismuth; vonoprazan; dyspepsia

1. Introduction

Hp is a Gram-negative, characteristically curved bacteria that was first observed to be present in the stomach lining in the 19th century [1,2]. It was not until 40 years ago that its association with gastric inflammation was demonstrated [3]. The finding that *Hp* could cause gastritis earned the investigators the Nobel Prize in 2005 for its myriad implications [2]. This discovery generated a massive body of research into the manifestations, treatments, and associations of *Hp* infection and revolutionized our understanding of the role of pathogens in disease [2,4].

Why Is H. Pylori Important?

Hp is strongly associated with duodenal ulcers (present in as many as 90% of cases), gastric ulcers (up to 80%), and malignancy; it can lead to mucosa-associated lymphoid tissue (MALT) lymphoma, as well as gastric cancer in as many as 90% of cases [5]. In 2014, the World Health Organization (WHO) called for the elimination of *Hp* as a means to decrease gastric cancer mortality worldwide, and in 2017. it deemed clarithromycin-resistant *Hp* strains a serious threat to public health [6]. In this review, we will present an overview of *H. pylori* disease characteristics, including epidemiology and clinical presentation, and discuss the most recent advances in evaluation and management of this entity.

2. Epidemiology

Helicobacter pylori is highly ubiquitous [7], colonizing roughly half of the world's population [7,8]. The primary mechanism of transmission is yet to be identified but is presumed to involve person-to-person transmission [9] through fecal/oral exposure. The prevalence of *Hp* varies widely by region; Asia, Latin America, and Africa tend to have higher rates (up to 80% in some countries), whereas North America and Oceania have the lowest rates (as low as 24%) [10,11]; those born in the 1930s have a much higher prevalence than those born in the 1970s [10]. One meta-analysis estimated the global prevalence of *Hp* at 44.3%, ranging from 34.7% in developed countries to 50.8% in developing countries [12], and most recent studies show a continuous decline in *Hp* prevalence over the years [13]. Despite this trend, there is a worrisome increase in antibiotic-resistant *Hp* strains [14].

2.1. Antibiotic Resistance

Unsuccessful eradication has been a recurrent issue over the years; treatment failure rates are continuously on the rise, in large part due to the increasing prevalence of antibiotic-resistant *Hp* strains [14–18]. This is a global phenomenon affecting most countries, although specific resistance rates vary by region and antibiotic type [19]. One meta-analysis found that clarithromycin resistance reached as high as 35% in eastern Mediterranean, European, and western Pacific regions, whereas it was the lowest in Africa, the Americas, and southeast Asia, at around 15% [14]. Levofloxacin showed a somewhat similar trend, with 14% resistance in the Americas, Africa, and Europe; and around 25% in Mediterranean, southeast Asian, and western Pacific regions. Reported metronidazole rates were much higher in this study, ranging from 30 to 91%, whereas amoxicillin resistance was negligible in most regions, except for Africa, where it was 38% [14]. To put these numbers into perspective, a local resistance of >15% is the common threshold for choosing alternate treatment regimens [19,20]. In reality, the epidemiology of antibiotic resistance is far more complex, as there considerable variation within the countries of each region. This obstacle is compounded by the fact that in most regions worldwide, studies are focused primarily on a handful of countries [19]. In the US, for instance, national data are scarce, and fewer than half the states are routinely included in studies [21,22]. Better data are available from Europe, where various studies have been conducted in individual countries, as well as larger-scale projects. One study on 3974 patients by the European Registry of *Helicobacter pylori* Management (*Hp*-EuReg) found that resistance rates to clarithromycin and levofloxacin were significantly higher in southern Europe (e.g., Italy, Spain, and Greece) as opposed to northern Europe (e.g., Norway) [23]. Alarmingly, strains collected from 52% of *Hp*-naïve and 80% of non-naïve patients exhibited some form of antibiotic resistance in this study [23]. Antibiotic resistance may, in part, be influenced by treatment for previous *Hp* infections. This entity recurs in around 4% of cases annually [24,25], and various risk factors have been identified that contribute to this phenomenon.

2.2. Risk Factors

Risk factors can be categorized on a societal or individual level. The former encompasses geographic location; economic development; and sanitation, including access to clean food and water [26]. Low familial socioeconomic status and overcrowding (i.e., crowded living conditions and large family sizes) are also associated with increased *Hp* prevalence [26]. Consumption of unpasteurized dairy products [27], sheepherding [28], high-risk occupations (healthcare) [29], obesity [30], male gender [31], and the gut microbiome [32] pose an increased risk of infection. Smoking and alcohol are two variables that are controversial with respect to their role in *Hp* infections [33–43].

3. Etiopathogenesis

The pathogenesis of *Hp* infection can be divided into distinct steps, whereby the bacteria (1) attaches to and colonizes the gastric mucosa, (2) evokes and evades an immune response, and (3) induces disease. Once present in the stomach, *H. pylori* swims toward the mucous lining the epithelial layer, showing a tropism for sites of injury along the stomach wall [44]. This chemotaxis relies on Tlp receptors (mainly TlpB) to direct flagellar motion in response to chemical signals in the cell environment [45]. Urea, gastric acid, lactate, and reactive oxygen species have all been identified as signals for these receptors; urea in particular is secreted by the gastric epithelium and is thought to play a significant role in bacterial colonization [45]. However, undiscovered chemicals may also be implicated in this process [46]. *Hp* utilizes urease to protect itself from the surrounding acid environment. Urease breaks urea down into ammonia and other useful metabolites, increasing the pH in the microenvironment to create a thin, pH-neutral layer around the bacterial cell, allowing it to survive the gastric acid. This barrier reduces the viscosity of the mucin gel lining the stomach wall and allows the bacteria to move freely through the mucous toward the gastric glands that it will ultimately colonize [46,47].

Bacterial attachment to gastric epithelial cells is a complex process that involves the synergistic interaction of several elements and relies heavily on Lewis (Le) antigens. Lewis antigens are cell-surface glycoproteins that mediate cell-to-cell adhesion by binding to selectins on target cells [48]. The lipopolysaccharide (LPS) component of the *Hp* cell wall has been found to express Lewis-like antigens, among which Le^X, in particular, has been shown to play a minor role in adhesion [49].

Bacterial outer membrane proteins (OMPs), on the other hand, operate as binding sites to which host Lewis antigens can bind, facilitating attachment. The OMPs on *Hp* can be divided into five genomic families [50], of which *H. pylori* OMP (Hop) and *Helicobacter* outer membrane (Hom) play the largest roles [51]. Blood antigen-binding adhesin A (BabA) and sialic acid-binding adherence (SabA) are members of the Hop family and are the most well-studied of all OMPs [52]. BabA promotes cell-to-cell adhesion by binding to host Le^B [53], whereas SabA binds to sialylated Le^X (sLe^X) to facilitate cell adhesion [54]. SabA additionally stimulates a neutrophil response by binding neutrophil sLe^X and activating a G-protein-coupled, receptor-mediated signaling cascade [55]. Interestingly, sLe^X is up-regulated upon the occurrence of *Hp* infection and gastric inflammation, which suggests that SabA may be involved in strengthening and maintaining adhesion, as opposed to initiating it [54]. MUC5a and MUC1 mucin receptors are the primary target for these OMPs and can expedite and hinder infection, respectively [56–58]. Whereas BabA and SabA are the main adhesins involved, several other OMPs, such as outer inflammatory protein A (OipA), HopQ, HopZ, and the Hom family, improve *Hp* adhesion and promote inflammation by prompting the transcription of virulence factors and the secretion of inflammatory cytokines [52].

Certain virulence factors involved in pathogenicity also contribute to adhesion. BabA-Le^B binding has been shown to activate the type-four secretion system (T4SS), a pilus-like structure that allows for the translocation of effector proteins, such as cytotoxin-associated gene A (CagA) and vacuolating cytotoxin A (VacA) [54]. CagA binds to epithelial cell integrin-$\beta 1$ [59] to anchor *Hp* and hijack host signaling pathways to disrupt cell motility, proliferation, and cytoskeletal stability [60]. VacA, on the other hand, binds to a wide range of receptors, with numerous downstream effects. It primarily functions as a pore-forming toxin than acutely induces host cell apoptosis but plays a key role in evading the immune response in chronic infections. It carries out this latter role by impairing autophagy and forming intracellular vacuoles in the host cell in which *H. pylori* can survive. It also binds to the integrin $\beta 2$ subunit on T cells to inhibit their activation and proliferation and can induce macrophage apoptosis by inhibiting interferon-β signaling [61]. Together, these toxins are the major virulence factors expressed by *Hp* that are key to its pathogenicity. Whereas VacA is expressed by virtually all *Hp* cells, CagA is only present in specific strains; interestingly, CagA positivity is associated with more severe infection and worse clinical outcomes, including an increased risk of future malignancy [60,62]. Although these are the two major proteins involved in the pathogenesis of *Hp* infection, there are myriad others that similarly aid in adhesion, immune evasion, and provocation of inflammation [60].

4. Clinical Presentation

The presentation of *H. pylori* infection is highly variable. As many as 90% of individuals carrying the bacteria are asymptomatic [63]. It can present as dyspepsia, defined as an epigastric discomfort or pain lasting longer than one month that may be associated with nausea, early satiety, epigastric fullness, and bloating, among other symptoms [64], which is often presumed to be functional in etiology [65]. Gastrointestinal clinical symptomatology of *Hp* infection poorly correlates with severity of gastric mucosal injury upon endoscopy [19,64]. *Hp* can therefore go unnoticed and untreated, in which case it progresses to chronic gastritis [66]. This chronic inflammation of the gastric epithelium can promote intestinal metaplasia, which predisposes to gastric cancer [64]. Despite being asymptomatic for years, such patients may present with alarm symptoms of weight loss, iron deficiency anemia, dysphagia, vomiting, and the presence of an abdominal mass [19,64,65]. Similarly, MALT lymphomas may develop as a result of gastritis and present with dyspeptic or non-specific constitutional symptoms [64,67]. *Hp* can also cause peptic ulcer disease (PUD), with the risk of complications, such as gastrointestinal bleeding and perforation [64].

Rarely, *H. pylori* infection may present with extragastrointestinal manifestations, such as isolated iron deficiency anemia; idiopathic thrombocytopenic purpura; and ocular, dermatological, and metabolic diseases [65,68].

5. Evaluation and Management:

5.1. Indications for Testing

The American College of Gastroenterology (ACG) recommends testing in the following cases [65]:

(1) All patients with active PUD;
(2) All patients with a previous history of PUD (unless there is documentation of a resolved prior *Hp* infection), low-grade MALT lymphoma, or a history of endoscopic resection of early gastric cancer;
(3) Patients with uninvestigated dyspepsia under the age of 60;
(4) Patients initiating long-term, non-steroidal, anti-inflammatory drugs;
(5) Patients with unexplained iron deficiency anemia despite appropriate workup; and
(6) Adults with idiopathic thrombocytopenic purpura.

Other expert panels, including the global Taipei consensus [69] (TC) and the Houston conference [70] (HC), support guidelines similar to those outlined above, with the addition of a few other indications:

(7) Family members residing in the same household as patients with proven active *Hp* infection (HC);
(8) Patients with a family history of PUD or gastric cancer (HC);
(9) First-generation immigrants from high-prevalence areas *or* high-risk groups (HC); and
(10) Populations with a high incidence of gastric cancer (TC).

In all of the above cases, a "test-and-treat" strategy is recommended to ensure eradication of the bacteria and reduce the severity of symptoms and the risk for carcinogenesis. A variety of tests can be used to diagnose infection with *H. pylori*, and they can be divided into non-invasive and invasive tests, a summary of which can be found in Table 1.

5.2. Non-Invasive Tests

The most commonly used test to identify *H. pylori* is the urea breath test (UBT), which measures the difference in proportion of $^{13}C/^{14}C$ in exhaled air before and after the patient swallows radioactively labeled urea. This relies on the previously discussed *Hp* urease, which generates radiolabeled ^{13}C carbon dioxide as a result. Patients with active *Hp* infection exhale higher quantities of ^{13}C than healthy patients. Typically, four respiratory samples are collected (two before and two after ingestion of urea), and the labeled carbon dioxide is detected using mass spectrometry [71]. UBT is an accessible and commonly used tool to diagnose *Hp* infection, with a recent meta-analysis showing sensitivity and specificity of around 95% [72,73]. However, results can be influenced by concurrent medications, so patients are required to stop antibiotics 30 days prior to the test and proton pump inhibitors (PPIs) 15 days prior, as they may produce false negatives [71].

Stool antigen testing (SAT) is another low-cost and accurate means of diagnosing *Hp* infection that is often preferred by patients and physicians for its simplicity [71]. There are two main types of stool tests: enzyme immunoassays (EIAs) and immunochromatography assays (ICAs). Both tests operate under similar principles. In EIAs, a solution containing monoclonal or polyclonal antibodies is added to a diluted stool sample and processed, antigens detected through spectrometry [74]. In immunochromatography, antigen detection is made possible by a reaction caused by the antigen–antibody complex, producing a visible color change in the medium [75]. Between these two testing methods, EIA has proven to be a more effective diagnostic tool, although the accuracy of SATs varies widely depending on the detection kit used [76,77].

The final non-invasive method for diagnosing *H. pylori* is serological testing for immunoglobulin G (IgG) antibodies against *Hp* using an enzyme-linked immunosorbent assay that operates in a similar fashion to SAT. IgG antibodies appear about three weeks after infection and can remain detectable for several years thereafter. Serological tests have fallen out of favor for this reason, as they have trouble distinguishing past infections from recent or active infections and are associated with a risk of false positives [78]. Despite a high reported specificity and sensitivity for serologic antibody tests ranging from 80 to 95%, these values vary considerable depending on the testing kit used, with values reported as low as 55% [72,78]. This is especially true in the case of the newer latex agglutination immunoassay test. The latex or LZ test is increasingly used due to its low cost and rapid processing ability [79]. However, it relies on the agglutination of latex-bound antigens, and interpretation of results is highly subjective, potentially increasing the risk of false positives [79]. To their credit, serological tests are not affected by recent PPI or antibiotic use, making them an option for patients who have used either.

5.3. Invasive Tests

Endoscopic assessment is a critical component of invasive testing for *H. pylori* upon which all other invasive tests depend [71]. Conventional endoscopy alone is, for the most part, inadequate in diagnosing *Hp* infection, and a biopsy with histological assessment is still mandatory for evaluation [19]. However, advancements in endoscopic technology have allowed for image-enhanced scoping to improve the accuracy of endoscopic evaluation [19,80]. There is one scoring system currently in use called the Kyoto classification [81] that is used to evaluate active *H. pylori* infection and risk of gastric cancer. It consists of five endoscopic findings (atrophy, intestinal metaplasia, enlarged folds, nodularity, and diffuse redness), cumulating in a score ranging from 0 to 8. A Kyoto score ≥ 2 indicates *H. pylori* infection, whereas a score ≥ 4 suggests gastric cancer risk [80]. Whereas a few studies have supported the accuracy of the Kyoto classification in diagnosing active *H. pylori* infection [81,82], endoscopy is rarely the only diagnostic technique used to evaluate *Hp* infection. Instead, it is almost always paired with biopsies or alternative tests.

The gold standard for *H. pylori* diagnosis is histological examination. For this evaluation, at least six biopsies must be taken during biopsy targeting the antrum, large and small curvatures of the stomach, and the middle of the gastric body, as well as any suspicious lesions or ulcerations [71]. Hematoxylin–eosin and Giemsa stains are the most inexpensive and commonly used stains, but immunohistochemical staining is the most accurate (fluorescence in situ hybridization) and is recommended when histochemical methods fail [83]. The updated Sydney grading system relies on histopathological findings to assess the severity of chronic gastritis and categorizes the intensity of mononuclear inflammatory cellular infiltrates, polymorph activity, atrophy, intestinal metaplasia, and *Hp* density as mild, moderate, or severe [84]. The sensitivity and specificity of histological methods can range from 60% to 100% and depend on a variety of factors, including stain used; location, size, and quality of the sample; and the pathologist's experience [71].

Alternative testing methods include bacterial culture, molecular testing (polymerase chain reaction; PCR), and rapid urease test (RUT). Bacterial culture is a highly specific means of diagnosing *H. pylori* infection but, as mentioned earlier, can be an arduous task that requires well-equipped laboratories [71]. *Hp* is a notoriously difficult microorganism to grow and requires incubation for more than a week in selective blood agar (a detailed description of culture requirements can be found in the study by Blanchard and colleagues) [85]. It has the additional benefit of identifying antibiotic resistance, as does PCR testing, which is becoming increasingly necessary [71]. The RUT, on the other hand, relies on a pH indicator that changes color in response to the ammonia produced by *Hp* urease. Previous studies have shown it to be highly sensitive and specific, at ≥90%, and it has the added benefit of rapidly producing results (within 5 min with some tests). Given its ease of use, it is considered the first-line diagnostic method in cases for which endoscopy is indicated [71].

Table 1. Sensitivities and specificities of various diagnostic modalities.

Test	Sensitivity	Specificity	Cost [86]	Advantages [87]	Disadvantages [87]	Study
UBT	97%	96%	Cost-effective	Fast, simple, non-invasive, good for detecting eradication	Potential risk for false negatives in cases of bleeding and PPI or antibiotic use; low accuracy in atrophic gastritis and gastric malignancy	Abd Rahim et al., 2019 [72] Zhou et al., 2017 [88]
Fecal antigen test	94%	97%	Cost-effective	Fast, simple, inexpensive, can potentially be used to determine antibiotic sensitivity	False negatives in cases of low bacterial load; accuracy affected by recent antibiotic, bismuth, or PPI use; may be uncomfortable for patients; difficulty maintaining sample; and variable accuracy depending on commercial kit used	Gisbert et al., 2006 [89]
Serology	Variable (76–84%)	Variable (79–90%)	Cost-effective	Cheapest, widely available, can be used in patients with recent PPI or antibiotic use	Failure to distinguish between acute and previous infection; cannot confirm eradication	Thaker et al., 2016 [90]
Rapid Urease Test	Variable (80–99%)	Variable (92–100%)	Cost-effective	Fast, inexpensive, simple	Accuracy impaired by gastric ulcer bleeding or intestinal metaplasia; invasive	Roy et al., 2016 [91]
Bacterial Culture	Variable (70–80%)	100%	Expensive	Determination of antibiotic resistance and sensitivity	Expensive, time-consuming, requires a well-equipped lab	Thaker et al., 2016 [90]
PCR	96%	98%	Expensive	High sensitivity and specificity; effective, even at low bacterial loads	Expensive, requires a well-equipped lab, false-positive risk due to detection of DNA from dead bacteria	Pichon et al., 2020 [92]

5.4. Management

Most societies endorse the non-invasive "test-and-treat" method [93–95], and initial endoscopy is recommended for older patients and those who present with alarm symptoms (first-degree relative with upper GI malignancy, weight loss, GI bleeding, dysphagia, odynophagia, persistent vomiting, and abnormal imaging) [94,95].

The first-line management of confirmed *H. pylori* infections utilizes a PPI, alongside 2–3 antibiotics for periods ranging from 3 to 14 days [64]. A full breakdown of the available first- and second-line treatment modalities can be found in Table 2.

Local antibiotic resistance rates are a key factor in determining the most appropriate first-line of management, as reflected by several major guidelines [20,64,65,96,97]. Furthermore, reuse of antibiotics from first-line treatments in subsequent therapy can lead to secondary antibiotic resistance and should be avoided [98]. Resistance to nitroimidazole antibiotics, such as metronidazole, are interesting in that whereas resistance rates can be high, this resistance can be overcome with dose adjustments and the addition of bismuth, allowing for its reuse in new regimens after an initial failure [98]. Whereas guidelines are not clear on sensitivity testing for first-line management of Hp, susceptibility testing is recommended in refractory cases [98].

An important consideration in initial management of infection is that the most commonly used acid suppressants, PPIs, are metabolized by hepatic cytochrome P450 (CYP2C19) [99]. Genetic polymorphisms may limit the efficacy of treatment regimens with particular PPIs [100]. It may be advisable to rely on PPIs less affected by CYP metabolism, such as esomeprazole and rabeprazole, especially in non-Asian regions, where extensive metabolizers are common [66,98].

Table 2. Treatment options for Hp.

Regimen	Dosing Frequency	Duration	Indications	Notes	Study
First-Line Treatments					
Triple PPI (variable dose) [a] CA (500 mg) AM [b] (1 g) OR MZ (500 mg)	BID BID BID	14 days	First-line treatment in regions where CA resistance is low (<15%) or with high proven local eradication rates (>85%) and in patients with no previous macrolide exposure.	A few studies are listed to summarize global resistance rates [14,101]. Eradication rates of up to 92.6% have been reported with triple therapy when potent and long-lasting gastric acid inhibitors, such as K$^+$-competetive blocker vonoprazan, are used [102].	Maastricht ACG Toronto
Concomitant PPI (variable dose) [a] CA (500 mg) AM (1 g) MZ (500 mg)	BID BID BID BID	10–14 days	First-line treatment, especially in regions where CA resistance is high (>15%) and metronidazole resistance is low.		Maastricht ACG Toronto
Quadruple Bismuth PPI (variable dose) [a] Bismuth (variable dose and preparation) [c] AM MZ	QID BID TID or QID	10–14 days	First-line treatment, especially in regions where CA and MZ resistances are high.		Maastricht ACG Toronto Chinese Spanish
Second-line treatments					
Quadruple Bismuth PPI (high dose) [a] Bismuth (variable dose and preparation) [c] TZ (500 mg) MZ (500 mg)	BID QID QID TID to QID	10–14 days	Can be used as a first-line treatment. Used as a second-line treatment if: 1. Triple or concomitant treatment failed; or 2. Earlier bismuth quadruple treatment failed (two different antibiotics need to be used).	The list of antibiotics that can be used alongside bismuth includes [103]: Clarithromycin; Amoxicillin; Doxycycline; Nitroimidazole; Furazolidone; and Levofloxacin.	Maastricht ACG Toronto Chinese Spanish AGA

Table 2. Cont.

First-Line Treatments					
Regimen	Dosing Frequency	Duration	Indications	Notes	Study
Levofloxacin Regimens Levofloxacin (500 mg) Amoxicillin (1 g) PPI (high dose) [a]	QD BID BID	10–14 days	Potential first-line treatment in areas with low fluroquinolone resistance (reference to ACG). Second-line treatment after failure of a bismuth regimen.	Only ACG suggests this as a first-line treatment in regions where levofloxacin resistance is low. Levofloxacin can be replaced by sitofloxacin.	Maastricht ACG Toronto Chinese Spanish AGA
Rescue treatments [d]					
High-dose dual PPI (high dose) [a] AM (750 mg or 1 g)	BID QID or TID respectively	14 days	Salvage therapy after two eradication failures.	Amoxicillin resistance rates are still low globally.	ACG Toronto AGA
Rifabutin-based triple Rifabutin Amoxicillin PPI (high dose) [a]	QD TID BID	14 days	Salvage therapy after two (Malfertheimer) or three (fallone) eradication failures. AGA guidelines suggest use as a second-line treatment after failed Bismuth therapy.	There is some concern about increasing M. tuberculosis resistance as a result of this treatment.	Maastricht Toronto AGA Spanish
Alternative or adjunctive treatments					
Statins Atorvastatin (40 mg) Simvastatin (20 mg)	QD BID	14 days	Experimental use	Statins have been shown to have antibacterial and anti-inflammatory effects [104,105]. One study found that statins reduced Hp burden in macrophages and increased Hp-infected macrophage autophagy [106].	AGA
Probiotics [e]		14 days	Experimental use	Probiotic strains have been shown to have a beneficial effect on eradication and to reduce treatment adverse effects, including: Lactobacillus; Bifidobacterium; Lactiplantibacillus; and Saccharomyces	AGA Kyoto Viazis et al., 2022 [107]

Notes: Abbreviations: PPI—proton pump inhibitor; CA—clarithromycin; AM—amoxicillin; MZ—metronidazole; BID—bidaily; QID—quad daily; TID—tridaily; TZ—tetracycline; QD—once daily; [a] dose varies depending on PPI used. Standard doses include esomeprazole 20 mg, lansoprazole 30 mg, omeprazole 20 mg, pantoprazole 40 mg, and rabeprazole 20 mg. High dose implies double the standard dose. [b] In patients with a penicillin allergy, amoxicillin should be substituted for metronidazole. [c] Bismuth can come in multiple preparations; the most common preparations are: Bismuth subsalicylate (262 mg), two tablets QID; colloidal bismuth subcitrate (120 mg), one tablet QID; bismuth biskalcitrate (140 mg), three tablets QID; bismuth subcitrate potassium (140 mg), three tablets QID. [d] Alternative antibiotics that can be used in rescue treatments include sitafloxacin, tinidazole, and furazolidone. [e] Lactobacillus and Bifidobacterium are supported by a growing body of evidence, whereas the benefits of Lactiplantibacillus and Saccharomyces are supported by a limited number of studies.

The exact recommendation for treatment duration differs depending on the guidelines and treatment line (Table 2). However, there is a trend toward standardization of all treatment lines to 14 days [108].

Table 2 highlights various treatment strategies: sequential, hybrid, concomitant, and reverse hybrid. Sequential therapy involves initial dual treatment with a PPI and amoxicillin for 5–7 days, followed by standard triple therapy for the same amount of time [108]. Concomitant therapy is a non-bismuth quadruple therapy and involves the concurrent administration of four medications [109]. Hybrid therapy combines the two, initiating patients on dual therapy (PPI + amoxicillin) for 7 days, then adding two more antibiotics for the next 7 days. Reverse hybrid therapy follows the opposite order: three antibiotics and a PPI for 7 days, followed by only a PPI + amoxicillin [110]. Sequential therapy has fallen out of favor due to worse eradication rates [20,64,66,95,96,108,109]. Hybrid and reverse-hybrid treatment strategies have proven to be equivalent to concomitant across various studies but are of limited efficacy in areas of high dual resistance to clarithromycin and metronidazole [111,112]. Concomitant therapy is currently the most widely used treatment strategy.

5.5. Treatment Outcomes

The ultimate goal of treatment is documented eradication of the bacteria [20,65,96,97]. There is evidence for endoscopic and histologic remission of gastritis features, including intestinal metaplasia and reduction in recurrence following eradication therapy [69,113–120], as well as prevention of gastric adenocarcinoma and regression of gastric MALT lymphoma [121–127]. Treatment also resolves *H. pylori*-associated iron deficiency anemia [128] and ITP [129].

6. Long-Term Surveillance and Complications

6.1. Surveillance

It is currently recommended to retest at least 4 weeks after completion of the initial treatment regimen, with the patient stopping PPIs as many as 2 weeks prior [64]. All aforementioned diagnostic tests are suitable for confirmation of eradication.

Despite the lack of established evidence-based guidelines, a growing body of literature supports endoscopic surveillance following eradication, particularly in high-risk patients [130–133]. The "ABC method" relies on an investigation of anti-*H. pylori* antibodies and serum pepsinogen (PG), whereby patients are divided into four groups depending on the presence of either (group A, negative for both; group B, anti-*Hp*-positive and PG-negative; group C, positive for both; group D, anti-*Hp*-negative and PG-positive). Groups B, C, and D were found to be increasingly more likely to develop gastric cancer than group A and were therefore recommended triennial, biennial, and annual endoscopic follow-up based on the increased risk [134]. Nonetheless, regular endoscopy is invasive, costly, and impractical in certain settings. A recent study identified several biomarkers that could potentially be used in lieu of endoscopy for screening, detection, and monitoring of individuals at risk of gastric cancer (GC), namely virulence markers, genomic markers, transcriptomic markers, and inflammatory markers [135]. cagA and VacA-toxin expression; pepsinogen levels (PG1 and PG2); bacterial lipopolysaccharides; connexin expression; specific microRNA fragments; and cytokines, such as IL-1β, IL-6, IFN-γ, and IL-10, have been found to be significantly upregulated in cases of GC [136–139].

6.2. Complications

Treatment of *H. pylori* does not guarantee permanent eradication. One prospective study of 1050 patients estimated recurrence rates at one and three years to be 1.75% and 4.61%, respectively [140]. Recurrent infection necessitates alternative antibiotic treatment regimens to those used previously and may contribute to increased antibiotic resistance globally. Oral colonization of *H. pylori* is a potential source of reinfection that can often go undiagnosed by standard diagnostic methods for *Hp* and is unaffected by traditional treatment methods, requiring specific treatment strategies [141,142]. The existence of a secondary *H. pylori* colonization site is still highly controversial but may be a consideration in complex cases with frequent recurrences [141,142]. The main complications of untreated H. pylori infection were outlined above but include gastric ulceration; perforation; progression to gastric malignancy (adenocarcinoma or MALT lymphoma); and extragastrointestinal manifestations, such as ITP and iron deficiency anemia [65]. Other complications take the form of side effects to treatment and are listed in Table 3.

Table 3. Medication adverse events resulting from H. pylori treatment.

Adverse Effect	Reported Frequency *	Associated Treatment Group †
Taste disturbance/oral mucositis [143–145]	17–44%	Triple therapy
Nausea [143,144]	7–31%	Bismuth
Diarrhea [143–145]	7–33%	Triple
Dyspepsia [143,145]	3–11%	
Reduced appetite [143,144]	4–12%	
Vomiting [144,145]	3–6%	
Abdominal pain [144,145]	8–20%	
Headache [144,145]	7–31%	Bismuth
Rash [144]	3–7%	Bismuth
Discoloration of feces [144,145]	4–16%	Bismuth
Oral/vaginal candidiasis [143,145]	1–4%	

Notes: * frequencies represent a range report in the selected studies comparing different treatment modalities; † not based on statistical comparison between different treatments, rather an observed difference in frequency between different treatment modalities. However, Calvet et al. [143] showed that triple therapy was significantly associated with more frequent taste disturbance.

7. Treatment Challenges

H. pylori eradication rates may not be optimally attributed primarily to antibiotic resistance and patient noncompliance/adherence due to side effects and provider prescriptive error [146–148]. These data highlight the importance of improved awareness and strict adherence to existing guidelines.

8. Recent Advances

In the decades since its discovery, considerable progress has been made with regards to diagnostic and therapeutic modalities in the management of Hp infection. Nanotechnology is an exciting innovation in the realm of diagnosis and treatment that could eventually represent cost-efficient and less invasive alternative to current endoscopic measures. Biosensors are one such tool that can translate unique biological elements attached to a transducer surface into detectable signals [149]. This is accomplished without additional reagents, reactions, or sample pretreatment, contrary to other modalities, such as PCR or ELISA, while providing accurate and real-time monitoring of disease [149–151]. Whereas the process itself is complex, it relies on detecting bacterial antigens or patient Hp antibodies. Electrochemical sensors rely on a change in electric potential or conductance of a transducing surface upon element attachment, optical sensors rely on a change in fluorescence or color absorbance, piezoelectric sensors rely on a change in acoustics, and thermal sensors rely on a change in temperature to detect disease [151]. Yadav et al. (2022) mentioned the novel use of aptamers, single stranded nucleic acid sequences that are highly specific to target antigens, proteins, or antibodies, to diagnose disease and have high hopes for their clinical utility [152].

Recent advances in therapy make potential use of nanotechnology as auxiliary treatment, improving drug delivery, with a direct antibacterial effect [153]. The development of novel drugs can also improve treatment of Hp. A potassium-competitive acid blocker, vonoprazan (VPZ) has advantages over traditional acid suppression with PPIs, in that it does not require activation by gastric acid and has a longer half-life than PPIs [154].

It is also unaffected by genetic polymorphisms in CYP450 [99]. Genetic polymorphisms are receiving increasing attention for their potential role in treatment outcomes. A few studies to date have shown that eradication rates may be higher in slower CYP metabolizers [99,155,156], although this association has not always been statistically significant. Polymorphisms in immune response genes can similarly impact disease severity and predispose to complications [157–159]. VPZ was only recently introduced in east Asia, and several meta-analyses show the superior efficacy of VPZ relative to standard PPI-containing triple therapy [154,160–162]. A more recent meta-analysis of RCTs found that VPZ demonstrated comparable and even superior eradication rates relative to PPI across different treatment regimens and in both low- and high-clarithromycin-resistance areas [162]. A lower rate of adverse events was also reported among VPZ users [162].

Antimicrobial peptides are short, positively-charged peptide chains that disrupt the integrity of the negatively charged bacterial cell membrane, leading to cell lysis and disruption of intracellular processes [163]. Photodynamic therapy relies on microbial production of photosensitive molecules that use light to produce cytotoxic reactive oxygen species, leading to bacterial cell death [164]. Phage therapy uses bacteriophages specific to *H. pylori* to induce bacterial cell lysis, eliminating the pathogen [165]. Finally, vaccination is an attractive strategy for combatting *Hp* infection globally. Various attempts have been made to develop an *Hp* vaccine over the years, but the results have been disappointing [166]. Whereas some vaccine candidates have shown potential as an option for prophylaxis, none have yet shown a therapeutic effect [166,167].

9. Conclusions

H. pylori is a ubiquitous and complex organism that has rightfully received tremendous interest over the years. It can manifest in a variety of ways and increases the risk of severe complications, such as peptic ulceration and malignancy. Therefore, treatment with adequate follow-up is imperative. In the current era of antibiotic stewardship, it is important to be mindful of antibiotic resistance and susceptibility when selecting a treatment regimen. Extensive research has been conducted on the pathogenesis of *Hp* infection, which has aided in identifying diagnostic and therapeutic targets. However, there is still room to improve our knowledge. In particular, there is more to be gleaned regarding bacterial transmission, reinfection, and optimized surveillance. Finally, there have been numerous recent technological advances that hold promise for streamlining the management of this pathogen in the future.

Author Contributions: Conceptualization, M.S. and A.S.T.; writing—original draft preparation, M.S.; writing, M.S.; review and editing, A.S.T.; supervision, A.S.T. All authors have read and agreed to the published version of the manuscript.

Funding: This research received no external funding.

Institutional Review Board Statement: Not applicable.

Informed Consent Statement: Not applicable.

Data Availability Statement: Not applicable.

Conflicts of Interest: The authors declare no conflict of interest.

References

1. Bizzozero, G.; der Eidechsen, D. Ueber die schlauchförmigen Drüsen des Magendarmkanals und die Beziehungen ihres. *Arch. Mikrosk. Anat.* **1893**, *42*, 82. [CrossRef]
2. Krienitz, W. Ueber das Auftreten von Spirochäten verschiedener form im Mageninhalt bei Carcinoma ventriculi. *DMW Dtsch. Med. Wochenschr.* **1906**, *32*, 872. [CrossRef]
3. Watts, G. Nobel prize is awarded to doctors who discovered *H. pylori*. *BMJ* **2005**, *331*, 795. [CrossRef] [PubMed]
4. Sonnenberg, A. Epidemiology of Helicobacter pylori. *Aliment. Pharmacol. Ther.* **2022**, *55* (Suppl. 1), S1–S13. [CrossRef]
5. Fong, I.W. Helicobacter pylori Infection: When Should It Be Treated? In *Current Trends and Concerns in Infectious Diseases. Emerging Infectious Diseases of the 21st Century*; Springer: Cham, Switzerland, 2020. [CrossRef]

6. WHO. Media Centre. News Release. WHO Publishes List of Bacteria for Which New Antibiotics Are Urgently Needed. 2017. Available online: http://www.who.int/mediacentre/news/releases/2017/bacteria-antibiotics-needed/en/ (accessed on 27 August 2022).
7. Hooi, J.K.Y.; Lai, W.Y.; Ng, W.K.; Suen, M.M.Y.; Underwood, F.E.; Tanyingoh, D.; Malfertheiner, P.; Graham, D.Y.; Wong, V.W.S.; Wu, J.C.Y.; et al. Global Prevalence of *Helicobacter pylori* Infection: Systematic Review and Meta-Analysis. *Gastroenterology* 2017, 153, 420–429. [CrossRef]
8. Salama, N.R.; Hartung, M.L.; Müller, A. Life in the human stomach: Persistence strategies of the bacterial pathogen *Helicobacter pylori*. *Nat. Rev. Microbiol.* 2013, 11, 385–399. [CrossRef] [PubMed]
9. Kayali, S.; Manfredi, M.; Gaiani, F.; Bianchi, L.; Bizzarri, B.; Leandro, G.; Di Mario, F.; Angelis, G.L.D. *Helicobacter pylori*, transmission routes and recurrence of infection: State of the art. *Acta Bio Med. Atenei Parm.* 2018, 89, 72–76. [CrossRef]
10. FitzGerald, R.; Smith, S.M. An Overview of Helicobacter pylori Infection. In *Helicobacter pylori. Methods in Molecular Biology*; Smith, S.M., Ed.; Humana: New York, NY, USA, 2021; Volume 2283. [CrossRef]
11. Sjomina, O.; Pavlova, J.; Niv, Y.; Leja, M. Epidemiology of *Helicobacter pylori* infection. *Helicobacter* 2018, 23 (Suppl. 1), e12514. [CrossRef]
12. Zamani, M.; Ebrahimtabar, F.; Zamani, V.; Miller, W.H.; Alizadeh-Navaei, R.; Shokri-Shirvani, J.; Derakhshan, M.H. Systematic review with meta-analysis: The worldwide prevalence of *Helicobacter pylori* infection. *Aliment. Pharmacol. Ther.* 2018, 47, 868–876. [CrossRef]
13. Mezmale, L.; Coelho, L.G.; Bordin, D.; Leja, M. Review: Epidemiology of *Helicobacter pylori*. *Helicobacter* 2020, 25, e12734. [CrossRef]
14. Savoldi, A.; Carrara, E.; Graham, D.Y.; Conti, M.; Tacconelli, E. Prevalence of Antibiotic Resistance in *Helicobacter pylori*: A Systematic Review and Meta-analysis in World Health Organization Regions. *Gastroenterology* 2018, 155, 1372–1382.e17. [CrossRef] [PubMed]
15. Egan, B.J.; Katicic, M.; O'Connor, H.J.; O'Morain, C.A. Treatment of *Helicobacter pylori*. *Helicobacter* 2007, 12, 31–37. [CrossRef]
16. Selgrad, M.; Meile, J.; Bornschein, J.; Kandulski, A.; Langner, C.; Varbanova, M.; Wex, T.; Tammer, I.; Schlüter, D.; Malfertheiner, P. Antibiotic susceptibility of *Helicobacter pylori* in central Germany and its relationship with the number of eradication therapies. *Eur. J. Gastroenterol. Hepatol.* 2013, 25, 1257–1260. [CrossRef] [PubMed]
17. Zou, Y.; Qian, X.; Liu, X.; Song, Y.; Song, C.; Wu, S.; An, Y.; Yuan, R.; Wang, Y.; Xie, Y. The effect of antibiotic resistance on *Helicobacter pylori* eradication efficacy: A systematic review and meta-analysis. *Helicobacter* 2020, 25, e12714. [CrossRef]
18. Thung, I.; Aramin, H.; Vavinskaya, V.; Gupta, S.; Park, J.Y.; Crowe, S.E.; Valasek, M.A. Review article: The global emergence of *Helicobacter pylori* antibiotic resistance. *Aliment. Pharmacol. Ther.* 2016, 43, 514–533. [CrossRef] [PubMed]
19. Malfertheiner, P.; Megraud, F.; O'Morain, C.A.; Gisbert, J.P.; Kuipers, E.J.; Axon, A.T.; Bazzoli, F.; Gasbarrini, A.; Atherton, J.; European Helicobacter and Microbiota Study Group and Consensus panel; et al. Management of *Helicobacter pylori* infection—The Maastricht V/Florence Consensus Report. *Gut* 2017, 66, 6–30. [CrossRef]
20. Fallone, C.A.; Chiba, N.; van Zanten, S.V.; Fischbach, L.; Gisbert, J.P.; Hunt, R.H.; Jones, N.L.; Render, C.; Leontiadis, G.I.; Moayyedi, P.; et al. The Toronto Consensus for the Treatment of *Helicobacter pylori* Infection in Adults. *Gastroenterology* 2016, 151, 51–69.e14. [CrossRef]
21. Hulten, K.G.; Lamberth, L.B.; Kalfus, I.N.; Graham, D.Y. National and Regional US Antibiotic Resistance to *Helicobacter pylori*: Lessons from a Clinical Trial. *Gastroenterology* 2021, 161, 342–344.e1. [CrossRef]
22. Ho, J.J.C.; Navarro, M.; Sawyer, K.; Elfanagely, Y.; Moss, S.F. *Helicobacter pylori* Antibiotic Resistance in the United States Between 2011–2021: A Systematic Review and Meta-Analysis. *Am. J. Gastroenterol.* 2022, 117, 1221–1230. [CrossRef]
23. Bujanda, L.; Nyssen, O.P.; Vaira, D.; Saracino, I.M.; Fiorini, G.; Lerang, F.; Georgopoulos, S.; Tepes, B.; Heluwaert, F.; Gasbarrini, A.; et al. Antibiotic Resistance Prevalence and Trends in Patients Infected with *Helicobacter pylori* in the Period 2013–2020: Results of the European Registry on *H. pylori* Management (Hp-EuReg). *Antibiotics* 2021, 10, 1058. [CrossRef]
24. Hu, Y.; Wan, J.-H.; Li, X.-Y.; Zhu, Y.; Graham, D.Y.; Lu, N.-H. Systematic review with meta-analysis: The global recurrence rate of *Helicobacter pylori*. *Aliment. Pharmacol. Ther.* 2017, 46, 773–779. [CrossRef]
25. Zhao, H.; Yan, P.; Zhang, N.; Feng, L.; Chu, X.; Cui, G.; Qin, Y.; Yang, C.; Wang, S.; Yang, K. The recurrence rate of *Helicobacter pylori* in recent 10 years: A systematic review and meta-analysis. *Helicobacter* 2021, 26, e12852. [CrossRef] [PubMed]
26. Kotilea, K.; Bontems, P.; Touati, E. Epidemiology, Diagnosis and Risk Factors of Helicobacter pylori Infection. In *Helicobacter pylori in Human Diseases. Advances in Experimental Medicine and Biology*; Kamiya, S., Backert, S., Eds.; Springer: Cham, Switzerland, 2019; Volume 1149. [CrossRef]
27. Assaad, S.; Chaaban, R.; Tannous, F.; Costanian, C. Dietary habits and *Helicobacter pylori* infection: A cross sectional study at a Lebanese hospital. *BMC Gastroenterol.* 2018, 18, 48. [CrossRef] [PubMed]
28. Dore, M.P.; Bilotta, M.; Vaira, D.; Manca, A.; Massarelli, G.; Leandro, G.; Atzei, A.; Pisanu, G.; Graham, D.Y.; Realdi, G. High prevalence of *Helicobacter pylori* infection in shepherds. *Dig. Dis. Sci.* 1999, 44, 1161–1164. [CrossRef]
29. Mastromarino, P.; Conti, C.; Donato, K.; Strappini, P.; Cattaruzza, M.; Orsi, G. Does hospital work constitute a risk factor for *Helicobacter pylori* infection? *J. Hosp. Infect.* 2005, 60, 261–268. [CrossRef]
30. Baradaran, A.; Dehghanbanadaki, H.; Naderpour, S.; Pirkashani, L.M.; Rajabi, A.; Rashti, R.; Riahifar, S.; Moradi, Y. The association between *Helicobacter pylori* and obesity: A systematic review and meta-analysis of case–control studies. *Clin. Diabetes Endocrinol.* 2021, 7, 15. [CrossRef] [PubMed]

31. de Martel, C.; Parsonnet, J. *Helicobacter pylori* Infection and Gender: A Meta-Analysis of Population-Based Prevalence Surveys. *Am. J. Dig. Dis.* **2006**, *51*, 2292–2301. [CrossRef] [PubMed]
32. Wang, D.; Li, Y.; Zhong, H.; Ding, Q.; Lin, Y.; Tang, S.; Zong, Y.; Wang, Q.; Zhang, X.; Yang, H.; et al. Alterations in the human gut microbiome associated with *Helicobacter pylori* infection. *FEBS Open Bio.* **2019**, *9*, 1552–1560. [CrossRef]
33. Wang, W.; Jiang, W.; Zhu, S.; Sun, X.; Li, P.; Liu, K.; Liu, H.; Gu, J.; Zhang, S. Assessment of prevalence and risk factors of helicobacter pylori infection in an oilfield Community in Hebei, China. *BMC Gastroenterol.* **2019**, *19*, 186. [CrossRef]
34. Zhang, F.; Pu, K.; Wu, Z.; Zhang, Z.; Liu, X.; Chen, Z.; Ye, Y.; Wang, Y.; Zheng, Y.; Zhang, J.; et al. Prevalence and associated risk factors of *Helicobacter pylori* infection in the Wuwei cohort of north-western China. *Trop. Med. Int. Health* **2021**, *26*, 290–300. [CrossRef]
35. Zhu, Y.; Zhou, X.; Wu, J.; Su, J.; Zhang, G. Risk Factors and Prevalence of *Helicobacter pylori* Infection in Persistent High Incidence Area of Gastric Carcinoma in Yangzhong City. *Gastroenterol. Res. Pract.* **2014**, *2014*, 481365. [CrossRef] [PubMed]
36. Smith, S.; Jolaiya, T.; Fowora, M.; Palamides, P.; Ngoka, F.; Bamidele, M.; Lesi, O.; Onyekwere, C.; Ugiagbe, R.; Agbo, I.; et al. Clinical and Socio-Demographic Risk Factors for Acquisition of *Helicobacter pylori* Infection in Nigeria. *Asian Pac. J. Cancer Prev.* **2018**, *19*, 1851–1857. [CrossRef]
37. Zhang, L.; Eslick, G.D.; Xia, H.H.-X.; Wu, C.; Phung, N.; Talley, N.J. Relationship between Alcohol Consumption and Active *Helicobacter pylori* Infection. *Alcohol Alcohol.* **2010**, *45*, 89–94. [CrossRef] [PubMed]
38. Seid, A.; Demsiss, W. Feco-prevalence and risk factors of *Helicobacter pylori* infection among symptomatic patients at Dessie Referral Hospital, Ethiopia. *BMC Infect. Dis.* **2018**, *18*, 260. [CrossRef] [PubMed]
39. Wu, W.; Leja, M.; Tsukanov, V.; Basharat, Z.; Hua, D.; Hong, W. Sex differences in the relationship among alcohol, smoking, and *Helicobacter pylori* infection in asymptomatic individuals. *J. Int. Med. Res.* **2020**, *48*. [CrossRef] [PubMed]
40. Ogihara, A.; Kikuchi, S.; Hasegawa, A.; Kurosawa, M.; Miki, K.; Kaneko, E.; Mizukoshi, H. Relationship between *Helicobacter pylori* infection and smoking and drinking habits. *J. Gastroenterol. Hepatol.* **2000**, *15*, 271–276. [CrossRef]
41. Ozaydin, N.; A Turkyilmaz, S.; Cali, S. Prevalence and risk factors of helicobacter pylori in Turkey: A nationally-representative, cross-sectional, screening with the 13C-Urea breath test. *BMC Public Health* **2013**, *13*, 1215. [CrossRef] [PubMed]
42. de Jésus Ngoma, P.; Longo-Mbenza, B.; Tshibangu-Kabamba, E.; Matungo, B.; Lupande, D.; Malu, C.; Kengibe, P.; Yaba, A.T.W.; Nlombi, C.M.; Fiasse, R.; et al. Seroprevalence and Risk Factors of the *Helicobacter pylori* Infection in Bukavu City in the Democratic Republic of Congo. *OALib* **2021**, *8*, e8032. [CrossRef]
43. Sirkeci, Ö.; Sirkeci, E.E.; Ulas, T. Does waterpipe smoking increase the risk of *Helicobacter pylori* infection? *J. Res. Med. Sci.* **2022**, *27*, 7. [CrossRef]
44. Denic, M.; Touati, E.; De Reuse, H. Review: Pathogenesis of *Helicobacter pylori* infection. *Helicobacter* **2020**, *25*, e12736. [CrossRef]
45. Hanyu, H.; Engevik, K.A.; Matthis, A.L.; Ottemann, K.M.; Montrose, M.H.; Aihara, E. *Helicobacter pylori* Uses the TlpB Receptor to Sense Sites of Gastric Injury. *Infect. Immun.* **2019**, *87*, e00202-19. [CrossRef] [PubMed]
46. Idowu, S.; Bertrand, P.P.; Walduck, A.K. Gastric organoids: Advancing the study of *H. pylori* pathogenesis and inflammation. *Helicobacter* **2022**, *27*, e12891. [CrossRef] [PubMed]
47. Celli, J.P.; Turner, B.S.; Afdhal, N.H.; Keates, S.; Ghiran, I.; Kelly, C.P.; Ewoldt, R.H.; McKinley, G.H.; So, P.; Erramilli, S.; et al. *Helicobacter pylori* moves through mucus by reducing mucin viscoelasticity. *Proc. Natl. Acad. Sci. USA* **2009**, *106*, 14321–14326. [CrossRef]
48. Soejima, M.; Koda, Y. Molecular mechanisms of Lewis antigen expression. *Leg. Med.* **2005**, *7*, 266–269. [CrossRef]
49. Odenbreit, S.; Faller, G.; Haas, R. Role of the AlpAB proteins and lipopolysaccharide in adhesion of *Helicobacter pylori* to human gastric tissue. *Int. Med. Microbiol.* **2002**, *292*, 247–256. [CrossRef] [PubMed]
50. Alm, R.A.; Bina, J.; Andrews, B.M.; Doig, P.; Hancock, R.E.W.; Trust, T.J. Comparative Genomics of *Helicobacter pylori*: Analysis of the Outer Membrane Protein Families. *Infect. Immun.* **2000**, *68*, 4155–4168. [CrossRef]
51. Oleastro, M.; Ménard, A. The Role of *Helicobacter pylori* Outer Membrane Proteins in Adherence and Pathogenesis. *Biology* **2013**, *2*, 1110–1134. [CrossRef]
52. Xu, C.; Soyfoo, D.M.; Wu, Y.; Xu, S. Virulence of *Helicobacter pylori* outer membrane proteins: An updated review. *Eur. J. Clin. Microbiol. Infect. Dis.* **2020**, *39*, 1821–1830. [CrossRef]
53. Hage, N.; Howard, T.; Phillips, C.; Brassington, C.; Overman, R.; Debreczeni, J.; Gellert, P.; Stolnik, S.; Winkler, G.S.; Falcone, F.H. Structural basis of Lewis ^{b} antigen binding by the *Helicobacter pylori* adhesin BabA. *Sci. Adv.* **2015**, *1*, e1500315. [CrossRef]
54. Doohan, D.; Rezkitha, Y.A.A.; Waskito, L.A.; Yamaoka, Y.; Miftahussurur, M. *Helicobacter pylori* BabA–SabA Key Roles in the Adherence Phase: The Synergic Mechanism for Successful Colonization and Disease Development. *Toxins* **2021**, *13*, 485. [CrossRef]
55. Unemo, M.; Aspholm-Hurtig, M.; Ilver, D.; Bergström, J.; Borén, T.; Danielsson, D.; Teneberg, S. The Sialic Acid Binding SabA Adhesin of *Helicobacter pylori* Is Essential for Nonopsonic Activation of Human Neutrophils. *J. Biol. Chem.* **2005**, *280*, 15390–15397. [CrossRef] [PubMed]
56. Giraldi, L.; Michelazzo, M.B.; Arzani, D.; Persiani, R.; Pastorino, R.; Boccia, S. MUC1, MUC5AC, and MUC6 polymorphisms, Helicobacter pylori infection, and gastric cancer: A systematic review and meta-analysis. *Eur. J. Cancer Prevention* **2018**, *27*, 323–330. [CrossRef] [PubMed]
57. van de Bovenkamp, J.H.B.; Mahdavi, J.; Male, A.M.K.-V.; Buller, H.A.; Einerhand, A.W.C.; Boren, T.; Dekker, J. The MUC5AC Glycoprotein is the Primary Receptor for *Helicobacter pylori* in the Human Stomach. *Helicobacter* **2003**, *8*, 521–532. [CrossRef] [PubMed]

58. Lindén, S.K.; Sheng, Y.H.; Every, A.L.; Miles, K.M.; Skoog, E.C.; Florin, T.H.J.; Sutton, P.; McGuckin, M.A. MUC1 Limits *Helicobacter pylori* Infection both by Steric Hindrance and by Acting as a Releasable Decoy. *PLoS Pathog.* **2009**, *5*, e1000617. [CrossRef]
59. Backert, S.; Tegtmeyer, N. Type IV Secretion and Signal Transduction of *Helicobacter pylori* CagA through Interactions with Host Cell Receptors. *Toxins* **2017**, *9*, 115. [CrossRef]
60. Baj, J.; Forma, A.; Sitarz, M.; Portincasa, P.; Garruti, G.; Krasowska, D.; Maciejewski, R. *Helicobacter pylori* Virulence Factors—Mechanisms of Bacterial Pathogenicity in the Gastric Microenvironment. *Cells* **2021**, *10*, 27. [CrossRef]
61. Chauhan, N.; Tay, A.C.Y.; Marshall, B.J.; Jain, U. *Helicobacter pylori* VacA, a distinct toxin exerts diverse functionalities in numerous cells: An overview. *Helicobacter* **2019**, *24*, e12544. [CrossRef]
62. Sharndama, H.C.; Mba, I.E. *Helicobacter pylori*: An up-to-date overview on the virulence and pathogenesis mechanisms. *Braz. J. Microbiol.* **2022**, *53*, 33–50. [CrossRef]
63. Alexander, S.M.; Retnakumar, R.J.; Chouhan, D.; Devi, T.N.B.; Dharmaseelan, S.; Devadas, K.; Thapa, N.; Tamang, J.P.; Lamtha, S.C.; Chattopadhyay, S. *Helicobacter pylori* in Human Stomach: The Inconsistencies in Clinical Outcomes and the Probable Causes. *Front. Microbiol.* **2021**, *12*, 713955. [CrossRef]
64. Guevara, B.; Cogdill, A.G. *Helicobacter pylori*: A Review of Current Diagnostic and Management Strategies. *Am. J. Dig. Dis.* **2020**, *65*, 1917–1931. [CrossRef]
65. Chey, W.D.; Leontiadis, G.I.; Howden, C.W.; Moss, S.F. ACG Clinical Guideline: Treatment of *Helicobacter pylori* Infection. *Am. J. Gastroenterol.* **2017**, *112*, 212–239. [CrossRef] [PubMed]
66. Sugano, K.; Tack, J.; Kuipers, E.J.; Graham, D.Y.; El-Omar, E.M.; Miura, S.; Haruma, K.; Asaka, M.; Uemura, N.; Kyoto Global Consensus Conference; et al. Kyoto global consensus report on *Helicobacter pylori* gastritis. *Gut* **2015**, *64*, 1353–1367. [CrossRef] [PubMed]
67. Fischbach, W. Gastric Mucosal-Associated Lymphoid Tissue Lymphoma. *Gastroenterol. Clin. N. Am.* **2013**, *42*, 371–380. [CrossRef] [PubMed]
68. Gravina, A.G.; Priadko, K.; Ciamarra, P.; Granata, L.; Facchiano, A.; Miranda, A.; Dallio, M.; Federico, A.; Romano, M. Extra-Gastric Manifestations of *Helicobacter pylori* Infection. *J. Clin. Med.* **2020**, *9*, 3887. [CrossRef]
69. Liou, J.-M.; Malfertheiner, P.; Lee, Y.-C.; Sheu, B.-S.; Sugano, K.; Cheng, H.-C.; Yeoh, K.-G.; Hsu, P.-I.; Goh, K.-L.; Mahachai, V.; et al. Screening and eradication of *Helicobacter pylori* for gastric cancer prevention: The Taipei global consensus. *Gut* **2020**, *69*, 2093–2112. [CrossRef]
70. El-Serag, H.B.; Kao, J.Y.; Kanwal, F.; Gilger, M.; LoVecchio, F.; Moss, S.F.; Crowe, S.; Elfant, A.; Haas, T.; Hapke, R.J.; et al. Houston Consensus Conference on Testing for *Helicobacter pylori* Infection in the United States. *Clin. Gastroenterol. Hepatol.* **2018**, *16*, 992–1002.e6, Correction in *Clin. Gastroenterol. Hepatol.* **2019**, *17*, 801. [CrossRef]
71. Cardos, A.I.; Maghiar, A.; Zaha, D.C.; Pop, O.; Fritea, L.; Miere , F.; Cavalu, S. Evolution of Diagnostic Methods for *Helicobacter pylori* Infections: From Traditional Tests to High Technology, Advanced Sensitivity and Discrimination Tools. *Diagnostics* **2022**, *12*, 508. [CrossRef]
72. Rahim, M.A.A.; Johani, F.H.; Shah, S.A.; Hassan, M.R.; Manaf, M.R.A. 13C-Urea Breath Test Accuracy for *Helicobacter pylori* Infection in the Asian Population: A Meta-Analysis. *Ann. Glob. Health* **2019**, *85*, 110. [CrossRef]
73. O'Connor, A. The Urea Breath Test for the Noninvasive Detection of Helicobacter pylori. In *Helicobacter Pylori. Methods in Molecular Biology*; Smith, S.M., Ed.; Humana: New York, NY, USA, 2021; Volume 2283. [CrossRef]
74. Koletzko, S.; Konstantopoulos, N.; Bosman, D.; Feydt-Schmidt, A.; van der Ende, A.; Kalach, N.; Raymond, J.; Rüssmann, H. Evaluation of a novel monoclonal enzyme immunoassay for detection of *Helicobacter pylori* antigen in stool from children. *Gut* **2003**, *52*, 804–806. [CrossRef]
75. Gatta, L.; Perna, F.; Ricci, C.; Osborn, J.F.; Tampieri, A.; Bernabucci, V.; Miglioli, M.; Vaira, D. A rapid immunochromatographic assay for *Helicobacter pylori* in stool before and after treatment. *Aliment. Pharmacol. Ther.* **2004**, *20*, 469–474. [CrossRef]
76. Qiu, E.; Li, Z.; Han, S. Methods for detection of *Helicobacter pylori* from stool sample: Current options and developments. *Braz. J. Microbiol.* **2021**, *52*, 2057–2062. [CrossRef] [PubMed]
77. Shimoyama, T. Stool antigen tests for the management of *Helicobacter pylori* infection. *World J. Gastroenterol.* **2013**, *19*, 8188–8191. [CrossRef] [PubMed]
78. Dore, M.P.; Graham, D.Y. Modern approach to the diagnosis of *Helicobacter pylori* infection. *Aliment. Pharmacol. Ther.* **2022**, *55*, S14–S21. [CrossRef] [PubMed]
79. Stefano, K.; Rosalia, A.; Chiara, B.; Federica, G.; Marco, M.; Gioacchino, L.; Fabiola, F.; Francesco, D.M.; Gian, L.D.A. Non-invasive tests for the diagnosis of *helicobacter pylori*: State of the art. *Acta Biomed.* **2018**, *89* (Suppl. 8), 58–64. [CrossRef]
80. Toyoshima, O.; Nishizawa, T.; Koike, K. Endoscopic Kyoto classification of *Helicobacter pylori* infection and gastric cancer risk diagnosis. *World J. Gastroenterol.* **2020**, *26*, 466–477. [CrossRef]
81. Toyoshima, O.; Nishizawa, T.; Yoshida, S.; Matsuno, T.; Odawara, N.; Toyoshima, A.; Sakitani, K.; Watanabe, H.; Fujishiro, M.; Suzuki, H. Consistency between the endoscopic Kyoto classification and pathological updated Sydney system for gastritis: A cross-sectional study. *J. Gastroenterol. Hepatol.* **2022**, *37*, 291–300. [CrossRef]
82. Zhao, J.; Xu, S.; Gao, Y.; Lei, Y.; Zou, B.; Zhou, M.; Chang, D.; Dong, L.; Qin, B. Accuracy of Endoscopic Diagnosis of *Helicobacter pylori* Based on the Kyoto Classification of Gastritis: A Multicenter Study. *Front. Oncol.* **2020**, *10*, 599218. [CrossRef]

83. White, J.R.; Sami, S.S.; Reddiar, D.; Mannath, J.; Ortiz-Fernández-Sordo, J.; Beg, S.; Scott, R.; Thiagarajan, P.; Ahmad, S.; Parra-Blanco, A.; et al. Narrow Band Imaging and Serology in the Assessment of Premalignant Gastric Pathology. *Scand. J. Gastroenterol.* **2018**, *53*, 1611–1618. [CrossRef]
84. Hassan, T.M.M.; Al-Najjar, S.I.; Al-Zahrani, I.H.; Alanazi, F.I.B.; Alotibi, M.G. *Helicobacter pylori* chronic gastritis updated Sydney grading in relation to endoscopic findings and H. pylori IgG antibody: Diagnostic methods. *J. Microsc. Ultrastruct.* **2016**, *4*, 167–174. [CrossRef]
85. Blanchard, T.G.; Nedrud, J.G. Laboratory Maintenance of *Helicobacter* Species. *Curr. Protoc. Microbiol.* **2006**, 8B.1.1–8B.1.13. [CrossRef]
86. Sulo, P.; Šipková, B. DNA diagnostics for reliable and universal identification of *Helicobacter pylori*. *World J. Gastroenterol.* **2021**, *27*, 7100–7112. [CrossRef] [PubMed]
87. Sabbagh, P.; Mohammadnia-Afrouzi, M.; Javanian, M.; Babazadeh, A.; Koppolu, V.; Vasigala, V.R.; Nouri, H.R.; Ebrahimpour, S. Diagnostic methods for *Helicobacter pylori* infection: Ideals, options, and limitations. *Eur. J. Clin. Microbiol.* **2019**, *38*, 55–66. [CrossRef]
88. Zhou, Q.; Li, L.; Ai, Y.; Pan, Z.; Guo, M.; Han, J. Diagnostic accuracy of the ^{14}C-urea breath test in *Helicobacter pylori* infections: A meta-analysis. *Wien Klin Wochenschr* **2017**, *129*, 38–45. [CrossRef] [PubMed]
89. Gisbert, J.P.; de la Morena, F.; Abraira, V. Accuracy of monoclonal stool antigen test for the diagnosis of H. pylori infection: A systematic review and meta-analysis. *Am. J. Gastroenterol.* **2006**, *101*, 1921. [CrossRef] [PubMed]
90. Thaker, Y.; Moon, A.; Afzali, A. *Helicobacter pylori*: A review of epidemiology, treatment, and management. *J. Clin. Gastroenterol. Treat.* **2016**, *2*, 1–5. [CrossRef]
91. Roy, A.D.; Deuri, S.; Dutta, U.C. The diagnostic accuracy of rapid urease biopsy test compared to histopathology in implementing "test and treat" policy for *Helicobacter pylori*. *Int. J. Appl. Basic Med. Res.* **2016**, *6*, 18–22. [CrossRef]
92. Pichon, M.; Pichard, B.; Barrioz, T.; Plouzeau, C.; Croquet, V.; Fotsing, G.; Chéron, A.; Vuillemin, É.; Wangermez, M.; Haineaux, P.-A.; et al. Diagnostic Accuracy of a Noninvasive Test for Detection of *Helicobacter pylori* and Resistance to Clarithromycin in Stool by the Amplidiag H. pylori + ClariR Real-Time PCR Assay. *J. Clin. Microbiol.* **2020**, *58*, e01787-19. [CrossRef]
93. Ford, A.C.; Qume, M.; Moayyedi, P.; Arents, N.L.; Lassen, A.T.; Logan, R.F.; McColl, K.E.; Myres, P.; Delaney, B.C. *Helicobacter pylori* "Test and Treat" or Endoscopy for Managing Dyspepsia: An Individual Patient Data Meta-analysis. *Gastroenterology* **2005**, *128*, 1838–1844. [CrossRef]
94. ASGE Standards of Practice Committee; Shaukat, A.; Wang, A.; Acosta, R.D.; Bruining, D.H.; Chandrasekhara, V.; Chathadi, K.V.; Eloubeidi, M.A.; Fanelli, R.D.; Faulx, A.L.; et al. The role of endoscopy in dyspepsia. *Gastrointest. Endosc.* **2015**, *82*, 227–232. [CrossRef]
95. Moayyedi, P.M.; E Lacy, B.; Andrews, C.N.; Enns, R.A.; Howden, C.W.; Vakil, N. ACG and CAG Clinical Guideline: Management of Dyspepsia. *Am. J. Gastroenterol.* **2017**, *112*, 988–1013. [CrossRef]
96. Liu, W.Z.; Xie, Y.; Lu, H.; Cheng, H.; Zeng, Z.R.; Zhou, L.Y.; Chen, Y.; Bin Wang, J.; Du, Y.Q.; Lu, N.H.; et al. Fifth Chinese National Consensus Report on the management of *Helicobacter pylori* infection. *Helicobacter* **2018**, *23*, e12475. [CrossRef] [PubMed]
97. Gisbert, J.P.; Alcedo, J.; Amador, J.; Bujanda, L.; Calvet, X.; Castro-Fernández, M.; Fernández-Salazar, L.; Gené, E.; Lanas, Á.; Lucendo, A.J.; et al. V Conferencia Española de Consenso sobre el tratamiento de la infección por *Helicobacter pylori*. *Gastroenterol. Hepatol.* **2022**, *45*, 392–417. [CrossRef] [PubMed]
98. Shah, S.C.; Iyer, P.G.; Moss, S.F. AGA Clinical Practice Update on the Management of Refractory *Helicobacter pylori* Infection: Expert Review. *Gastroenterology* **2021**, *160*, 1831–1841. [CrossRef] [PubMed]
99. Argueta, E.A.; Moss, S.F. How We Approach Difficult to Eradicate *Helicobacter pylori*. *Gastroenterology* **2022**, *162*, 32–37. [CrossRef] [PubMed]
100. Kuo, C.-H.; Lu, C.-Y.; Shih, H.-Y.; Liu, C.-J.; Wu, M.-C.; Hu, H.-M.; Hsu, W.-H.; Yu, F.-J.; Wu, D.-C.; Kuo, F.-C. CYP2C19 polymorphism influences *Helicobacter pylori* eradication. *World J. Gastroenterol.* **2014**, *20*, 16029–16036. [CrossRef]
101. Suzuki, H.; Mori, H. World trends for H. pylori eradication therapy and gastric cancer prevention strategy by H. pylori test-and-treat. *J. Gastroenterol.* **2018**, *53*, 354–361. [CrossRef]
102. Murakami, K.; Sakurai, Y.; Shiino, M.; Funao, N.; Nishimura, A.; Asaka, M. Vonoprazan, a novel potassium-competitive acid blocker, as a component of first-line and second-line triple therapy for *Helicobacter pylori* eradication: A phase III, randomised, double-blind study. *Gut* **2016**, *65*, 1439–1446. [CrossRef]
103. Lu, H.; Zhang, W.; Graham, D.Y. Bismuth-containing quadruple therapy for *Helicobacter pylori*: Lessons from China. *Eur. J. Gastroenterol. Hepatol.* **2013**, *25*, 1134–1140. [CrossRef]
104. Hassan, A.M.; Shawky, M.A.E.-G.; Mohammed, A.Q.; Haridy, M.A.; Eid, K.A.-E. Simvastatin improves the eradication rate of *Helicobacter pylori*: Upper Egypt experience. *Infect. Drug Resist.* **2019**, *12*, 1529–1534. [CrossRef]
105. Sarkeshikian, S.S.; Ghadir, M.R.; Alemi, F.; Jalali, S.M.; Hormati, A.; Mohammadbeigi, A. Atorvastatin in combination with conventional antimicrobial treatment of *Helicobacter pylori* eradication: A randomized controlled clinical trial. *J. Gastroenterol. Hepatol.* **2020**, *35*, 71–75. [CrossRef]
106. Liao, W.-C.; Huang, M.-Z.; Wang, M.L.; Lin, C.-J.; Lu, T.-L.; Lo, H.-R.; Pan, Y.-J.; Sun, Y.-C.; Kao, M.-C.; Lim, H.-J.; et al. Statin Decreases *Helicobacter pylori* Burden in Macrophages by Promoting Autophagy. *Front. Cell. Infect. Microbiol.* **2017**, *6*, 203. [CrossRef] [PubMed]

107. Viazis, N.; Argyriou, K.; Kotzampassi, K.; Christodoulou, D.K.; Apostolopoulos, P.; Georgopoulos, S.D.; Liatsos, C.; Giouleme, O.; Koustenis, K.; Veretanos, C.; et al. A Four-Probiotics Regimen Combined with A Standard *Helicobacter pylori*-Eradication Treatment Reduces Side Effects and Increases Eradication Rates. *Nutrients* **2022**, *14*, 632. [CrossRef] [PubMed]
108. Graham, D.Y.; Liou, J.-M. Primer for Development of Guidelines for *Helicobacter pylori* Therapy Using Antimicrobial Stewardship. *Clin. Gastroenterol. Hepatol.* **2022**, *20*, 973–983.e1. [CrossRef] [PubMed]
109. Wang, Y.; Zhao, R.; Wang, B.; Zhao, Q.; Li, Z.; Zhu-Ge, L.; Yin, W.; Xie, Y. Sequential versus concomitant therapy for treatment of *Helicobacter pylori* infection: An updated systematic review and meta-analysis. *Eur. J. Clin. Pharmacol.* **2018**, *74*, 1–13. [CrossRef] [PubMed]
110. Georgopoulos, S.; Papastergiou, V. An update on current and advancing pharmacotherapy options for the treatment of H. pylori infection. *Expert Opin. Pharmacother.* **2021**, *22*, 729–741. [CrossRef]
111. Du, L.-J.; Chen, B.-R.; Kim, J.J.; Kim, S.; Shen, J.-H.; Dai, N. *Helicobacter pylori* eradication therapy for functional dyspepsia: Systematic review and meta-analysis. *World J. Gastroenterol.* **2016**, *22*, 3486–3495. [CrossRef]
112. Hsu, P.; Tsay, F.; Kao, J.Y.; Peng, N.; Tsai, K.; Tsai, T.; Kuo, C.; Kao, S.; Wang, H.; Chen, Y.; et al. Equivalent efficacies of reverse hybrid and concomitant therapies in first-line treatment of *Helicobacter pylori* infection. *J. Gastroenterol. Hepatol.* **2020**, *35*, 1731–1737. [CrossRef]
113. Zhao, B.; Zhao, J.; Cheng, W.-F.; Shi, W.-J.; Liu, W.; Pan, X.-L.; Zhang, G.-X. Efficacy of *Helicobacter pylori* Eradication Therapy on Functional Dyspepsia. *J. Clin. Gastroenterol.* **2014**, *48*, 241–247. [CrossRef]
114. Kim, S.E.; Park, Y.S.; Kim, N.; Kim, M.S.; Jo, H.J.; Shin, C.M.; Lee, S.H.; Hwang, J.-H.; Kim, J.-W.; Jeong, S.-H.; et al. Effect of *Helicobacter pylori* Eradication on Functional Dyspepsia. *J. Neurogastroenterol. Motil.* **2013**, *19*, 233–243. [CrossRef]
115. Harvey, R.F.; Lane, A.; Nair, P.; Egger, M.; Harvey, I.; Donovan, J.; Murray, L. Clinical trial: Prolonged beneficial effect of *Helicobacter pylori* eradication on dyspepsia consultations—The Bristol Helicobacter Project. *Aliment. Pharmacol. Ther.* **2010**, *32*, 394–400. [CrossRef]
116. Ford, A.C.; Tsipotis, E.; Yuan, Y.; I Leontiadis, G.; Moayyedi, P. Efficacy of *Helicobacter pylori* eradication therapy for functional dyspepsia: Updated systematic review and meta-analysis. *Gut* **2021**, *2021*, 326583. [CrossRef] [PubMed]
117. Hwang, Y.J.; Choi, Y.J.; Kim, N.; Lee, H.S.; Yoon, H.; Shin, C.M.; Park, Y.S.; Lee, D.H. The Difference of Endoscopic and Histologic Improvements of Atrophic Gastritis and Intestinal Metaplasia After *Helicobacter pylori* Eradication. *Am. J. Dig. Dis.* **2021**, *67*, 3055–3066. [CrossRef] [PubMed]
118. Toyoshima, O.; Nishizawa, T.; Sakitani, K.; Yamakawa, T.; Takahashi, Y.; Kinoshita, K.; Torii, A.; Yamada, A.; Suzuki, H.; Koike, K. *Helicobacter pylori* eradication improved the Kyoto classification score on endoscopy. *JGH Open* **2020**, *4*, 909–914. [CrossRef]
119. Hwang, Y.-J.; Kim, N.; Lee, H.S.; Lee, J.B.; Choi, Y.J.; Yoon, H.; Shin, C.M.; Park, Y.S.; Lee, D.H. Reversibility of atrophic gastritis and intestinal metaplasia after *Helicobacter pylori* eradication—A prospective study for up to 10 years. *Aliment. Pharmacol. Ther.* **2018**, *47*, 380–390. [CrossRef] [PubMed]
120. Ford, A.C.; Gurusamy, K.S.; Delaney, B.; Forman, D.; Moayyedi, P. Eradication therapy for peptic ulcer disease in *Helicobacter pylori*-positive people. *Cochrane Database Syst. Rev.* **2016**, *4*, CD003840. [CrossRef]
121. Lee, Y.-C.; Chiang, T.-H.; Chou, C.-K.; Tu, Y.-K.; Liao, W.-C.; Wu, M.-S.; Graham, D.Y. Association Between *Helicobacter pylori* Eradication and Gastric Cancer Incidence: A Systematic Review and Meta-analysis. *Gastroenterology* **2016**, *150*, 1113–1124.e5. [CrossRef]
122. Tsukamoto, T.; Nakagawa, M.; Kiriyama, Y.; Toyoda, T.; Cao, X. Prevention of Gastric Cancer: Eradication of *Helicobacter pylori* and Beyond. *Int. J. Mol. Sci.* **2017**, *18*, 1699. [CrossRef]
123. Ford, A.C.; Yuan, Y.; Moayyedi, P. *Helicobacter pylori* eradication therapy to prevent gastric cancer: Systematic review and meta-analysis. *Gut* **2020**, *69*, 2113–2121. [CrossRef]
124. Doorakkers, E.; Lagergren, J.; Engstrand, L.; Brusselaers, N. Eradication of *Helicobacter pylori* and Gastric Cancer: A Systematic Review and Meta-analysis of Cohort Studies. *J. Natl. Cancer Inst.* **2016**, *108*, djw132. [CrossRef]
125. Nakamura, S.; Sugiyama, T.; Matsumoto, T.; Iijima, K.; Ono, S.; Tajika, M.; Tari, A.; Kitadai, Y.; Matsumoto, H.; Nagaya, T.; et al. Long-term clinical outcome of gastric MALT lymphoma after eradication of *Helicobacter pylori*: A multicentre cohort follow-up study of 420 patients in Japan. *Gut* **2012**, *61*, 507–513. [CrossRef]
126. Hu, Q.; Zhang, Y.; Zhang, X.; Fu, K. Gastric mucosa-associated lymphoid tissue lymphoma and *Helicobacter pylori* infection: A review of current diagnosis and management. *Biomark. Res.* **2016**, *4*, 15. [CrossRef] [PubMed]
127. Filip, P.V.; Cuciureanu, D.; Diaconu, L.S.; Vladareanu, A.M.; Pop, C.S. MALT lymphoma: Epidemiology, clinical diagnosis and treatment. *J. Med. Life* **2018**, *11*, 187–193. [CrossRef] [PubMed]
128. Kim, B.J.; Kim, H.S.; Jang, H.J.; Kim, J.H. *Helicobacter pylori* Eradication in Idiopathic Thrombocytopenic Purpura: A Meta-Analysis of Randomized Trials. *Gastroenterol. Res. Pract.* **2018**, *2018*, 6090878. [CrossRef] [PubMed]
129. Sapmaz, F.; Basyigit, S.; Kısa, Ü.; Kavak, E.E.; Guliter, S.; Kalkan, I.H. The impact of *Helicobacter pylori* eradication on serum hepcidin-25 level and iron parameters in patients with iron deficiency anemia. *Wien. Klin. Wochenschr.* **2016**, *128*, 335–340. [CrossRef] [PubMed]
130. Kishikawa, H.; Ojiro, K.; Nakamura, K.; Katayama, T.; Arahata, K.; Takarabe, S.; Miura, S.; Kanai, T.; Nishida, J. Previous *Helicobacter pylori* infection-induced atrophic gastritis: A distinct disease entity in an understudied population without a history of eradication. *Helicobacter* **2020**, *25*, e12669. [CrossRef]

131. Shichijo, S.; Hirata, Y. Characteristics and predictors of gastric cancer after *Helicobacter pylori* eradication. *World J. Gastroenterol.* **2018**, *24*, 2163–2172. [CrossRef]
132. Sakitani, K.; Nishizawa, T.; Arita, M.; Yoshida, S.; Kataoka, Y.; Ohki, D.; Yamashita, H.; Isomura, Y.; Toyoshima, A.; Watanabe, H.; et al. Early detection of gastric cancer after *Helicobacter pylori* eradication due to endoscopic surveillance. *Helicobacter* **2018**, *23*, e12503. [CrossRef]
133. Take, S.; Mizuno, M.; Ishiki, K.; Kusumoto, C.; Imada, T.; Hamada, F.; Yoshida, T.; Yokota, K.; Mitsuhashi, T.; Okada, H. Risk of gastric cancer in the second decade of follow-up after *Helicobacter pylori* eradication. *J. Gastroenterol.* **2020**, *55*, 281–288. [CrossRef]
134. Mizuno, S.; Miki, I.; Ishida, T.; Yoshida, M.; Onoyama, M.; Azuma, T.; Habu, Y.; Inokuchi, H.; Ozasa, K.; Miki, K.; et al. Prescreening of a High-Risk Group for Gastric Cancer by Serologically Determined *Helicobacter pylori* Infection and Atrophic Gastritis. *Am. J. Dig. Dis.* **2010**, *55*, 3132–3137. [CrossRef]
135. Dang, Y.; Dong, Y.; Mu, Y.; Yan, J.; Lu, M.; Zhu, Y.; Zhang, G. Identification of gastric microbiota biomarker for gastric cancer. *Chin. Med. J.* **2021**, *133*, 2765–2767. [CrossRef]
136. Boubrik, F.; Belmouden, A.; El-Kadmiri, N. Potential Non-invasive Biomarkers of *Helicobacter pylori*—Associated Gastric Cancer. *J. Gastrointest. Cancer* **2021**, 1–8. [CrossRef] [PubMed]
137. Link, A.; Kupcinskas, J. MicroRNAs as non-invasive diagnostic biomarkers for gastric cancer: Current insights and future perspectives. *World J. Gastroenterol.* **2018**, *24*, 3313–3329. [CrossRef] [PubMed]
138. Sepulveda, J.L.; Gutierrez-Pajares, J.L.; Luna, A.; Yao, Y.; Tobias, J.W.; Thomas, S.; Woo, Y.; Giorgi, F.; Komissarova, E.V.; Califano, A.; et al. High-definition CpG methylation of novel genes in gastric carcinogenesis identified by next-generation sequencing. *Mod. Pathol. Off. J. U. S. Can. Acad. Pathol. Inc.* **2016**, *29*, 182–193. [CrossRef] [PubMed]
139. Sánchez-Zauco, N.; Torres, J.; Gómez, A.; Camorlinga-Ponce, M.; Muñoz-Pérez, L.; Herrera-Goepfert, R.; Medrano-Guzmán, R.; Giono-Cerezo, S.; Maldonado-Bernal, C. Circulating blood levels of IL-6, IFN-γ, and IL-10 as potential diagnostic biomarkers in gastric cancer: A controlled study. *BMC Cancer* **2017**, *17*, 384.
140. Xue, Y.; Zhou, L.-Y.; Lu, H.-P.; Liu, J.-Z. Recurrence of *Helicobacter pylori* infection. *Chin. Med. J.* **2019**, *132*, 765–771. [CrossRef]
141. Yee, J.K. *Helicobacter pylori* colonization of the oral cavity: A milestone discovery. *World J. Gastroenterol.* **2016**, *22*, 641–648. [CrossRef]
142. Alkhaldi, N.K.; Alghamdi, W.K.; Alharbi, M.H.; Almutairi, A.S.; Alghamdi, F.T. The Association Between Oral *Helicobacter pylori* and Gastric Complications: A Comprehensive Review. *Cureus* **2022**, *14*, e24703. [CrossRef]
143. Calvet, X.; Ducons, J.; Guardiola, J.; Tito, L.; Andreu, V.; Bory, F.; Guirao, R.; The Group for Eradication Studies from Catalonia and Aragón (Gresca). One-week triple vs. quadruple therapy for *Helicobacter pylori* infection—A randomized trial. *Aliment. Pharmacol. Ther.* **2002**, *16*, 1261–1267. [CrossRef]
144. Katelaris, P.H.; Forbes, G.M.; Talley, N.J.; Crotty, B. A randomized comparison of quadruple and triple therapies for *Helicobacter pylori* eradication: The QUADRATE study. *Gastroenterology* **2002**, *123*, 1763–1769. [CrossRef]
145. Xie, Y.; Pan, X.; Li, Y.; Wang, H.; Du, Y.; Xu, J.; Wang, J.; Zeng, Z.; Chen, Y.; Zhang, G.; et al. New single capsule of bismuth, metronidazole and tetracycline given with omeprazole versus quadruple therapy consisting of bismuth, omeprazole, amoxicillin and clarithromycin for eradication of *Helicobacter pylori* in duodenal ulcer patients: A Chinese prospective, randomized, multicentre trial. *J. Antimicrob. Chemother.* **2018**, *73*, 1681–1687. [CrossRef]
146. Luo, M.; Hao, Y.; Tang, M.; Shi, M.; He, F.; Xie, Y.; Chen, W. Application of a social media platform as a patient reminder in the treatment of *Helicobacter pylori*. *Helicobacter* **2020**, *25*, e12682. [CrossRef] [PubMed]
147. Nyssen, O.P.; Vaira, D.; Tepes, B.; Kupcinskas, L.; Bordin, D.; Pérez-Aisa, Á.; Gasbarrini, A.; Castro-Fernández, M.; Bujanda, L.; Garre, A.; et al. Room for Improvement in the Treatment of *Helicobacter pylori* Infection: Lessons from the European Registry on H. pylori Management (Hp-EuReg). *J. Clin. Gastroenterol.* **2022**, *56*, e98–e108. [CrossRef] [PubMed]
148. Murakami, T.T.; Scranton, R.A.; Brown, H.E.; Harris, R.B.; Chen, Z.; Musuku, S.; Oren, E. Management of Helicobacter Pylori in the United States: Results from a national survey of gastroenterology physicians. *Prev. Med.* **2017**, *100*, 216–222. [CrossRef] [PubMed]
149. Saxena, K.; Chauhan, N.; Jain, U. Advances in diagnosis of *Helicobacter pylori* through biosensors: Point of care devices. *Anal. Biochem.* **2021**, *630*, 114325. [CrossRef]
150. Prasad, S. Nanobiosensors: The future for diagnosis of disease? *Configurations* **2014**, *3*, 1–10. [CrossRef]
151. Pramanik, P.K.D.; Solanki, A.; Debnath, A.; Nayyar, A.; El-Sappagh, S.; Kwak, K.S. Advancing modern healthcare with nanotechnology, nanobiosensors, and internet of nano things: Taxonomies, applications, architecture, and challenges. *IEEE Access* **2020**, *8*, 65230–65266. [CrossRef]
152. Yadav, A.K.; Verma, V.; Chaudhary, N.; Kumar, A.; Solanki, P.R. Aptamer based switches: A futuristic approach for *Helicobacter pylori* detection. *Mater. Lett.* **2022**, *308*, 131239. [CrossRef]
153. Safarov, T.; Kıran, B.; Bagirova, M.; Allahverdiyev, A.M.; Abamor, E.S. An overview of nanotechnology-based treatment approaches against *Helicobacter pylori*. *Expert Rev. Anti-Infect. Ther.* **2019**, *17*, 829–840. [CrossRef]
154. Rokkas, T.; Gisbert, J.P.; Malfertheiner, P.; Niv, Y.; Gasbarrini, A.; Leja, M.; Megraud, F.; O'morain, C.; Graham, D.Y. Comparative Effectiveness of Multiple Different First-Line Treatment Regimens for *Helicobacter pylori* Infection: A Network Meta-analysis. *Gastroenterology* **2021**, *161*, 495–507.e494. [CrossRef]

155. Fu, J.; Sun, C.-F.; He, H.-Y.; Ojha, S.C.; Shi, H.; Deng, C.-L.; Sheng, Y.-J. The effect of *CYP2C19* gene polymorphism on the eradication rate of *Helicobacter pylori* by proton pump inhibitors-containing regimens in Asian populations: A meta-analysis. *Pharmacogenomics* **2021**, *22*, 859–879. [CrossRef]
156. Zihlif, M.; Bashaireh, B.; Rashid, M.; Almadani, Z.; Jarrar, Y. Effect of major CYP2C19 genetic polymorphisms on *Helicobacter pylori* eradication based on different treatment regimens. *Biomed. Rep.* **2022**, *16*, 1485. [CrossRef]
157. Clyne, M.; Rowland, M. The Role of Host Genetic Polymorphisms in *Helicobacter pylori* Mediated Disease Outcome. *Adv. Exp. Med. Biol.* **2019**, *1149*, 151–172. [CrossRef] [PubMed]
158. Karbalaei, M.; Khorshidi, M.; Sisakht-Pour, B.; Ghazvini, K.; Farsiani, H.; Youssefi, M.; Keikha, M. What are the effects of IL-1β (rs1143634), IL-17A promoter (rs2275913) and TLR4 (rs4986790) gene polymorphism on the outcomes of infection with H. pylori within as Iranian population; A systematic review and meta-analysis. *Gene Rep.* **2020**, *20*, 100735. [CrossRef]
159. Eed, E.M.; Hawash, Y.A.; Khalifa, A.S.; Alsharif, K.F.; Alghamdi, S.A.; Almalki, A.A.; Almehmadi, M.M.; Ismail, K.A.; Taha, A.A.; Saber, T. Association of Toll-Like Receptors 2, 4, 9 and 10 Genes Polymorphisms and *Helicobacter pylori*-Related Gastric Diseases in Saudi Patients. *Indian J. Med. Microbiol.* **2020**, *38*, 94–100. [CrossRef]
160. Shinozaki, S.; Kobayashi, Y.; Osawa, H.; Sakamoto, H.; Hayashi, Y.; Lefor, A.K.; Yamamoto, H. Effectiveness and Safety of Vonoprazan versus Proton Pump Inhibitors for Second-Line *Helicobacter pylori* Eradication Therapy: Systematic Review and Meta-Analysis. *Digestion* **2021**, *102*, 319–325. [CrossRef]
161. Lyu, Q.J.; Pu, Q.H.; Zhong, X.F.; Zhang, J. Efficacy and safety of vonoprazan-based versus proton pump inhibitor-based triple therapy for *Helicobacter pylori* eradication: A meta-analysis of randomized clinical trials. *Biomed. Res. Int.* **2019**, *2019*, 9781212.
162. Kiyotoki, S.; Nishikawa, J.; Sakaida, I. Efficacy of Vonoprazan for *Helicobacter pylori* Eradication. *Intern. Med.* **2020**, *59*, 153–161. [CrossRef]
163. Brogden, K.A. Antimicrobial peptides: Pore formers or metabolic inhibitors in bacteria? *Nat. Rev. Microbiol.* **2005**, *3*, 238–250.
164. Castano, A.P.; Demidova, T.N.; Hamblin, M.R. Mechanisms in photodynamic therapy: Part two-cellular signaling, cell metabolism and modes of cell death. *Photodiagn. Photodyn. Ther.* **2005**, *2*, 1–23.
165. Viertel, T.M.; Ritter, K.; Horz, H.P. Viruses versus bacteria-novel approaches to phage therapy as a tool against multi-drug-resistant pathogens. *J. Antimicrob. Chemother.* **2014**, *69*, 2326–2336.
166. Sousa, C.; Ferreira, R.; Azevedo, N.F.; Oleastro, M.; Azeredo, J.; Figueiredo, C.; Melo, L.D.R. *Helicobacter pylori* infection: From standard to alternative treatment strategies. *Crit. Rev. Microbiol.* **2022**, *48*, 376–396. [CrossRef]
167. Sutton, P.; Boag, J.M. Status of vaccine research and development for *Helicobacter pylori*. *Vaccine* **2018**, *37*, 7295–7299. [CrossRef] [PubMed]

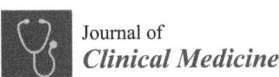

Article

Comparative Study of *Helicobacter pylori*-Infected Gastritis in Okinawa and Tokyo Based on the Kyoto Classification of Gastritis

Shotaro Oki [1], Tsutomu Takeda [1,*], Mariko Hojo [1], Ryota Uchida [1], Nobuyuki Suzuki [1], Daiki Abe [1], Atsushi Ikeda [1], Yoichi Akazawa [1], Hiroya Ueyama [1], Shuko Nojiri [2], Shinichi Hoshino [3], Hayashi Shokita [4] and Akihito Nagahara [1]

1. Department of Gastroenterology, Juntendo University School of Medicine, 2-1-1 Hongo, Bunkyo-ku, Tokyo 113-8421, Japan
2. Medical Technology Innovation Center, Juntendo University School of Medicine, 2-1-1 Hongo, Bunkyo-ku, Tokyo 113-8421, Japan
3. Department of Gastroenterology, Okinawa Prefectural Hokubu Hospital, 2-12-3 Oonaka, Nagoshi 905-8512, Japan
4. Department of Gastroenterology, Northern Okinawa Medical Center, 1712-3 Umusa, Nagoshi 905-8611, Japan
* Correspondence: t-takeda@juntendo.ac.jp; Tel.: +81-(0)3-5803-1060

Abstract: The incidence of gastric cancer in Okinawa Prefecture is the lowest in Japan, which is attributed to differences in strains of *Helicobacter pylori* in Okinawa and other prefectures in Japan. Our aim was to compare the endoscopic findings of *H. pylori*-infected gastric mucosa in Okinawa and Tokyo. Patients who underwent upper gastrointestinal endoscopy (UGI) at Northern Okinawa Medical Center (Okinawa group) and Juntendo University Hospital (Tokyo group) from April 2019 to March 2020 were included. Patients diagnosed with *H. pylori*-infected gastric mucosa were retrospectively compared between the Okinawa and Tokyo groups according to the Kyoto Classification of Gastritis. The numbers of subjects (Okinawa/Tokyo) were 435/352, male/female ratio was 247:188/181:171, and age was 53.3 ± 14.7/64.6 ± 14.3 (mean ± standard deviation) years. Regarding the Kyoto Classification of Gastritis, the prevalence (Okinawa/Tokyo) of the closed type of atrophic gastritis was 73%/37% ($p < 0.001$), diffuse redness 80%/84% ($p = 0.145$), mucosal swelling 46%/46% ($p = 0.991$), enlarged fold 26%/32% ($p = 0.048$), spotty redness 77%/68% ($p = 0.002$), sticky mucus 17%/36% ($p < 0.001$), and intestinal metaplasia 32%/42% ($p < 0.001$). Age analysis also revealed that closed-type atrophy and spotty redness were more frequent in the Okinawa group than in the Tokyo group. There may be regional differences in endoscopic findings of *H. pylori*-infected gastric mucosa between Okinawa and Tokyo.

Keywords: *Helicobacter pylori*; Kyoto Classification of Gastritis; *cagA*; Okinawa; endoscopic findings

1. Introduction

Helicobacter pylori (*H. pylori*) infection is known to be an important pathogenic factor for gastric cancer [1–4]. The incidence of gastric cancer is generally higher in East Asia, while it is lower in North America, Northern Europe, and Africa, suggesting regional differences throughout the world [5]. The prevalence of *H. pylori* in Okinawa is not significantly different from that in other regions of Japan [1,6,7]. However, the age-standardized incidence rate of gastric cancer in Japan is 43.1%, while the rate in Okinawa is 20.4%, the lowest age-standardized incidence rate among prefectures in Japan [8]. Even within Japan, regional differences are recognized. This may be due to differences in the cagA gene of *H. pylori* [9–12]. Regional differences and polymorphisms in *H. pylori* genotypes also differ in their influence as virulence factors, which has been studied in recent years as one of the factors contributing to regional differences in gastric cancer incidence.

In addition, in routine endoscopic practice, the risk of gastric cancer is approximately 20 times higher in *H. pylori*-infected patients than in *H. pylori*-uninfected patients [13], and it is important to determine the *H. pylori* infection status from the background mucosa. Therefore, in 2014, the Kyoto Classification of Gastritis was published to systematically summarize the findings of *H. pylori*-associated gastritis for the first time [14]. The English version was published in 2017, and the second edition with new findings was published in 2018 [15,16]. Many Japanese studies have evaluated the Kyoto Classification of Gastritis, but recently some reports have confirmed its usefulness in European countries [17]. The Kyoto Classification of Gastritis allows efficient evaluation of gastric cancer risk based on the state of the background mucosa with 19 endoscopic findings. In particular, diffuse redness, mucosal swelling, enlarged fold, sticky mucus, and spotty redness are considered findings suggestive of *H. pylori* infection [14–16,18–22].

Although differences in gastric cancer incidence rates and strains of *H. pylori* are observed between Okinawa and other regions of Japan, there have been no reports comparing gastritis findings in Okinawa with those in other regions of Japan. The purpose of this study was to clarify the differences and characteristics of endoscopic findings of *H. pylori*-infected gastric mucosa between Okinawa and Tokyo on the mainland of Japan.

2. Materials and Methods

2.1. Patients

Patients who underwent upper gastrointestinal endoscopy (UGI) at Northern Okinawa Medical Center (Okinawa Group) and Juntendo University Hospital (Tokyo Group) from April 2019 to March 2020 were included in this retrospective study. Inclusion criteria were patients who were 18 years old or older, and who were infected with *H. pylori* at the time of UGI. Patients were considered to be infected with *H. pylori* when at least one of the urea breath tests with cutoff value of 2.5 per 1000, serum *H. pylori* antibody test with cutoff value of 10 U/mL (E-plate; Eiken Chemical, Tokyo, Japan), and stool *H. pylori* antigen test was positive from April 2017 to March 2020.

Exclusion criteria were patients who had undergone gastrectomy, those whose mucosa was poorly observed due to food residues, those who did not have pure *H. pylori*-infected gastric mucosa due to coexistence of liver cirrhosis and/or autoimmune gastritis, and those who had undergone *H. pylori* eradication. This retrospective study was conducted according to the guidelines of the Helsinki Declaration and was approved by the Ethics Committee of Northern Okinawa Medical Center (2019-5) and the Ethics Committee of Juntendo University Hospital (E21-0335-H01). Patient consent was waived because the design of this study was a retrospective clinical documentation study.

2.2. Methods

This retrospective cross-sectional study investigated the endoscopic findings of patients with *H. pylori*-infected gastric mucosa according to the Kyoto Classification of Gastritis in Okinawa and Tokyo. Six expert endoscopists in Tokyo and two expert endoscopists in Okinawa who each have performed more than 1500 UGIs, independently and retrospectively reviewed all photographs of endoscopic examinations performed at the Okinawa and Tokyo hospitals during the study period, and evaluated the endoscopic findings in the photographs according to the Kyoto Classification of Gastritis [14–16]. Regarding atrophy, the Kimura-Takemoto classification [23] was used to evaluate the degree of spread of gastric mucosal atrophy. C-1, C-2, and C-3 were classified as the closed type of atrophy, and O-1, O-2, and O-3 as the open type.

2.3. Statistical Analysis

All data on patients' background characteristics and endoscopic findings according to the Kyoto Classification of Gastritis in each group were expressed as mean and standard deviation (SD) for continuous variables and as the number (percentage) for categorical variables. The prevalence of each characteristic was examined using the *t*-test, chi-square test or Fisher's exact test, with $p < 0.05$ being considered statistically significant. In addition, the number of gastric cancer cases in patients over 65 years of age has been increasing in Japan [8]. Therefore, in order to analyze the risk of gastric cancer and age changes, we conducted subgroup analyses in patients under 65 years of age and in patients 65 years of age or older. We compared the distribution of endoscopic features in the Kyoto Classification of Gastritis between the patients in Tokyo and patients in Okinawa using the logistic regression model adjusting for age and sex. All analyses were conducted using SAS software (SAS Institute, Cary, NC, USA). Odds ratio (OR) value was presented with the 95% confidence interval (CI). All tests were two-sided and statistical significance was set at $p < 0.05$.

3. Results
3.1. Patients Studied

Patient flow is shown in Figure 1. During the study period, 7261 patients at the hospital in Tokyo and 3159 patients at the hospital in Okinawa underwent UGI and had been tested for *H. pylori*. Of these, 390 patients were 18 years of age or older and infected with *H. pylori* at the hospital in Tokyo, and 437 patients were 18 years of age or older and infected with *H. pylori* at the hospital in Okinawa. Based on the exclusion criteria, 38 cases at the hospital in Tokyo (6 patients after gastrectomy, 8 patients with liver cirrhosis, 11 foreigners, 1 patient with autoimmune gastritis, 3 patients with insufficient observation of the gastric mucosa, and 9 patients after *H. pylori* eradication) and 2 cases at the hospital in Okinawa (2 patients with liver cirrhosis) were excluded. Therefore, the Tokyo group included 352 cases and the Okinawa group included 435 cases. The mean ($\pm$ standard deviation) age of the 352 patients in the Tokyo group and the 435 patients in the Okinawa group was 64.6 $\pm$ 14.3 and 53.3 $\pm$ 14.7, respectively ($p < 0.001$). There was no difference in sex distribution (male/female) between the Tokyo group (181/171) and the Okinawa group (247/188) ($p = 0.133$) (Table 1). The numbers of patients under 65 years old (Tokyo/Okinawa group) were 156/327 patients and the numbers of patients 65 years old or older (Tokyo/Okinawa group) were 196/108 patients (Table 2).

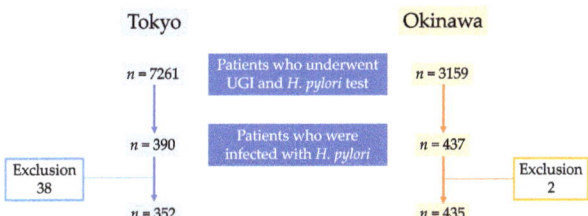

Figure 1. Flow diagram of the patients.

Table 1. Baseline characteristics.

		Tokyo Group	Okinawa Group	*p*-Value
Number of patients		352	435	
Age (yr; mean $\pm$ SD)		64.6 $\pm$ 14.3	53.3 $\pm$ 14.7	<0.001
Sex	male	181	247	0.133
	female	171	188	

SD, standard deviation.

Table 2. Baseline characteristics of the patients under 65 years old and patients 65 years old or older.

		Tokyo Group	Okinawa Group	*p*-Value
Group of patients under 65 years old	Number of patients	156	327	
	Age (yr; mean ± SD)	52.0 ± 11.3	46.9 ± 10.5	<0.001
	Male/female	72/84	181/146	0.058
Group of patients 65 years old or older	Number of patients	196	108	
	Age (yr; mean ± SD)	74.6 ± 6.1	72.7 ± 5.6	0.006
	Male/female	109/87	66/42	0.353

3.2. Endoscopic Findings of H. pylori Gastritis Based on the Kyoto Classification of Gastritis

Typical endoscopic findings in the Tokyo and Okinawa groups are shown in Figures 2–4.

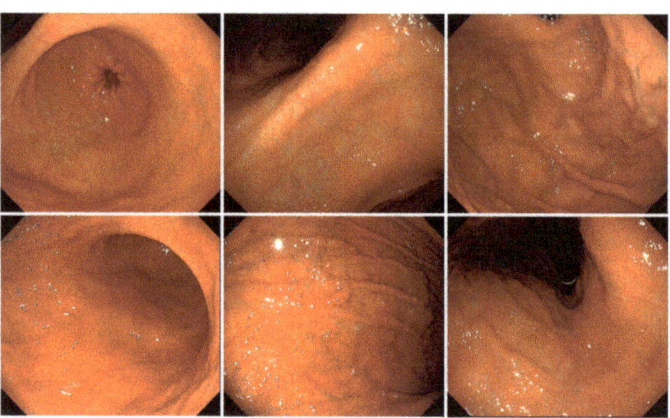

Figure 2. Typical endoscopic images of *H. pylori*-infected gastric mucosa in the Tokyo group. The patient is a 75-year-old woman. O-1 atrophy is observed, with diffuse redness, spotty redness, and mucosal swelling. Overall, it has a reddish tint.

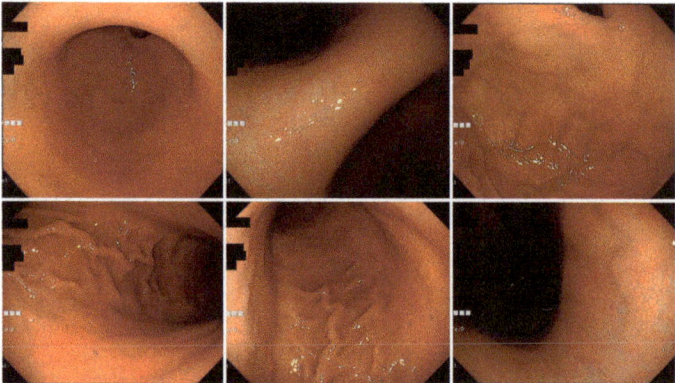

Figure 3. Typical endoscopic images of *H. pylori*-infected gastric mucosa in the Okinawa group. This patient is an 83-year-old woman. O-2 atrophy is observed, and there are only a few findings of *H. pylori* infection. Mild spotty redness on the posterior wall of the gastric body is observed.

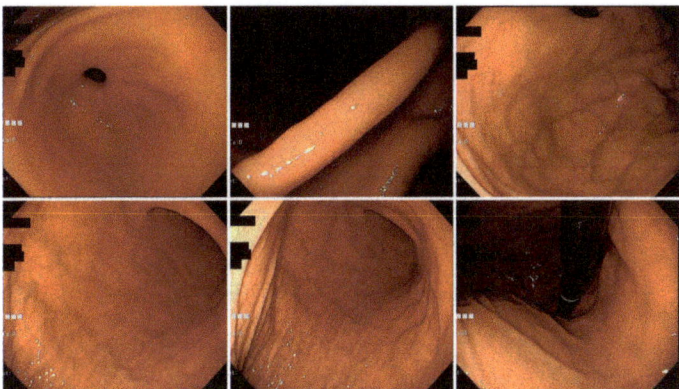

Figure 4. Typical endoscopic images of *H. pylori*-infected gastric mucosa in the Okinawa group. This patient is a 46-year-old woman. C-1 atrophy is observed, and there are few findings of *H. pylori* infection.

Closed-type atrophy was more common in the Okinawa group than in the Tokyo group [318/435 (73.1%) vs. 131/352 (37.2%)] ($p < 0.001$). Diffuse redness, mucosal swelling, enlarged fold, spotty redness, and sticky mucus are the findings of *H. pylori*-infected gastric mucosa. The following characteristics were significantly more common in the Tokyo group than in the Okinawa group: enlarged fold [114/352 (32.4%) vs. 113/435 (26.0%), $p = 0.048$], sticky mucus [125/352 (35.5%) vs. 73/435 (16.8%), $p < 0.001$], foveolar-hyperplastic polyp [50/352 (14.2%) vs. 39/435 (8.97%), $p = 0.021$], intestinal metaplasia [147/352 (41.8%) vs. 142/435 (32.6%), $p = 0.007$], and xanthoma [33/352 (9.38%) vs. 20/435 (4.60%), $p < 0.001$]. The following characteristics were significantly less common in the Tokyo group than in the Okinawa group: spotty redness [239/352 (67.9%) vs. 338/435 (77.7%), $p = 0.002$], patchy redness [29/352 (8.24%) vs. 59/435 (13.6%), $p = 0.018$], and hematin [6/352 (1.70%) vs. 28/435 (6.44%), $p = 0.001$] (Table 3).

Table 3. Comparison of endoscopic findings according to the Kyoto Classification of Gastritis between the Tokyo and Okinawa groups.

Kyoto Classification of Gastritis		Tokyo Group (%) $n = 352$	Okinawa Group (%) $n = 435$	*p*-Value
Atrophy [1]	closed	131 (37.2) [2]	318 (73.1)	<0.001
	open	221 (62.8)	117 (26.9)	
diffuse redness		298 (84.7)	351 (80.7)	0.145
mucous swelling		165 (46.9)	212 (48.7)	0.696
enlarged fold		114 (32.4)	113 (26.0)	0.048
spotty redness		239 (67.9)	338 (77.7)	0.002
sticky mucus		125 (35.5)	73 (16.8)	<0.001
foveolar-hyperplastic polyp		50 (14.2)	39 (8.97)	0.021
patchy redness		29 (8.24)	59 (13.6)	0.018
intestinal metaplasia		147 (41.8)	142 (32.6)	0.007
nodularity		23 (6.53)	37 (8.51)	0.300
xanthoma		33 (9.38)	20 (4.60)	0.007
hematin		6 (1.70)	28 (6.44)	0.001

[1] Kimura-Takemoto classification. [2] Data are expressed as the number of patients (%).

3.3. Age Analysis

Among patients with *H. pylori*-infected gastric mucosa under 65 years of age, closed-type atrophy was more common in the Okinawa group than in the Tokyo group [270/327 (82.6%) vs. 82/156 (52.6%), $p < 0.001$]. Similar to the results of the main analysis, enlarged fold [51/156 (32.7%) vs. 76/327(23.2%), Tokyo group vs. Okinawa group, $p = 0.027$], sticky mucus [58/156 (37.2%) vs. 45/327 (13.7%), $p < 0.001$], foveolar-hyperplastic polyp [21/156 (13.5%) vs. 23/327 (7.03%), $p = 0.021$], and xanthoma [9/156 (5.77%) vs. 7/327 (2.14%), $p = 0.037$] were more common in the Tokyo group. Spotty redness [100/156 (64.1%) vs. 248/327 (75.8%), Tokyo group vs. Okinawa group, $p = 0.007$], patchy redness [7/156 (4.48%) vs. 39/327 (11.9%), $p = 0.009$], and hematin [2/156 (1.28%) vs. 23/327 (7.03%), $p = 0.008$] were less common in the Tokyo group than in the Okinawa group (Table 4).

Table 4. Subgroup analyses in each age group below and above 65 years of age between the Tokyo and Okinawa patients. (**a**) The under-65-years age group; (**b**) the 65-years-and-older age group.

(a) The under-65-years age group				
Kyoto Classification of Gastritis		Tokyo Group (%) $n = 156$	Okinawa Group (%) $n = 327$	*p*-Value
Atrophy	closed	82 (52.6)	270 (82.6)	<0.001
	open	74 (47.4)	57 (17.4)	
diffuse redness		132 (84.6)	260 (79.6)	0.180
mucosal swelling		71 (45.5)	149 (45.6)	0.991
enlarged fold		51 (32.7)	76 (23.2)	0.027
spotty redness		100 (64.1)	248 (75.8)	0.007
sticky mucus		58 (37.2)	45 (13.7)	<0.001
foveolar-hyperplastic polyp		21 (13.5)	23 (7.03)	0.021
patchy redness		7 (4.48)	39 (11.9)	0.009
intestinal metaplasia		48 (30.8)	89 (27.2)	0.340
nodularity		19 (12.2)	36 (11.0)	0.705
xanthoma		9 (5.77)	7 (2.14)	0.037
hematin		2 (1.28)	23 (7.03)	0.008
(b) The 65-years-and-older age group				
Kyoto Classification of Gastritis		Tokyo Group (%) $n = 196$	Okinawa Group (%) $n = 108$	*p*-Value
Atrophy	closed	49 (25.0)	48 (44.4)	<0.001
	open	147 (75.0)	60 (55.6)	
diffuse redness		166 (84.7)	91 (84.3)	0.920
mucosal swelling		94 (48.0)	63 (58.3)	0.083
enlarged fold		63 (32.1)	37 (34.3)	0.707
spotty redness		139 (70.9)	90 (83.3)	0.016
sticky mucus		67 (34.2)	28 (26.0)	0.137
foveolar-hyperplastic polyp		29 (14.8)	16 (14.8)	0.966
patchy redness		22 (11.2)	20 (18.5)	0.078
intestinal metaplasia		99 (50.5)	53 (49.1)	0.811
nodularity		4 (2.04)	1 (0.93)	0.659
xanthoma		24 (12.2)	13 (12.0)	0.958
hematin		4 (2.04)	5 (4.63)	0.288

Even among patients aged 65 years or older, closed-type atrophy was more frequent in the Okinawa group than in the Tokyo group [48/108 (44.4%) vs. 49/196 (25.0%), $p < 0.001$]. In terms of *H. pylori*-infected gastric mucosa findings, spotty redness was less common in the Tokyo group than in the Okinawa group [139/196 (70.9%) vs. 90/108 (83.3%), $p = 0.016$]. The frequencies of other findings of *H. pylori*-infected gastric mucosa were not significantly different between the Tokyo and Okinawa groups (Table 4).

3.4. Age-Adjusted Analysis

The data were age-adjusted as the Okinawa group was significantly younger than the Tokyo group. In the Okinawa group, closed-type atrophy (closed:1, open:0) (OR [95%CI] = 2.843 [2.032–3.985], $p < 0.001$), spotty redness (OR [95%CI] = 1.947 [1.379–2.761], $p < 0.001$), patchy redness (OR [95%CI] = 2.336 [1.421–3.917], $p = 0.001$), and hematin (OR [95%CI] = 3.526 [1.471–9.849], $p = 0.008$) were more common and sticky mucus was less common (OR [95%CI] = 0.439 [0.306–0.626], $p < 0.001$) (Table 5).

Table 5. Odds ratios of each endoscopic feature in the Kyoto Classification of Gastritis between the Tokyo and Okinawa groups in logistic regression analysis.

Kyoto Classification of Gastritis	OR *	95%CI	p-Value
atrophy (closed 1; open 0)	2.843	2.032–3.985	<0.001
diffuse redness	0.787	0.524–1.174	0.244
mucosal swelling	1.221	0.900–1.658	0.200
enlarged fold	0.816	0.583–1.141	0.234
spotty redness	1.947	1.379–2.761	<0.001
sticky mucus	0.439	0.306–0.626	<0.001
foveolar hyperplastic polyp	0.816	0.504–1.317	0.406
patchy redness	2.336	1.421–3.917	0.001
intestinal metaplasia	0.975	0.708–1.346	0.876
nodularity	0.601	0.318–1.142	0.117
xanthoma	0.731	0.390–1.344	0.319
hematin	3.526	1.471–9.849	0.008

* OR: Odds Ratio (reference: Tokyo prefecture) adjusting for age and sex.

4. Discussion

Comparison of the endoscopic findings of the gastric mucosa of *H. pylori*-infected patients according to the Kyoto Classification of Gastritis suggested that there may be regional differences in endoscopic findings of *H. pylori*-infected mucosa between the Okinawa and Tokyo groups. In addition, spotty redness in the Kyoto Classification of Gastritis was useful for the endoscopic diagnosis of *H. pylori* infection in the Okinawa group. To our knowledge, this is the first study to compare regional differences in endoscopic findings of *H. pylori*-infected gastric mucosa according to the Kyoto Classification of Gastritis.

In the Kyoto Classification of Gastritis, atrophy, intestinal metaplasia, diffuse redness, and nodularity are risk factors for gastric cancer [22,24–28]. Enlarged fold has also been weakly associated with undifferentiated gastric carcinoma [26]. Regarding the inhibitory effect of *H. pylori* eradication on gastric carcinogenesis, the greater the extent of mucosal atrophy, the lower the inhibitory effect of eradication on carcinogenesis [29]. In the present study, the Okinawa group had a higher frequency of closed-type atrophy than the Tokyo group, and lower frequencies of enlarged fold and intestinal metaplasia, suggesting that the risk of gastric cancer according to the Kyoto Classification of Gastritis was low in Okinawa.

The prevalence of diffuse redness was not significantly different between the two groups, but was less common in the Okinawa group. In addition, the degree of atrophy was weaker in the Okinawa group, and the presence of *H. pylori* infection findings such as enlarged fold and sticky mucus was less conspicuous, making the endoscopic diagnosis of *H. pylori*-infected gastric mucosa more difficult than in the Tokyo group. The Okinawa group showed predominantly more spotty redness as a finding of *H. pylori*-infected gastric mucosa. It is considered that diffuse redness was less noticeable in the Okinawa group than in the Tokyo group, and therefore, it was inferred that the spotty redness was relatively easy to see endoscopically in the Okinawa group. Spotty redness was considered to be helpful in the diagnosis of *H. pylori*-infected gastric mucosa among the endoscopic findings in Okinawa.

Diffuse redness is a basic finding of *H. pylori* infection as well as mucosal swelling, and correlates predominantly with the degree of neutrophilic and mononuclear cell infiltration caused by *H. pylori* infection [19]. The diffuse redness in the Okinawa group was weak and difficult to diagnose endoscopically, which means that the *H. pylori* strains in Okinawa are less inflammatory. In addition, more hematin adherence was observed in the Okinawa group than in the Tokyo group. Hematin is considered to appear when the intragastric pH is highly acidic [30], and it has been reported that *H. pylori*-uninfected individuals have a higher acid secretory capacity than *H. pylori*-infected individuals [31–33]. In the age-adjusted analysis, the Okinawa group had significantly fewer cases of sticky mucus, foveolar hyperplastic polyp, and enlarged fold in those under 65 years of age, but in those 65 years of age and older, these frequencies increased to the same levels as those in the Tokyo group, and the differences were no longer significant. This suggests that the inflammation caused by *H. pylori* was stronger in the Tokyo group and weaker in the Okinawa group, and that the mucosal findings were therefore less noticeable in the younger age group in Okinawa. On the other hand, the elderly group showed changes due to long-term inflammation, and the difference in mucosal findings between the Tokyo group and the Okinawa group became smaller, although not regarding the extent of atrophy.

Okinawa is an island far from the mainland of Japan, and one of the reasons for the low incidence of gastric cancer in Okinawa is thought to be the different environmental factors and dietary habits compared to those in the rest of Japan [34]. Furthermore, genetic analysis of *H. pylori* has pointed to differences in *H. pylori* strains in Okinawa compared to those in other regions of Japan as a cause for the different incidence of gastric cancer [9–12]. The *cagA* gene is known to be a representative pathogenic factor for gastric cancer in *H. pylori*, but the CagA protein itself is not essential for the survival of the bacteria, and there are *cagA*-positive and *cagA*-negative strains. *cagA*-positive strains are more pathogenic than *cagA*-negative strains and are reported to increase the risk of peptic ulcers and gastric cancer [35,36]. *cagA*-negative strains are more common in South Africa, with a higher proportion of *cagA*-positive strains in the Asian region. Among *cagA* strains, East Asian-type *cagA* strains are considered to be more virulent compared to Western-type *cagA* strains [37]. In Japan, almost 100% of the *H. pylori* strains are East Asian-type *cagA* strains, except in Okinawa. In Okinawa, about 15% of *H. pylori* strains are *cagA*-negative and about 15% of strains are Western-type *cagA* strains, and this difference in *H. pylori* strains is thought to be the reason that the gastric cancer incidence rate is lowest in Okinawa Prefecture among prefectures in Japan [9–12].

About 50% of the world's population is a carrier of *H. pylori*. Because *H. pylori* is transmitted mainly by vertical transmission from parent to child and has a high mutation rate compared to human genes, recent studies have shown that it is possible to estimate not only the diversity of its pathogenicity but also the history of human migration by studying its genotypes in various regions of the world [12,38–40]. Genetic analysis of *H. pylori* by the multi locus sequence typing (MLST) method has demonstrated the existence of two new types unique to Okinawa, not found in other regions, one of which diverged from other strains tens of thousands of years ago [12]. It has been speculated that there were multiple waves of human migration starting in Africa [12,38–42], and the Okinawa-specific *H. pylori* strains are thought to be the result of early migratory people. At present, the route of arrival of the new type of *H. pylori* strains recognized in Okinawa is unknown, but Okinawa has its own strains of *H. pylori*, and it is possible that regional differences in gastritis findings were observed due to differences in these *H. pylori* strains.

There are several limitations in this study. Because this was a retrospective cross-sectional study and *H. pylori* gene analysis was not performed, the *H. pylori* strains could not be identified. In addition, each endoscopist evaluated the endoscopic findings independently, which may have resulted in interobserver variability. The methods used to diagnose *H. pylori* infection were different in each group, and the accuracy, sensitivity, and specificity of each *H. pylori* test varied, which may have affected the results of this study. The present study did not consider the effects of drugs that alter the gastric mucosa and duodeno-gastric reflux, and age stratification analysis was not performed. As the number of hospitals surveyed in this study was limited, we have not been able to examine whether the study is representative of the general population in Japan. Among patients who underwent UGI, the Okinawa group underwent endoscopy based on medical checkup, whereas the Tokyo group underwent endoscopy based on disease, suggesting selection bias. Therefore, a prospective study considering other factors that may affect the gastric mucosa and combining *H. pylori* gene analysis and age stratification analysis will be required to confirm our findings.

5. Conclusions

When the endoscopic findings according to the Kyoto Classification of Gastritis were compared between the Okinawa and Tokyo groups, the Okinawa group showed a higher percentage of closed-type atrophy and a difference in inflammation-related findings of *H. pylori*-infected gastric mucosa compared with the Tokyo group. Among the endoscopic features in the Kyoto Classification of Gastritis, spotty redness was considered to be useful for the diagnosis of *H. pylori* infection in the Okinawa group. Our results suggested the possibility of regional differences in endoscopic findings of *H. pylori*-infected gastric mucosa between Okinawa and Tokyo.

Author Contributions: Conceptualization, T.T. and A.N.; Methodology, M.H., A.I., S.H. and H.S.; Software, M.H.; Validation, T.T.; Formal Analysis, T.T., M.H. and S.N.; Investigation, S.O., M.H., R.U., D.A., N.S., A.I., Y.A. and H.U.; Resources, S.O., R.U., D.A., N.S., A.I., M.H., S.H. and H.S.; Data Curation, S.O., T.T. and S.N.; Writing—Original Draft Preparation, S.O.; Writing—Review and Editing, T.T.; Visualization, T.T. and S.O.; Supervision, A.N.; Project Administration, T.T.; Funding Acquisition, T.T. All authors have read and agreed to the published version of the manuscript.

Funding: This research received no external funding.

Institutional Review Board Statement: The study was conducted in accordance with the Declaration of Helsinki, and approved by the Ethics Committee of Juntendo University Hospital (protocol code E21-0335-H01) and the Ethics Committee of Northern Okinawa Medical Center (protocol code 2019-5).

Informed Consent Statement: Patient consent was waived because the design of this study was a retrospective clinical documentation study.

Data Availability Statement: All data supporting this study are available in the article.

Acknowledgments: We thank all members of the Department of Gastroenterology of Juntendo University School of Medicine, Medical Technology Innovation Center of Juntendo University School of Medicine, Department of Gastroenterology of Okinawa Prefectural Hokubu Hospital, and Department of Gastroenterology of Northern Okinawa Medical Center for helping us to conduct this study.

Conflicts of Interest: The authors declare no conflict of interest.

References

1. Warren, J.R.; Marshall, B. Unidentified curved bacilli on gastric epithelium in active chronic gastritis. *Lancet* **1983**, *1*, 1273–1275.
2. NIH Consensus Conference. *Helicobacter pylori* in peptic ulcer disease. NIH Consensus Development Panel on *Helicobacter pylori* in Peptic Ulcer Disease. *JAMA* **1994**, *272*, 65–69. [CrossRef]
3. Marshall, B.J.; Goodwin, C.S.; Warren, J.R.; Murray, R.; Blincow, E.D.; Blackbourn, S.J.; Phillips, M.; Waters, T.E.; Sanderson, C.R. Prospective double-blind trial of duodenal ulcer relapse after eradication of *Campylobacter pylori*. *Lancet* **1988**, *2*, 1437–1442. [CrossRef]
4. Parsonnet, J.; Friedman, G.D.; Vandersteen, D.P.; Chang, Y.; Vogelman, J.H.; Orentreich, N.; Sibley, R.K. *Helicobacter pylori* infection and the risk of gastric carcinoma. *N. Engl. J. Med.* **1991**, *325*, 1127–1131. [CrossRef] [PubMed]
5. Bray, F.; Ferlay, J.; Soerjomataram, I.; Siegel, R.L.; Torre, L.A.; Jemal, A. Global cancer statistics 2018: GLOBOCAN estimates of incidence and mortality worldwide for 36 cancers in 185 countries. *CA Cancer J. Clin.* **2018**, *68*, 394–424. [CrossRef] [PubMed]

6. Ito, S.; Azuma, T.; Murakita, H.; Hirai, M.; Miyaji, H.; Ito, Y.; Ohtaki, Y.; Yamazaki, Y.; Kuriyama, M.; Keida, Y.; et al. Profile of *Helicobacter pylori* cytotoxin derived from two areas of Japan with different prevalence of atrophic gastritis. *Gut* **1996**, *39*, 800–806. [CrossRef] [PubMed]
7. Jones, K.R.; Joo, Y.M.; Jang, S.; Yoo, Y.J.; Lee, H.S.; Chung, I.S.; Olsen, C.H.; Whitmire, J.M.; Merrell, D.S.; Cha, J.H. Polymorphism in the CagA EPIYA motif impacts development of gastric cancer. *J. Clin. Microbiol.* **2009**, *47*, 959–968. [CrossRef]
8. Cancer Statistics. Cancer Information Service, National Cancer Center, Japan (National Cancer Registry, Ministry of Health, Labour and Welfare). 2018. Available online: https://ganjoho.jp/reg_stat/statistics/data/dl/en.html (accessed on 8 April 2022).
9. Azuma, T.; Yamakawa, A.; Yamazaki, S.; Ohtani, M.; Ito, Y.; Muramatsu, A.; Suto, H.; Yamazaki, Y.; Keida, Y.; Higashi, H.; et al. Distinct diversity of the cag pathogenicity island among *Helicobacter pylori* strains in Japan. *J. Clin. Microbiol.* **2004**, *42*, 2508–2517. [CrossRef]
10. Satomi, S.; Yamakawa, A.; Matsunaga, S.; Masaki, R.; Inagaki, T.; Okuda, T.; Suto, H.; Ito, Y.; Yamazaki, Y.; Kuriyama, M.; et al. Relationship between the diversity of the cagA gene of *Helicobacter pylori* and gastric cancer in Okinawa, Japan. *J. Gastroenterol.* **2006**, *41*, 668–673. [CrossRef]
11. Yamazaki, S.; Yamakawa, A.; Okuda, T.; Ohtani, M.; Suto, H.; Ito, Y.; Yamazaki, Y.; Keida, Y.; Higashi, H.; Hatakeyama, M.; et al. Distinct diversity of vacA, cagA, and cagE genes of *Helicobacter pylori* associated with peptic ulcer in Japan. *J. Clin. Microbiol.* **2005**, *43*, 3906–3916. [CrossRef]
12. Matsunari, O.; Shiota, S.; Suzuki, R.; Watada, M.; Kinjo, N.; Murakami, K.; Fujioka, T.; Kinjo, F.; Yamaoka, Y. Association between *Helicobacter pylori* virulence factors and gastroduodenal diseases in Okinawa, Japan. *J. Clin. Microbiol.* **2012**, *50*, 876–883. [CrossRef]
13. Ekström, A.M.; Held, M.; Hansson, L.E.; Engstrand, L.; Nyrén, O. *Helicobacter pylori* in gastric cancer established by CagA immunoblot as a marker of past infection. *Gastroenterology* **2001**, *121*, 784–791. [CrossRef]
14. Kato, M.; Inoue, K.; Murakami, K.; Kamada, T.; Haruma, K. *Kyoto Classification of Gastritis*; Nihon Medical Center: Singapore, 2014. (In Japanese)
15. Kato, M.; Inoue, K.; Murakami, K.; Kamada, T.; Haruma, K. *Kyoto Classification of Gastritis*; Nihon Medical Center: Singapore, 2017. (In English)
16. Kato, M.; Inoue, K.; Murakami, K.; Kamada, T.; Haruma, K. *Kyoto Classification of Gastritis*, 2nd ed.; Nihon Medical Center: Singapore, 2018. (In Japanese)
17. Ebigbo, A.; Marienhagen, J.; Messmann, H. Regular arrangement of collecting venules and the Kimura-Takemoto classification for the endoscopic diagnosis of *Helicobacter pylori* infection: Evaluation in a Western setting. *Dig. Endosc.* **2021**, *33*, 587–591. [CrossRef]
18. Glover, B.; Teare, J.; Ashrafian, H.; Patel, N. The endoscopic predictors of *Helicobacter pylori* status: A meta-analysis of diagnostic performance. *Ther. Adv. Gastrointest. Endosc.* **2020**, *13*, 2631774520950840. [CrossRef]
19. Nomura, S.; Terao, S.; Adachi, K.; Kato, T.; Ida, K.; Watanabe, H.; Shimbo, T. Endoscopic diagnosis of gastric mucosal activity and inflammation. *Dig. Endosc.* **2013**, *25*, 136–146. [CrossRef]
20. Kato, T.; Yagi, N.; Kamada, T.; Shimbo, T.; Watanabe, H.; Ida, K. Diagnosis of *Helicobacter pylori* infection in gastric mucosa by endoscopic features: A multicenter prospective study. *Dig. Endosc.* **2013**, *25*, 508–518. [CrossRef]
21. Kato, M.; Terao, S.; Adachi, K.; Nakajima, S.; Ando, T.; Yoshida, N.; Uedo, N.; Murakami, K.; Ohara, S.; Ito, M.; et al. Changes in endoscopic findings of gastritis after cure of *H. pylori* infection: Multicenter prospective trial. *Dig. Endosc.* **2013**, *25*, 264–273. [CrossRef]
22. Nagahara, A.; Shiotani, A.; Iijima, K.; Kamada, T.; Fujiwara, Y.; Kasugai, K.; Kato, M.; Higuchi, K. The role of advanced endoscopy in the management of inflammatory digestive diseases (upper gastrointestinal tract). *Dig. Endosc.* **2022**, *34*, 63–72. [CrossRef]
23. Kimura, K.; Takemoto, T. An endoscopic recognition of atrophic border and its significance in chronic gastritis. *Endocopy* **1969**, *1*, 87–97. [CrossRef]
24. Ohno, A.; Miyoshi, J.; Kato, A.; Miyamoto, N.; Yatagai, T.; Hada, Y.; Kusuhara, M.; Jimbo, Y.; Ida, Y.; Tokunaga, K.; et al. Endoscopic severe mucosal atrophy indicates the presence of gastric cancer after *Helicobacter pylori* eradication -analysis based on the Kyoto classification. *BMC Gastroenterol.* **2020**, *20*, 232. [CrossRef]
25. Sakitani, K.; Nishizawa, T.; Toyoshima, A.; Yoshida, S.; Matsuno, T.; Yamada, T.; Irokawa, M.; Takahashi, Y.; Nakai, Y.; Toyoshima, O.; et al. Kyoto classification in patients who developed multiple gastric carcinomas after *Helicobacter pylori* eradication. *World J. Gastrointest. Endosc.* **2020**, *12*, 276–284. [CrossRef]
26. Shichijo, S.; Hirata, Y.; Niikura, R.; Hayakawa, Y.; Yamada, A.; Koike, K. Association between gastric cancer and the Kyoto classification of gastritis. *J. Gastroenterol. Hepatol.* **2017**, *32*, 1581–1586. [CrossRef]
27. Sugimoto, M.; Ban, H.; Ichikawa, H.; Sahara, S.; Otsuka, T.; Inatomi, O.; Bamba, S.; Furuta, T.; Andoh, A. Efficacy of the Kyoto Classification of Gastritis in Identifying Patients at High Risk for Gastric Cancer. *Intern. Med.* **2017**, *56*, 579–586. [CrossRef]
28. Majima, A.; Dohi, O.; Takayama, S.; Hirose, R.; Inoue, K.; Yoshida, N.; Kamada, K.; Uchiyama, K.; Ishikawa, T.; Takagi, T.; et al. Linked color imaging identifies important risk factors associated with gastric cancer after successful eradication of *Helicobacter pylori*. *Gastrointest. Endosc.* **2019**, *90*, 763–769. [CrossRef]
29. Take, S.; Mizuno, M.; Ishiki, K.; Yoshida, T.; Ohara, N.; Yokota, K.; Oguma, K.; Okada, H.; Yamamoto, K. The long-term risk of gastric cancer after the successful eradication of *Helicobacter pylori*. *J. Gastroenterol.* **2011**, *46*, 318–324. [CrossRef]

30. Hatta, W.; Iijima, K.; Koike, T.; Kondo, Y.; Ara, N.; Asanuma, K.; Uno, K.; Asano, N.; Imatani, A.; Shimosegawa, T. Endoscopic findings for predicting gastric acid secretion status. *Dig. Endosc.* **2015**, *27*, 582–589.
31. Haruma, K.; Kamada, T.; Kawaguchi, H.; Okamoto, S.; Yoshihara, M.; Sumii, K.; Inoue, M.; Kishimoto, S.; Kajiyama, G.; Miyoshi, A. Effect of age and *Helicobacter pylori* infection on gastric acid secretion. *J. Gastroenterol. Hepatol.* **2000**, *15*, 277–283. [CrossRef]
32. Haruma, K.; Mihara, M.; Okamoto, E.; Kusunoki, H.; Hananoki, M.; Tanaka, S.; Yoshihara, M.; Sumii, K.; Kajiyama, G. Eradication of *Helicobacter pylori* increases gastric acidity in patients with atrophic gastritis of the corpus-evaluation of 24-h pH monitoring. *Aliment Pharm. Ther.* **1999**, *13*, 155–162. [CrossRef]
33. Koike, T.; Ohara, S.; Sekine, H.; Iijima, K.; Kato, K.; Toyota, T.; Shimosegawa, T. Increased gastric acid secretion after *Helicobacter pylori* eradication may be a factor for developing reflux oesophagitis. *Aliment. Pharm. Ther.* **2001**, *15*, 813–820. [CrossRef]
34. Willcox, D.C.; Willcox, B.J.; Todoriki, H.; Suzuki, M. The Okinawan diet: Health implications of a low-calorie, nutrient-dense, antioxidant-rich dietary pattern low in glycemic load. *J. Am. Coll. Nutr.* **2009**, *28*, 500s–516s. [CrossRef]
35. Parsonnet, J.; Friedman, G.D.; Orentreich, N.; Vogelman, H. Risk for gastric cancer in people with CagA positive or CagA negative *Helicobacter pylori* infection. *Gut* **1997**, *40*, 297–301. [CrossRef] [PubMed]
36. Yamaoka, Y.; Kikuchi, S.; el-Zimaity, H.M.; Gutierrez, O.; Osato, M.S.; Graham, D.Y. Importance of *Helicobacter pylori* oipA in clinical presentation, gastric inflammation, and mucosal interleukin 8 production. *Gastroenterology* **2002**, *123*, 414–424. [CrossRef] [PubMed]
37. Yamaoka, Y. Mechanisms of disease: Helicobacter pylori virulence factors. *Nat. Rev. Gastroenterol. Hepatol.* **2010**, *7*, 629–641. [CrossRef] [PubMed]
38. Falush, D.; Wirth, T.; Linz, B.; Pritchard, J.K.; Stephens, M.; Kidd, M.; Blaser, M.J.; Graham, D.Y.; Vacher, S.; Perez-Perez, G.I.; et al. Traces of human migrations in *Helicobacter pylori* populations. *Science* **2003**, *299*, 1582–1585. [CrossRef]
39. Linz, B.; Balloux, F.; Moodley, Y.; Manica, A.; Liu, H.; Roumagnac, P.; Falush, D.; Stamer, C.; Prugnolle, F.; van der Merwe, S.W.; et al. An African origin for the intimate association between humans and *Helicobacter pylori*. *Nature* **2007**, *445*, 915–918. [CrossRef]
40. Moodley, Y.; Linz, B.; Yamaoka, Y.; Windsor, H.M.; Breurec, S.; Wu, J.Y.; Maady, A.; Bernhöft, S.; Thiberge, J.M.; Phuanukoonnon, S.; et al. The peopling of the Pacific from a bacterial perspective. *Science* **2009**, *323*, 527–530. [CrossRef]
41. Yamaoka, Y.; Orito, E.; Mizokami, M.; Gutierrez, O.; Saitou, N.; Kodama, T.; Osato, M.S.; Kim, J.G.; Ramirez, F.C.; Mahachai, V.; et al. *Helicobacter pylori* in North and South America before Columbus. *FEBS Lett.* **2002**, *517*, 180–184. [CrossRef]
42. Kersulyte, D.; Mukhopadhyay, A.K.; Velapatiño, B.; Su, W.; Pan, Z.; Garcia, C.; Hernandez, V.; Valdez, Y.; Mistry, R.S.; Gilman, R.H.; et al. Differences in genotypes of *Helicobacter pylori* from different human populations. *J. Bacteriol.* **2000**, *182*, 3210–3218. [CrossRef]

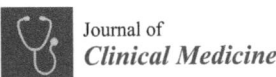

Review

Multiple Bismuth Quadruple Therapy Containing Tetracyclines Combined with Other Antibiotics and *Helicobacter pylori* Eradication Therapy

Yingchao Sun [1], Mengjia Zhu [1], Lei Yue [1] and Weiling Hu [1,2,3,*]

1 Department of Gastroenterology, Sir Run Run Shaw Hospital, Medical School, Zhejiang University, Hangzhou 310016, China
2 Institute of Gastroenterology, Zhejiang University (IGZJU), Hangzhou 310027, China
3 Zhejiang University Cancer Center, Hangzhou 310029, China
* Correspondence: huweiling@zju.edu.cn; Tel.: +86-135-1680-0685

Abstract: *Helicobacter pylori* (HP) infection is closely associated with the development of chronic gastritis, peptic ulcer, and gastric cancer. However, the resistance rate of *H. pylori* strains to antibiotics such as clarithromycin, metronidazole, and levofloxacin has increased significantly, resulting in a significant decrease in the eradication efficacy of commonly used regimens. Tetracycline has received the attention of domestic and foreign scholars because of its low resistance. The purpose of this review is to provide an update on the tetracycline-containing bismuth quadruple eradication therapy for *H. pylori* infection and review the efficacy and safety of the regimens, hoping to provide guidance for clinical practice.

Keywords: Helicobacter infection; tetracycline; eradication; penicillin allergy; furazolidone; metronidazole; amoxicillin

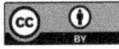

1. Introduction

Helicobacter pylori (HP) infection is closely associated with the development of chronic gastritis, peptic ulcers, dyspepsia, gastric mucosa-associated lymphoid tissue lymphoma, and gastric cancer, and approximately 75% of gastric cancers worldwide can be attributed to *Helicobacter pylori*-induced inflammation and injury [1]. China is a country with a dual high incidence of *Helicobacter pylori* infection and gastric cancer, with a current infection rate as high as 50%, and the number of cases of gastric cancer accounts for about 44% worldwide [2]. The Kyoto Global Consensus on HP Gastritis proposes that HP infection is an infectious disease, and all those who are positive for HP infection should receive eradication therapy [3]. However, the resistance rate of *H. pylori* strains to antibiotics such as clarithromycin, metronidazole, and levofloxacin has increased significantly, resulting in a significant decrease in the eradication efficacy of commonly used regimens [4].

Tetracycline was discovered in the 1940s and exhibited activity against a wide range of microorganisms, including *Helicobacter pylori*. It binds reversibly to a pocket in the 30S subunit of bacterial ribosomes containing 16S rRNA, causing bacteriostatic and bactericidal effects by inhibiting protein synthesis and bacterial growth [5]. Tetracycline has received the attention of domestic and foreign scholars because of its low resistance and high eradication efficacy; therefore, the Maastricht VI consensus recommended in 2022 that PPI-bismuth-tetracycline-metronidazole be used to eradicate HP during first-line treatment regardless of clarithromycin resistance [6]. According to Italy's latest guidelines, bismuth-based quadruple therapy (BQT) should be used as first-line treatment for *H. pylori* in Italy for patients with high (>15%) or unknown prevalence of clarithromycin resistance [7]. The sixth expert consensus in China also recommends a bismuth quadruple regimen as the first and rescue therapy for HP-infected individuals, and the non-bismuth quadruple regimen (concomitant regimen, heterozygous regimen, and sequential regimen) is no longer recommended. Bismuth is a mucosal protective agent that can eradicate HP by inhibiting the adhesion of HP and inhibiting its protease, urokinase and phospholipase [8]. Bismuth has no drug resistance and has high safety in short-term applications. Recommended tetracycline-containing bismuth quadruple regimens include tetracycline (500 mg three times daily/four times daily) combined with metronidazole (400 mg three times daily/four times daily) or amoxicillin (1000 mg twice daily).

The purpose of this review is to provide a summary of the tetracycline-containing bismuth quadruple eradication therapy used to treat HP infection. In the last decade, the importance of the infection and the advantages associated with its eradication have become increasingly recognized [9,10]. Treatment regimens for HP infection with eradication rates greater than 90% are generally regarded as successful [11]. As resistance to other antibiotics increases, tetracycline has been increasingly investigated for its effectiveness in eradication therapy, but it also has a higher incidence of adverse effects. Therefore, this article also reviews the safety of tetracycline-containing bismuth quadruple regimens, hoping to provide guidance for clinical practice.

2. Eradication Rates, Safety, and Compliance with Bismuth-Containing Tetracycline Quadruple Therapy

2.1. Tetracycline + Metronidazole

Due to the low rate of HP resistance to tetracycline, several countries or regions in Europe and the United States recommend bismuth quadruple therapy, commonly known as classical quadruple therapy, including PPI-bismuth-tetracycline-metronidazole, as a first or rescue therapy for HP eradication [6]. It has been shown that *H. pylori* eradication rates were less than 80% with the 7-day regimen, 88.9% with the 10-day regimen for the intention-to-treat (ITT) analysis, and 91.6% for the per-protocol (PP) analysis [12,13]. In 2020, the Spanish team explored the effectiveness of metronidazole combined with tetracycline as a third-line treatment in patients with refractory infections who had failed both clarithromycin and levofloxacin, with eradication rates of 82% and 83% by ITT and PP analysis, respectively. These rates were decreased by 5–10% in patients who had previously used metronidazole [14]. In 2013, a single-center randomized controlled trial (RCT) in China using tetracycline combined with furazolidone or amoxicillin or metronidazole for 14 days achieved an eradication rate of more than 90% in rescue therapy patients with HP infection [15]. Among them, the ITT and PP analysis of tetracycline combined with metronidazole regimen were 87.9% and 93.1%, and tetracycline combined with furazolidone achieved higher eradication rates with ITT and PP values of 91.6% and 96.7%, respectively. However, tetracycline combined with furazolidone also had a higher incidence of adverse events in patients compared with the other two regimens (33.6%). A real-life study has been conducted in Italy where BQT provided eradication rates higher than 90%, even in areas with high clarithromycin resistance, with an ITT and PP of 91.5% and 95.8%, respectively [16]. A single-center retrospective study in the northeast region of Poland investigated the effectiveness of BQT 10-day therapy in the eradication of *H. pylori* infection, resulting in an eradication rate of 89.4% (84/94), which also provided a good efficacy [17].

Pylera is a 3-in-1 capsule containing 140 mg bismuth subcitrate, 125 mg metronidazole, and 125 mg tetracycline. In a meta-analysis of 21 studies, Pylera, as a first-line therapy, resulted in approximately 90% eradication in an ITT analysis [18]. The incidence of clarithromycin resistance is approximately 30% in some regions of central and southern Italy, and several studies conducted in Italy have confirmed the high efficacy of Pylera across a high prevalence of clarithromycin (CLA) resistance regions [19–21]. A prospective, uncontrolled, single-center observational study of 200 treatment-naïve HP-infected patients conducted by the Spanish team achieved high eradication rates with four times daily Pylera capsules combined with PPI twice in the morning and evening for 10 consecutive days, with rates of 91.5% and 95.2% in the ITT and PP analyses [22]. A real-life study conducted in Italy drew a similar conclusion that BQT using Pylera is an effective treatment strategy, with ITT eradication rates higher than 90%, even in areas with high resistance rates to *H. pylori* strains CLA or CLA + metronidazole resistance [23].

2.2. Tetracycline + Furazolidone

Furazolidone is a nitrofuran antibiotic with strong antioxidant activity and good absorption and distribution characteristics. In addition, antibiotic resistance is unlikely to develop. Other regimens containing furazolidone have previously been reported to achieve relatively high eradication rates [24,25]. Previous retrospective studies have shown that bismuth quadruple therapy containing tetracycline and furazolidone regimens could provide good eradication, with eradication rates of 91.74% and 95.24% in ITT and PP analyses, but retrospective studies have a low level of evidence [26]. In northwest China, a multicenter RCT study was conducted in 2020 to investigate the non-inferiority of amoxicillin plus berberine vs. tetracycline plus furazolidone quadruple therapy for HP rescue therapy, and the ITT and PP analyses were 77.5% and 85% [27]. Previous Chinese studies have also reported 7-day therapy with tetracycline (750 mg twice daily) combined with furazolidone (1000 mg twice daily), but good eradication rates have not been achieved, with ITT and PP only 68.6% and 72.7% [28]. Another retrospective study using Lactobacillus acidophilus (1 g three times daily) for 2 weeks followed by a bismuth-containing quadruple regimen (tetracycline 750 mg twice daily + furazolidone 100 mg twice daily) for 10 days as rescue therapy in patients who had previously eradicated *H. pylori* twice or more showed values of 92% and 91.8% in ITT and PP analyses, respectively, suggesting that patients with multiple eradications of infection may benefit from probiotic therapy [29].

2.3. Tetracycline + Amoxicillin

A meta-analysis explored the efficacy of tetracycline combined with amoxicillin for *H. pylori* eradication and included 33 studies, with ITT and PP analysis of 78.1% and 84.5%, and the relative risk (OR) of this regimen was 0.9 compared with other regimens, suggesting that tetracycline plus amoxicillin may not be inferior to other studies, but more clinical studies are needed to verify this [30]. In 2018, a randomized controlled trial (RCT) in China using rabeprazole (10 mg twice daily), bismuth, amoxicillin (1000 mg twice daily), and tetracycline (750 mg twice daily) 10-day quadruple therapy as first-line treatment for *H. pylori* eradication showed eradication rates of 87.2% and 91.9% in ITT and PP analyses, respectively, and efficacy was not affected by antibiotic resistance [31]. Although some studies have shown that amoxicillin combined with tetracycline is pharmacologically resistant, this clinical study still achieved a high eradication rate. Several studies previously also reported that the efficacy of tetracycline combined with an amoxicillin bismuth quadruple regimen is unsatisfactory. In a 2016 Korean study using pantoprazole 40 mg, bismuth 600 mg, tetracycline 1 g, and amoxicillin 1 g twice daily as first-line therapy for HP infection, the ITT and PP analyses were only 68.7% and 76.5%, and there was a 36.9% incidence of adverse events [32].

2.4. Tetracycline + Levofloxacin

In China, due to the many clinical applications of quinolones, there is cross-resistance with levofloxacin. At present, the resistance rate of levofloxacin in China has reached more than 20% [33]. Therefore, the guidelines do not recommend levofloxacin-containing regimens as first-line treatments unless applied to patients allergic to penicillin [34]. The Maastricht VI consensus indicated in 2022 that, regardless of clarithromycin resistance, eradication of HP with PPI-bismuth-tetracycline-levofloxacin is recommended when rescue therapy is given [6]. The Taiwan team has explored that a 10-day tetracycline (500 mg four times daily) regimen combined with levofloxacin (500 mg once daily) quadruple bismuth-containing regimen for HP-infected patients who failed sequential therapy provides a better eradication rate, achieving values of 95.8% in both ITT and PP analyses, but the sample size was small, with only 24 patients, and more studies are needed to confirm these findings [35]. In a 2019 RCT study (NCT02978157) conducted by the CHINA Taiwan team,

50 patients were treated for second-line HP infection with esomeprazole 40 mg twice daily, bismuth 120 mg once daily, tetracycline 500 mg once daily, and levofloxacin 500 mg every other day. There was a 22% rate of adverse events, primarily nausea and dizziness, but results regarding eradication rates were not published.

In Table 1, we summarize the efficacy and safety of tetracycline-containing bismuth quadruple regimens and list the specific study regimens, durations, and sample sizes.

Table 1. Studies of tetracycline-containing bismuth quadruple regimens in HP-infected patients.

Year	Author	Study	Regimen	Duration (d)	Sample Size	ER (ITT/PP, %)	AE (%)	Compliance (%)	Ref
2020	Nyssen et al.	Rescue, RCT	O + T + M + B	14	45	82/83	63	96	[14]
2018	Xie et al.	1, RCT	R + T + A + B	14	109	87.2/91.9	5.5	97.2	[31]
			L + T + A + B	14	105	83.8/94.6	16.2	88.6	
2013	Lu et al.	Rescue, RCT	L + T + M + B		107	87.9/93.1	33.6	94.4	[15]
			L + T + F + B		108	91.7/96.1	17.6	95.4	
2020	Zhang et al.	Rescue, RCT	E + T + F + B	14	329	77.5/85	26.1	90	[27]
2014	Zhang et al.	Rescue, R	R + T + F + B	14	109	91.74/95.24	32.1	/	[26]
2014	Hsu et al.	Rescue, RCT	E + T + L + B	10	24	95.4/95.4	25	100	[35]
2016	Lee et al.	1, RCT	P + T + A + B	14	195	68.7/76.5	36.9	87.2	[32]
2020	Kim et al.	Rescue, R	P + T + M + B	7	98	92.9	36.7	/	[36]
2020	Fernandez et al.	1, RCT	PPI + Pylera®	10	200	91.5/95.2	28.5	96	[22]

R, rabeprazole; L, lansoprazole; E, esomeprazole; O, omeprazole; T, tetracycline; M, metronidazole; F, furazolidone; A, amoxicillin; L, levofloxacin; B, bismuth; ITT, intention-to-treat analysis; PP, per protocol analysis; RCT, randomized controlled trial; R, retrospective study; AE, adverse event; ER, eradication rate.

3. Tetracycline Regimen Selection for Penicillin-Allergic Patients

Amoxicillin is one of the most effective antibiotics against *Helicobacter pylori*, and the resistance rate is low, but about 10% of patients are allergic to penicillin, making it difficult to use these drugs in these patients. Maastricht VI consensus and the sixth Chinese consensus recommended that PPI-bismuth-tetracycline-metronidazole was first recommended to eradicate HP in patients allergic to penicillin during first-line treatment [6]. In 2018, a retrospective study in China using tetracycline (500 mg three times daily) combined with metronidazole (400 mg three times daily) as the first-line regimen included 120 patients with penicillin allergy and achieved a high eradication rate of 86.7% and 94.5% in ITT and PP analyses, respectively [37]. However, the incidence of adverse reactions was 44%, and 10 patients discontinued treatment due to adverse reactions. Although the total dosage of tetracycline and metronidazole in this study was lower than the dosage of antibiotics used in previous domestic studies, the efficacy was not disappointing [13]. In the past, two groups applied first-line 10-day regimens of PPI, tetracycline, and metronidazole in 5 and 17 patients with penicillin allergy, respectively, and reported eradication rates of 80–85%, but the number of patients was small, and more studies are needed to verify the reliability of this conclusion [38,39]. Quadruple therapy (PPI, bismuth, tetracycline, and metronidazole) is generally recommended as the best second-line therapy for HP infection after the failure of standard PPI-based triple therapy [40]. The Spanish team treated patients with penicillin allergy with tetracycline combined with metronidazole in a 10-day regimen for first-line treatment; 50 patients were included, but the eradication rate was less than 80% [41].

Although both the Maastricht consensus and the American Gastroenterological Association consensus recommend tetracycline combined with bismuth metronidazole quadruple regimen for rescue therapy, most retrospective studies have a low level of evidence and generally small sample size, and more studies are needed to verify its efficacy. In 2020, the Spanish team used data from the European *Helicobacter pylori* Administrative Registry to reassess the efficacy and safety of first and rescue therapy for HP-infected patients, and the classical bismuth quadruple regimen achieved a high eradication rate in first-line therapy in 250 patients, with values of 91% and 92% in the ITT and PP analyses. Classical bismuth quadruple therapy as second-line therapy also provided eradication rates of 78% and 82% in patients previously treated with triple therapy (PPI + clarithromycin + metronidazole).

The eradication rate of this regimen was 77.8% at third-line treatment. Adverse events were higher with bismuth quadruple therapy in the first-line setting (29% of cases). Dysgeusia, diarrhea, and nausea were the most common adverse events, and the duration varied from 5 to nearly 10 days [42]. In Table 2, we summarize the efficacy and safety of tetracycline-containing bismuth quadruple therapy for penicillin-allergic patients and list the specific treatment lines, regimens, durations, and sample sizes.

Table 2. Summary of studies with tetracycline-containing regimens in patients with penicillin allergy.

Year	Author	Treatment Line	Regimen	Duration (d)	Sample Size	ER (ITT/PP, %)	AE (%)	Ref
2020	Nyssen OP et al., RCT	1	PPI + T + M + B	14	250	91/92	29	[42]
		2		14	69	78.2/81.8	32	
		3		14	18	77.8/93.4	39	
2015	Gisbert et al., RCT	1	O + T + M + B	10	50	74/75	14	[41]
		2			24	37	58	
		3			3	100	67	
2018	Gao et al., R	1	R + T + A + B	14	120	86.7/94.5	47	[37]
2005	Rodrigue et al., R	1	E + T + M	10	17	82	/	[39]
		2			3	100	/	
2006	Matsushima et al., R	1	PPI + T + M	7–14	5	80	/	[38]
2005	Gisbert et al., RCT	2	RBC + T + M	7	17	47	53	[43]

R, rabeprazole; E, esomeprazole; O, omeprazole; PPI, proton pump inhibitors; RBC, ranitidine bismuth citrate; T, tetracycline; M, metronidazole; A, amoxicillin; B, bismuth; ITT, intention-to-treat analysis; PP, per protocol analysis; RCT, randomized controlled trial; R, retrospective study; AE, adverse event; ER, eradication rate.

4. Precautions for Using Tetracycline

Tetracycline is a broad-spectrum antibiotic produced by actinomycetes that inhibits bacterial reproduction and viability by interfering with protein synthesis. However, previous studies have shown that the incidence of individual adverse reactions is unsatisfied, and common adverse drug reactions to tetracycline include gastrointestinal symptoms (nausea, vomiting, and epigastric discomfort), photosensitivity reactions, allergy, anaphylactic shock, asthma, and hemolytic anemia. Loss of appetite, severe liver damage, and affected tooth and bone growth have been reported in studies. In previous studies, quadruple therapy with (PPI + bismuth + tetracycline + furazolidone) in penicillin-allergic patients developed more severe adverse reactions (drug fever, rash) in 5.5% of patients, although the eradication rate of the regimen (ITT 91.7%, PP 95.2%) exceeded 90% [26]. Tetracycline–metronidazole-containing quadruple regimens had a lower incidence of serious adverse reactions compared with tetracycline–furazolidone-containing quadruple regimens. Bismuth quadruple therapy with tetracycline 1000 mg twice daily combined with metronidazole 500 mg three times daily for seven days is as effective and safe as quadruple therapy with conventional doses (tetracycline 500 mg four times daily combined with metronidazole 500 mg three times daily) as rescue therapy [36]. Abdominal pain, bloating, and other discomforts were less frequent with twice-daily doses [36]. Common adverse events and the reported frequency of each regimen are listed in Table 3.

Table 3. Adverse events of tetracycline-containing bismuth quadruple eradication therapy.

Adverse Effect	Reported Frequency			
	T + M [14,15]	T + A [15,31,32,37]	T + F [15,26,27]	T + L [35]
Taste disturbance	1.9–35%	5.6%	0–19.8%	4.2%
Nausea	15.9–41%	2.9–8.3%	2.8–33.7%	4.2%
Diarrhea	2.8–15%	0.46–16.7%	0.9–18.6%	4.2%
Reduced appetite	7.1–8.4%	1.4–1.9%	0–2.8%	4.2%
Vomiting	18%	2.8%	0–17.4%	4.2%
Abdominal pain	5.9–8.4%	1.9–9.2%	0–23.3%	4.2%

Table 3. Cont.

Adverse Effect	T + M [14,15]	T + A [15,31,32,37]	T + F [15,26,27]	T + L [35]
Headache/dizziness	3.7%	2.76–10%	1.9–9.3%	8.4%
Rash	0	1.9–3.3%	1.9–3.67%	4.2%
Fatigue	7.5–12%	1–5%	6.5–10.5%	4.2%
Fever	0	0.8–1.9%	1.9–5.5%	0
Bloating	0	15.3%	9.3%	0

T, tetracycline; M, metronidazole; F, furazolidone; A, amoxicillin; L, levofloxacin.

5. Recent Advances

Following the formal recognition of HP gastritis as an infectious disease in 2015, it was recommended that all patients should undertake eradication medication [3,9]. With infectious diseases, it is generally possible to reliably cure almost 100% of cases; however, the eradication rates reported in current studies are still far from this goal. In the future, *H. pylori* treatment trials will focus on actual cure rates, and comparisons will be restricted to deciding which of two highly successful therapies (average cure rate of at least 90%, preferably ≥95%) is best [11].

H. pylori therapies should be susceptibility based, relying either on susceptibility testing or on proven high local success rates. The prevalence of antibiotic resistance has increased such that clarithromycin, metronidazole, or fluoroquinolone triple therapies can no longer be used empirically. The first step in identifying and prescribing an effective therapy is to exclude antibiotics where preexisting resistance is likely. This can be accomplished by history and/or susceptibility testing, such as real-time PCR and even next-generation sequencing (NGS). Susceptibility-guided therapy (SGT) is an effective way to achieve high efficacy and avoid unnecessary antibiotic use while ensuring cost-effectiveness. Several clinical trials [44,45] were conducted to evaluate whether SGT shows a superior or similar efficacy in comparison with bismuth-containing quadruple therapy. It is necessary to carry out susceptibility-guided *H. pylori* eradication therapy versus empirical tetracycline-bismuth containing quadruple regimen in terms of eradication rate and cost in the future.

Vonoprazan (VPZ), a reversible H+-K+ ATPase inhibitor, has a fast and sustained acid suppression action that is unaffected by diet or polymorphisms in genes [46,47]. Vonoprazan increased the intragastric pH to over 4.0 within 4 h, which allowed the opportunity to achieve a shorter treatment duration [48]. VPZ-based regimens appear to be more effective than PPI-based regimens according to a present meta-analysis [49]. Vonoprazan is typically used in combination with amoxicillin or clarithromycin for *H. pylori* eradication therapy, and there have been no clinical trials involving its use in combination with tetracycline. VPZ's excellent acid-suppressive ability combined with low tetracycline resistance will result in high eradication rates, but safety needs to be further evaluated in randomized controlled trials.

6. Conclusions

The HP infection rate is high, and drug resistance is prevalent worldwide. It is urgent to explore eradication regimens with high eradication rates, good safety, and good compliance. Tetracycline resistance is low in many countries, and tetracycline-containing bismuth quadruple regimens such as tetracycline combined with metronidazole or furazolidone or amoxicillin or levofloxacin can achieve better eradication rates. Especially in penicillin-allergic patients, tetracycline-containing bismuth quadruple regimens could be recommended as first-line therapy. However, current tetracycline-related studies were conducted mainly in Asia and Europe, and there are many retrospective studies. The efficacy and safety still need to be further evaluated by large-sample, multicenter prospective studies and more real-world data. Tetracycline has higher rates of adverse effects than other antibiotics, and current guidelines still recommend 1.5–2.0 g of tetracycline daily for eradication therapy. It is necessary to explore the effectiveness of lower doses of tetracycline-containing bismuth quadruple regimens in the future.

Author Contributions: Conceptualization, Y.S. and W.H.; writing—original draft preparation, Y.S. and L.Y.; writing, M.Z.; review and editing, Y.S., L.Y. and M.Z.; supervision, W.H. All authors have read and agreed to the published version of the manuscript.

Funding: This work was supported by the Medical and Health Science and Technology Project of Zhejiang Province (grant no. 2020RC064).

Institutional Review Board Statement: Not applicable.

Informed Consent Statement: Not applicable.

Data Availability Statement: Not applicable.

Conflicts of Interest: The authors declare no conflict of interest.

References

1. Amieva, M.; Peek, R.M., Jr. Pathobiology of *Helicobacter pylori*-Induced Gastric Cancer. *Gastroenterology* **2016**, *150*, 64–78. [CrossRef] [PubMed]
2. Gaskin, T.A.; Isobe, J.H.; Mathews, J.L.; Dillard, D.R. The peel away introducer for the peritoneal limb of peritoneal venous shunt placement. *Surg. Gynecol. Obstet.* **1988**, *166*, 352–353. [PubMed]
3. Sugano, K.; Tack, J.; Kuipers, E.J.; Graham, D.Y.; El-Omar, E.M.; Miura, S.; Haruma, K.; Asaka, M.; Uemura, N.; Malfertheiner, P.; et al. Kyoto global consensus report on *Helicobacter pylori* gastritis. *Gut* **2015**, *64*, 1353–1367. [CrossRef]
4. Undar, A.; Wang, S. Translational research is a necessity for selecting the best components of the extracorporeal circuitry for neonatal and pediatric CPB patients. *Perfusion* **2013**, *28*, 171–172. [CrossRef] [PubMed]
5. Chopra, I.; Roberts, M. Tetracycline antibiotics: Mode of action, applications, molecular biology, and epidemiology of bacterial resistance. *Microbiol. Mol. Biol. Rev.* **2001**, *65*, 232–260. [CrossRef] [PubMed]
6. Malfertheiner, P.; Megraud, F.; Rokkas, T.; Gisbert, J.P.; Liou, J.M.; Schulz, C.; Gasbarrini, A.; Hunt, R.H.; Leja, M.; O'Morain, C.; et al. Management of *Helicobacter pylori* infection: The Maastricht VI/Florence consensus report. *Gut* **2022**, *71*, 1724–1762. [CrossRef] [PubMed]
7. Romano, M.; Gravina, A.G.; Eusebi, L.H.; Pellegrino, R.; Palladino, G.; Frazzoni, L.; Dajti, E.; Gasbarrini, A.; Di Mario, F.; Zagari, R.M.; et al. Management of *Helicobacter pylori* infection: Guidelines of the Italian Society of Gastroenterology (SIGE) and the Italian Society of Digestive Endoscopy (SIED). *Dig. Liver Dis.* **2022**, *54*, 1153–1161. [CrossRef] [PubMed]
8. Lambert, J.R.; Midolo, P. The actions of bismuth in the treatment of *Helicobacter pylori* infection. *Aliment. Pharmacol. Ther.* **1997**, *11* (Suppl. S1), 27–33. [CrossRef] [PubMed]
9. El-Serag, H.B.; Kao, J.Y.; Kanwal, F.; Gilger, M.; LoVecchio, F.; Moss, S.F.; Crowe, S.E.; Elfant, A.; Haas, T.; Hapke, R.J.; et al. Houston Consensus Conference on Testing for *Helicobacter pylori* Infection in the United States. *Clin. Gastroenterol. Hepatol.* **2018**, *16*, 992–1002.e6. [CrossRef] [PubMed]
10. Liou, J.M.; Malfertheiner, P.; Lee, Y.C.; Sheu, B.S.; Sugano, K.; Cheng, H.C.; Yeoh, K.G.; Hsu, P.I.; Goh, K.L.; Mahachai, V.; et al. Screening and eradication of *Helicobacter pylori* for gastric cancer prevention: The Taipei global consensus. *Gut* **2020**, *69*, 2093–2112. [CrossRef] [PubMed]
11. Lee, Y.C.; Dore, M.P.; Graham, D.Y. Diagnosis and Treatment of *Helicobacter pylori* Infection. *Annu. Rev. Med.* **2022**, *73*, 183–195. [CrossRef] [PubMed]
12. Lu, H.; Zhang, W.; Graham, D.Y. Bismuth-containing quadruple therapy for *Helicobacter pylori*: Lessons from China. *Eur. J. Gastroenterol. Hepatol.* **2013**, *25*, 1134–1140. [CrossRef] [PubMed]
13. Zheng, Q.; Chen, W.J.; Lu, H.; Sun, Q.J.; Xiao, S.D. Comparison of the efficacy of triple versus quadruple therapy on the eradication of *Helicobacter pylori* and antibiotic resistance. *J. Dig. Dis.* **2010**, *11*, 313–318. [CrossRef] [PubMed]
14. Nyssen, O.P.; Perez-Aisa, A.; Rodrigo, L.; Castro, M.; Mata Romero, P.; Ortuno, J.; Barrio, J.; Huguet, J.M.; Modollel, I.; Alcaide, N.; et al. Bismuth quadruple regimen with tetracycline or doxycycline versus three-in-one single capsule as third-line rescue therapy for *Helicobacter pylori* infection: Spanish data of the European *Helicobacter pylori* Registry (Hp-EuReg). *Helicobacter* **2020**, *25*, e12722. [CrossRef]
15. Liang, X.; Xu, X.; Zheng, Q.; Zhang, W.; Sun, Q.; Liu, W.; Xiao, S.; Lu, H. Efficacy of bismuth-containing quadruple therapies for clarithromycin-, metronidazole-, and fluoroquinolone-resistant *Helicobacter pylori* infections in a prospective study. *Clin. Gastroenterol. Hepatol.* **2013**, *11*, 802–807.e1. [CrossRef]
16. Romano, M.; Gravina, A.G.; Nardone, G.; Federico, A.; Dallio, M.; Martorano, M.; Mucherino, C.; Romiti, A.; Avallone, L.; Granata, L.; et al. Non-bismuth and bismuth quadruple therapies based on previous clarithromycin exposure are as effective and safe in an area of high clarithromycin resistance: A real-life study. *Helicobacter* **2020**, *25*, e12694. [CrossRef] [PubMed]

17. Wasielica-Berger, J.; Gugnacki, P.; Mlynarczyk, M.; Rogalski, P.; Swidnicka-Siergiejko, A.; Antonowicz, S.; Krzyzak, M.; Maslach, D.; Dabrowski, A.; Daniluk, J. Comparative Effectiveness of Various Eradication Regimens for *Helicobacter pylori* Infection in the Northeastern Region of Poland. *Int. J. Environ. Res. Public Health* **2022**, *19*, 6921. [CrossRef] [PubMed]
18. Nyssen, O.P.; McNicholl, A.G.; Gisbert, J.P. Meta-analysis of three-in-one single capsule bismuth-containing quadruple therapy for the eradication of *Helicobacter pylori*. *Helicobacter* **2019**, *24*, e12570. [CrossRef] [PubMed]
19. Zagari, R.M.; Romiti, A.; Ierardi, E.; Gravina, A.G.; Panarese, A.; Grande, G.; Savarino, E.; Maconi, G.; Stasi, E.; Eusebi, L.H.; et al. The "three-in-one" formulation of bismuth quadruple therapy for *Helicobacter pylori* eradication with or without probiotics supplementation: Efficacy and safety in daily clinical practice. *Helicobacter* **2018**, *23*, e12502. [CrossRef] [PubMed]
20. Tursi, A.; Franceschi, M.; Allegretta, L.; Savarino, E.; De Bastiani, R.; Elisei, W.; Baldassarre, G.; Ferronato, A.; Scida, S.; Miraglia, C.; et al. Effectiveness and Safety of Pylera(R) in Patients Infected by *Helicobacter pylori*: A Multicenter, Retrospective, Real Life Study. *Dig. Dis.* **2018**, *36*, 264–268. [CrossRef] [PubMed]
21. Di Ciaula, A.; Scaccianoce, G.; Venerito, M.; Zullo, A.; Bonfrate, L.; Rokkas, T.; Portincasa, P. Eradication rates in Italian subjects heterogeneously managed for *Helicobacter pylori* infection. Time to abandon empiric treatments in Southern Europe. *J. Gastrointest. Liver Dis.* **2017**, *26*, 129–137. [CrossRef] [PubMed]
22. Castro Fernandez, M.; Romero Garcia, T.; Keco Huerga, A.; Pabon Jaen, M.; Lamas Rojas, E.; Llorca Fernandez, R.; Grande Santamaria, L.; Rojas Feria, M. Compliance, adverse effects and effectiveness of first line bismuth-containing quadruple treatment (Pylera(R)) to eradicate *Helicobacter pylori* infection in 200 patients. *Rev. Esp. Enferm. Dig.* **2019**, *111*, 467–470. [CrossRef] [PubMed]
23. Gravina, A.G.; Priadko, K.; Granata, L.; Facchiano, A.; Scida, G.; Cerbone, R.; Ciamarra, P.; Romano, M. Single Capsule Bismuth Quadruple Therapy for Eradication of *H. pylori* Infection: A Real-Life Study. *Front. Pharmacol.* **2021**, *12*, 667584. [CrossRef] [PubMed]
24. Cheng, H.; Hu, F.L. Furazolidone, amoxicillin, bismuth and rabeprazole quadruple rescue therapy for the eradication of *Helicobacter pylori*. *World J. Gastroenterol.* **2009**, *15*, 860–864. [CrossRef] [PubMed]
25. Eisig, J.N.; Silva, F.M.; Barbuti, R.C.; Rodriguez, T.N.; Malfertheiner, P.; Moraes Filho, J.P.; Zaterka, S. Efficacy of a 7-day course of furazolidone, levofloxacin, and lansoprazole after failed *Helicobacter pylori* eradication. *BMC Gastroenterol.* **2009**, *9*, 38. [CrossRef] [PubMed]
26. Zhang, Y.; Gao, W.; Cheng, H.; Zhang, X.; Hu, F. Tetracycline- and furazolidone-containing quadruple regimen as rescue treatment for *Helicobacter pylori* infection: A single center retrospective study. *Helicobacter* **2014**, *19*, 382–386. [CrossRef] [PubMed]
27. Zhang, J.; Han, C.; Lu, W.Q.; Wang, N.; Wu, S.R.; Wang, Y.X.; Ma, J.P.; Wang, J.H.; Hao, C.; Yuan, D.H.; et al. A randomized, multicenter and noninferiority study of amoxicillin plus berberine vs tetracycline plus furazolidone in quadruple therapy for *Helicobacter pylori* rescue treatment. *J. Dig. Dis.* **2020**, *21*, 256–263. [CrossRef]
28. Yang, J.C.; Lu, C.W.; Lin, C.J. Rescue therapy for treatment failure of *Helicobacter pylori* infection. *Chin. J. Gastroenterol.* **2002**, *7*, 347–349.
29. Liu, A.; Wang, Y.; Song, Y.; Du, Y. Treatment with compound Lactobacillus acidophilus followed by a tetracycline- and furazolidone-containing quadruple regimen as a rescue therapy for *Helicobacter pylori* infection. *Saudi J. Gastroenterol.* **2020**, *26*, 78–83. [CrossRef]
30. Lv, Z.F.; Wang, F.C.; Zheng, H.L.; Wang, B.; Xie, Y.; Zhou, X.J.; Lv, N.H. Meta-analysis: Is combination of tetracycline and amoxicillin suitable for *Helicobacter pylori* infection? *World J. Gastroenterol.* **2015**, *21*, 2522–2533. [CrossRef]
31. Xie, Y.; Zhu, Z.; Wang, J.; Zhang, L.; Zhang, Z.; Lu, H.; Zeng, Z.; Chen, S.; Liu, D.; Lv, N. Ten-Day Quadruple Therapy Comprising Low-Dose Rabeprazole, Bismuth, Amoxicillin, and Tetracycline Is an Effective and Safe First-Line Treatment for *Helicobacter pylori* Infection in a Population with High Antibiotic Resistance: A Prospective, Multicenter, Randomized, Parallel-Controlled Clinical Trial in China. *Antimicrob. Agents Chemother.* **2018**, *62*, e00432-18. [CrossRef]
32. Lee, J.Y.; Kim, N.; Park, K.S.; Kim, H.J.; Park, S.M.; Baik, G.H.; Shim, K.N.; Oh, J.H.; Choi, S.C.; Kim, S.E.; et al. Comparison of sequential therapy and amoxicillin/tetracycline containing bismuth quadruple therapy for the first-line eradication of *Helicobacter pylori*: A prospective, multi-center, randomized clinical trial. *BMC Gastroenterol.* **2016**, *16*, 79. [CrossRef] [PubMed]
33. Su, P.; Li, Y.; Li, H.; Zhang, J.; Lin, L.; Wang, Q.; Guo, F.; Ji, Z.; Mao, J.; Tang, W.; et al. Antibiotic resistance of *Helicobacter pylori* isolated in the Southeast Coastal Region of China. *Helicobacter* **2013**, *18*, 274–279. [CrossRef] [PubMed]
34. Liu, W.Z.; Xie, Y.; Lu, H.; Cheng, H.; Zeng, Z.R.; Zhou, L.Y.; Chen, Y.; Wang, J.B.; Du, Y.Q.; Lu, N.H.; et al. Fifth Chinese National Consensus Report on the management of *Helicobacter pylori* infection. *Helicobacter* **2018**, *23*, e12475. [CrossRef]
35. Hsu, P.I.; Chen, W.C.; Tsay, F.W.; Shih, C.A.; Kao, S.S.; Wang, H.M.; Yu, H.C.; Lai, K.H.; Tseng, H.H.; Peng, N.J.; et al. Ten-day Quadruple therapy comprising proton-pump inhibitor, bismuth, tetracycline, and levofloxacin achieves a high eradication rate for *Helicobacter pylori* infection after failure of sequential therapy. *Helicobacter* **2014**, *19*, 74–79. [CrossRef]
36. Kim, J.Y.; Lee, S.Y.; Kim, J.H.; Sung, I.K.; Park, H.S. Efficacy and safety of twice a day, bismuth-containing quadruple therapy using high-dose tetracycline and metronidazole for second-line *Helicobacter pylori* eradication. *Helicobacter* **2020**, *25*, e12683. [CrossRef]
37. Gao, W.; Zheng, S.H.; Cheng, H.; Wang, C.; Li, Y.X.; Xu, Y.; Hu, F.L. Tetracycline and metronidazole based quadruple regimen as first line treatment for penicillin allergic patients with *Helicobacter pylori* infection. *Zhonghua Yi Xue Za Zhi* **2019**, *99*, 1536–1540.
38. Matsushima, M.; Suzuki, T.; Kurumada, T.; Watanabe, S.; Watanabe, K.; Kobayashi, K.; Deguchi, R.; Masui, A.; Takagi, A.; Shirai, T.; et al. Tetracycline, metronidazole and amoxicillin-metronidazole combinations in proton pump inhibitor-based triple therapies are equally effective as alternative therapies against *Helicobacter pylori* infection. *J. Gastroenterol. Hepatol.* **2006**, *21*, 232–236. [CrossRef]

39. Rodriguez-Torres, M.; Salgado-Mercado, R.; Rios-Bedoya, C.F.; Aponte-Rivera, E.; Marxuach-Cuetara, A.M.; Rodriguez-Orengo, J.F.; Fernandez-Carbia, A. High eradication rates of *Helicobacter pylori* infection with first- and second-line combination of esomeprazole, tetracycline, and metronidazole in patients allergic to penicillin. *Dig. Dis. Sci.* **2005**, *50*, 634–639. [CrossRef]
40. Gisbert, J.P.; Pajares, J.M. Review article: *Helicobacter pylori* "rescue" regimen when proton pump inhibitor-based triple therapies fail. *Aliment. Pharmacol. Ther.* **2002**, *16*, 1047–1057. [CrossRef]
41. Gisbert, J.P.; Barrio, J.; Modolell, I.; Molina-Infante, J.; Aisa, A.P.; Castro-Fernandez, M.; Rodrigo, L.; Cosme, A.; Gisbert, J.L.; Fernandez-Bermejo, M.; et al. *Helicobacter pylori* first-line and rescue treatments in the presence of penicillin allergy. *Dig. Dis. Sci.* **2015**, *60*, 458–464. [CrossRef] [PubMed]
42. Nyssen, O.P.; Perez-Aisa, A.; Tepes, B.; Rodrigo-Saez, L.; Romero, P.M.; Lucendo, A.; Castro-Fernandez, M.; Phull, P.; Barrio, J.; Bujanda, L.; et al. *Helicobacter pylori* first-line and rescue treatments in patients allergic to penicillin: Experience from the European Registry on *H pylori* management (Hp-EuReg). *Helicobacter* **2020**, *25*, e12686. [CrossRef] [PubMed]
43. Gisbert, J.P.; Gisbert, J.L.; Marcos, S.; Olivares, D.; Pajares, J.M. *Helicobacter pylori* first-line treatment and rescue options in patients allergic to penicillin. *Aliment. Pharmacol. Ther.* **2005**, *22*, 1041–1046. [CrossRef] [PubMed]
44. Zhou, L.; Zhang, J.; Song, Z.; He, L.; Li, Y.; Qian, J.; Bai, P.; Xue, Y.; Wang, Y.; Lin, S. Tailored versus Triple plus Bismuth or Concomitant Therapy as Initial *Helicobacter pylori* Treatment: A Randomized Trial. *Helicobacter* **2016**, *21*, 91–99. [CrossRef] [PubMed]
45. Chen, Q.; Long, X.; Ji, Y.; Liang, X.; Li, D.; Gao, H.; Xu, B.; Liu, M.; Chen, Y.; Sun, Y.; et al. Randomised controlled trial: Susceptibility-guided therapy versus empiric bismuth quadruple therapy for first-line *Helicobacter pylori* treatment. *Aliment. Pharmacol. Ther.* **2019**, *49*, 1385–1394. [CrossRef]
46. Sue, S.; Maeda, S. Is a Potassium-Competitive Acid Blocker Truly Superior to Proton Pump Inhibitors in Terms of *Helicobacter pylori* Eradication? *Gut Liver* **2021**, *15*, 799–810. [CrossRef]
47. Kiyotoki, S.; Nishikawa, J.; Sakaida, I. Efficacy of Vonoprazan for *Helicobacter pylori* Eradication. *Intern. Med.* **2020**, *59*, 153–161. [CrossRef]
48. Jenkins, H.; Sakurai, Y.; Nishimura, A.; Okamoto, H.; Hibberd, M.; Jenkins, R.; Yoneyama, T.; Ashida, K.; Ogama, Y.; Warrington, S. Randomised clinical trial: Safety, tolerability, pharmacokinetics and pharmacodynamics of repeated doses of TAK-438 (vonoprazan), a novel potassium-competitive acid blocker, in healthy male subjects. *Aliment. Pharmacol. Ther.* **2015**, *41*, 636–648. [CrossRef]
49. Jung, Y.S.; Kim, E.H.; Park, C.H. Systematic review with meta-analysis: The efficacy of vonoprazan-based triple therapy on *Helicobacter pylori* eradication. *Aliment. Pharmacol. Ther.* **2017**, *46*, 106–114. [CrossRef]

Review

Helicobacter pylori-Associated Iron Deficiency Anemia in Childhood and Adolescence-Pathogenesis and Clinical Management Strategy

Seiichi Kato [1,*], Benjamin D. Gold [2] and Ayumu Kato [3]

1. Kato Children's Clinic, Natori 981-1227, Japan
2. Gi Care for Kids, Children's Center for Digestive Healthcare, LLC, Atlanta, GA 30342, USA
3. Department of General Pediatrics and Miyagi Children's Hospital, Sendai 989-3126, Japan
* Correspondence: skato@kato-kidsclinic.jp; Tel.: +81-22-399-9152; Fax: +81-22-399-9153

Citation: Kato, S.; Gold, B.D.; Kato, A. Helicobacter pylori-Associated Iron Deficiency Anemia in Childhood and Adolescence-Pathogenesis and Clinical Management Strategy. *J. Clin. Med.* **2022**, *11*, 7351. https://doi.org/10.3390/jcm11247351

Academic Editors: Mariko Hojo and Tamaki Ikuse

Received: 31 October 2022
Accepted: 8 December 2022
Published: 10 December 2022

Publisher's Note: MDPI stays neutral with regard to jurisdictional claims in published maps and institutional affiliations.

Copyright: © 2022 by the authors. Licensee MDPI, Basel, Switzerland. This article is an open access article distributed under the terms and conditions of the Creative Commons Attribution (CC BY) license (https://creativecommons.org/licenses/by/4.0/).

Abstract: Many epidemiological studies and meta-analyses show that persistent *Helicobacter pylori* infection in the gastric mucosa can lead to iron deficiency or iron deficiency anemia (IDA), particularly in certain populations of children and adolescents. Moreover, it has been demonstrated that *H. pylori* infection can lead to and be closely associated with recurrent and/or refractory iron deficiency and IDA. However, the pathogenesis and specific risk factors leading to this clinical outcome in *H. pylori*-infected children remain poorly understood. In general, most of pediatric patients with *H. pylori*-associated IDA do not show evidence of overt blood loss due to gastrointestinal hemorrhagic lesions. In adult populations, *H. pylori* atrophic gastritis is reported to cause impaired iron absorption due to impaired gastric acid secretion, which, subsequently, results in IDA. However, significant gastric atrophy, and the resultant substantial reduction in gastric acid secretion, has not been shown in *H. pylori*-infected children. Recently, it has been hypothesized that competition between *H. pylori* and humans for iron availability in the upper gastrointestinal tract could lead to IDA. Many genes, including those encoding major outer membrane proteins (OMPs), are known to be involved in iron-uptake mechanisms in *H. pylori*. Recent studies have been published that describe *H. pylori* virulence factors, including specific OMP genes that may be associated with the pathogenesis of IDA. Daily iron demand substantively increases in children as they begin pubertal development starting with the associated growth spurt, and this important physiological mechanism may play a synergistic role for the microorganisms as a host pathogenetic factor of IDA. Like in the most recent pediatric guidelines, a test-and-treat strategy in *H. pylori* infection should be considered, especially for children and adolescents in whom IDA is recurrent or refractory to iron supplementation and other definitive causes have not been identified. This review will focus on providing the evidence that supports a clear biological plausibility for *H. pylori* infection and iron deficiency, as well as IDA.

Keywords: child; gastritis; *Helicobacter pylori*; host genetic factor; iron deficiency anemia; iron demand; iron uptake; sports activity; virulence factor

1. Introduction

Helicobacter pylori infection is quite common and this organism colonizes an estimated fifty percent of the world's populations [1]. However, there is a wide difference in *H. pylori* prevalence among different countries, with infection rates in Latin America and Africa upwards of 70–80% of adults compared to infection prevalence of 20–30% of adults in Canada and U.S. [2]. Gastric colonization with *H. pylori* is usually life-long, which then, eventually, and inevitably, induces persistent mucosal inflammation. Long-term *H. pylori* infection can cause pre-cancerous pathology, including gastric atrophy and intestinal metaplasia in adulthood, leading to especially intestinal-type gastric cancer, particularly in at-risk populations [3,4]. Since 1994, *H. pylori* has been classified as a class I carcinogen associated with the development of gastric adenocarcinoma by the World Health Organization (WHO), as well as by the International Agency for Research on Cancer [5].

In the pediatric population, *H. pylori* is also associated with the development of gastritis, peptic ulcer disease (duodenal more than gastric ulcers), in rare cases mucosal-associated lymphoid-type tissue lymphoma, and extra-gastrointestinal diseases, including iron deficiency (ID)/iron deficiency anemia (IDA) and idiopathic thrombocytopenic purpura [6,7]. However, the majority of *H. pylori*-infected children remain relatively asymptomatic without any readily apparent clinical diseases. Significantly, atrophy and intestinal metaplasia are rarely found in *H. pylori*-infected children, and gastric cancer is extremely rare [6,7] (Figure 1). The fact that compared to adults, an abundance of *H. pylori*-infected children demonstrate less severe gastritis and the resultant outcome of severe clinical diseases indicates a down-regulation of host immune response in the early natural history of infection [8]. With data that suggests that *H. pylori* is an "old" pathogen with respect to human evolution, this dampening of the host response in the initial or early infection after gastric mucosal colonization makes biological sense in order to facilitate immune evasion and establish persistent infection in a unique biological niche. The knowledge that there is a wide difference in a clinical spectrum of *H. pylori*-associated disease, including *H. pylori*-associated IDA, between both pediatric and adult populations is very important in understanding the complex pathobiology of human *H. pylori* infection.

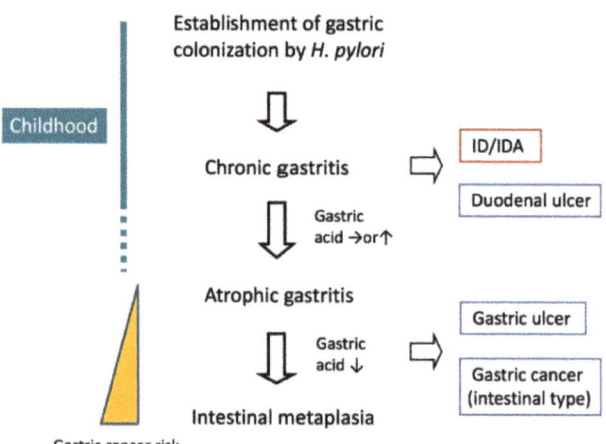

Figure 1. *H. pylori* infection and the related diseases.

It is known that *H. pylori* is closely associated with the development of IDA in children. Unlike in gastric cancer, *H. pylori*-associated IDA occurs commonly in children and adolescents [9]. Improvement of the associated IDA by eradication of *H. pylori* appears to be dependent primarily upon pediatric age groups, which might not be generalizable to adult populations [10]. These facts lead to a hypothesis that the pathogenesis of the IDA differs from that of gastric ulcer or cancer caused by long-term infection of *H. pylori* (Figure 1). There is a possibility that the development of *H. pylori*-associated IDA in children might not depend solely upon mucosal injury and pathologies such as gastric atrophy and intestinal metaplasia.

It is thought that the pathogenesis and clinical outcome of *H. pylori*-associated diseases, including IDA, depend upon multiple factors, including but not limited to bacterial virulence and environmental factors, as well as host genetic and acquired factors. Furthermore, it is the interaction between these bacterial and host factors and the modulation or influence by environmental exposures that affects the host microbiome, i.e., synergistic mechanisms that then result in gastro-duodenal mucosal disease outcome. However, the specific mechanisms underlying *H. pylori*-associated IDA remain poorly understood. In the present review, the biologically plausible and possible pathogenesis of *H. pylori*-associated IDA in childhood and adolescence and the clinical aspects, including management are discussed.

2. Clinical Aspects of *H. pylori*-Associated IDA

2.1. Iron Absorption in Humans

Non-heme iron accounts for >80% of dietary iron in developed countries [11]. Reduction from ferric (Fe^{+++}) to the ferrous (Fe^{++}) forms of iron is essential for intestinal absorption, and in this process gastric acid and ascorbic acid play important roles [11]. Non-heme iron is absorbed primarily in the proximal small intestine via the divalent metal transporter-1 expressed in the proximal duodenum mucosa [10]. On the other hand, the mechanism of absorption of heme iron remains to be poorly understood. Important regulators of hepcidin produced by hepatocytes, and, therefore, of systemic iron homeostasis, include the following components; plasma iron concentration, body iron stores, infection and inflammation, and erythropoiesis [10].

2.2. Clinical Evidence

It is reported that up to ID or IDA occurs in one-fourth of children with *H. pylori* infection [12]. *H. pylori* infection prevalence increases in the pre-teen and adolescent age groups, and IDA is also more prevalent in those age groups, irrespective of cause [6]. In a pediatric study in Alaska [13], ID was highly prevalent among school-aged children, and *H. pylori* infection was independently associated with ID and IDA. On the other hand, several studies showed no causal relationship between IDA and *H. pylori* infection in children [14–16]. In a randomized controlled study in Bangladeshi children [17], it was shown that *H. pylori* infection is neither a cause of ID/IDA nor a reason for treatment failure with iron supplementation.

However, many epidemiological and interventional studies have shown an association between *H. pylori* infection and ID/IDA in children [13,18,19]. In an international multi-center pediatric study [20], there was a significant association observed between *H. pylori* infection and low ferritin concentration in Chile and Brazil but not in United Kingdom. We speculate that these differences could be explained by different host factors in the populations infected in Chile and Brazil, compared to the U.K., and/or different environmental exposures in these geographically distinct populations, thereby leading to specific indigenous microbiome differences in these population, leading to ID/IDA in one and not in the other population. Meta-analyses have shown that a risk of ID and IDA, particularly that which is unexplained, is higher in individuals with *H. pylori* infection than in those without the infection [21,22]. *H. pylori* eradication can reduce the prevalence of ID in children [20]. It has been demonstrated that the eradication of *H. pylori* could improve iron status with IDA [23]. In a meta-analysis with 16 randomized controlled trials [24], it was demonstrated that *H. pylori* eradication therapy plus oral iron supplementation significantly increased levels of hemoglobin, serum iron, and ferritin more than iron supplementation alone. In particular, such effect for hematological indices with anti-*H. pylori* treatment was also shown in patients with moderate or severe IDA.

Recent studies have reported that *H. pylori*-associated IDA is frequently refractory to iron-supplementation therapy or shows recurrent episodes of the IDA once supplementation has been discontinued [25,26]. Such refractory or recurrent natures of *H. pylori*-associated IDA can be resolved by eradication of the bacteria [23,25,27]. Eradication of *H. pylori* results in reversal of long-standing IDA [28,29]. Furthermore, successful eradication of *H. pylori* leads to long-term resolution of refractory or recurrent IDA in Japanese teenagers [27]. Taking together the cumulative evidence described above, it is concluded that *H. pylori* causality on childhood IDA has been established. In addition, it is thought that *H. pylori* plays a central role in the pathogenesis of *H. pylori*-associated IDA.

3. Pathogenesis

3.1. Gastrointestinal Mucosal Lesions and IDA

IDA can be directly caused by blood loss from H. pylori-induced mucosal injury and gastroduodenal lesions such as erosions and ulcerations. A previous study showed that hemorrhagic gastritis was consistent and key finding in the Alaska native population who have a long history of refractory ID and in whom H. pylori infection is prevalent [30]. Moreover, some of H. pylori-infected Alaska native children had peptic ulcers with active bleeding that is clinically severe enough to require endoscopic hemostasis [31,32]. AGA technical review stresses that any gastrointestinal lesion that causes a mucosal defect can bleed enough to lead to both overt and/or occult blood loss and, therefore, cause IDA [10]. This review also mentioned that the clinical spectrum is broad because many different lesions in distinct gastrointestinal sites are capable of bleeding in an occult manner. In H. pylori-infected children, however, the most common clinical diagnosis at diagnostic upper endoscopy is chronic gastritis without any hemorrhagic mucosal lesions [32,33]. In a pediatric multi-center study in Japan [33], it is suggested that blood loss from the gastrointestinal tract rarely causes IDA in children with H. pylori infection. Children with H. pylori-associated IDA often have no endoscopic hemorrhagic lesions and negative results for fecal occult blood tests using ant-hemoglobin antibodies [27,34]. Blood loss from the gastrointestinal mucosa does not appear to be the primary pathogenetic cause of H. pylori-associated IDA /ID in Alaska native children. Thus, upper gastrointestinal mucosal lesions do not appear to play a direct or central role for IDA pathogenesis in H. pylori-infected children (Figure 2).

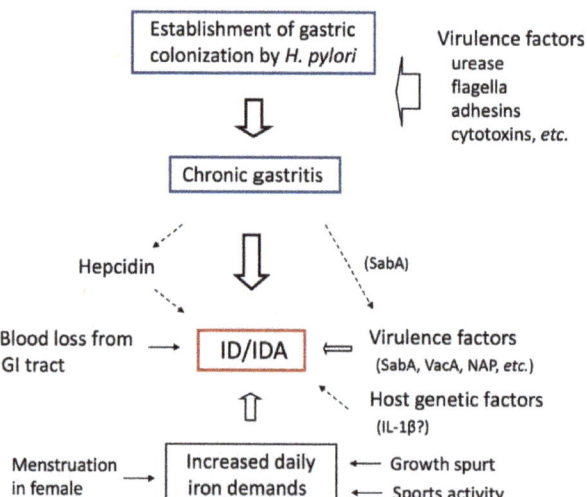

Figure 2. Possible pathogenesis of H. pylori-associated IDA in childhood and adolescence.

In some Western countries, Celiac disease is important as a cause of IDA, irrespective of H. pylori infection [20,35]. In developing countries, other non-H. pylori infections, in particular gastrointestinal parasitic infection, should be considered as risk factors of ID/IDA in addition to contributing factors of poor iron intake and low dietary iron bioavailability that occur in parasite endemic regions of the world [20].

3.2. Impaired Gastric Acid Secretion

Impaired iron absorption due to reduced gastric acidity and ascorbic acid concentration, both of which are related to H. pylori gastritis and, in particular, atrophic gastritis, are suggested as important pathogenetic factors of H. pylori-associated IDA in adults [36].

In addition, an association between transient hypochlorhydria often observed as a consequence of acute *H. pylori* infection and IDA is suggested [37,38]. However, *H. pylori* chronic gastritis is often not atrophic in the majority of the infected children [39] (Figure 1). In an international study with *H. pylori*-associated IDA, corpus atrophy was observed in only two patients and no intestinal metaplasia in any children studied [21]. In a recent Chinese study [40], chronic atrophic gastritis was observed in only 4.4% of *H. pylori*-infected children and neither marked atrophy nor intestinal metaplasia was detected in any patients. Conversely, it is reported that interleukin (IL)-1β may influence ID/IDA risk in *H. pylori*-infected children [41,42]. IL-1β is one of the earliest and most important pro-inflammatory cytokines, and has been detected in both in vitro and in vivo studies of *H. pylori* infection, and IL-1β is also a powerful inhibitor of gastric acid secretion [43]. However, gastric acid secretion is not universally impaired in children with *H. pylori* chronic gastritis, although the secretion is markedly increased in those with *H. pylori*-associated duodenal ulcers [44]. It can be concluded that impaired gastric acid secretion does not appear to be a primary or direct cause of *H. pylori*-associated IDA in childhood and adolescents.

3.3. Hepcidin

Hepcidin is an iron-regulatory hormone and inhibits macrophage iron release and intestinal absorption, leading to hypoferremia [45]. Hepcidin plays a key mediator of hypoferremia observed and associated with inflammation. Studies have demonstrated that IL-6 induces hepcidin expression in hepatic cells [46]. In *H. pylori*-infected children, IDA may be caused by increased serum hepcidin [47] (Figure 2). Anemia of chronic inflammation is mediated, in part, by the stimulation of hepcidin by cytokines [48]. Therefore, it has been suggested that refractory-increased hepcidin levels may be involved in the failure of patients with *H. pylori* infection to respond to iron [48].

3.4. Recent Pathogenetic Hypothesis

It has been recently hypothesized that competition between *H. pylori* and humans for iron availability could lead to IDA [9]. Iron is essential for cell growth and maintenance not only in human hosts but also in the principle metabolic processes of a number of bacteria, in particular *H. pylori*. Most strains of *H. pylori* likely perform some degree of iron metabolism necessary for their survival and reproduction in the gastric environment, may not, by themselves harm the health of most infected hosts. If this hypothesis is right, it is speculated that some of *H. pylori* strains are not harmful for the host [49], and the others aggressively steal bioavailable iron from the host, resulting in ID/IDA. It has been reported that *H. pylori* strains from IDA patients show more rapid growth and enhanced uptake of both ferrous and ferric ions compared to those from non-IDA patients [50]. In the other study [34], however, the degree of bacterial growth was not significantly different between the IDA and control strains. Thus, further studies will be needed to determine the specific phenotype(s) of the infecting *H. pylori* strains and whether the patient is then at risk for ID or IDA.

3.4.1. Iron-Uptake Mechanisms in *H. pylori*

Knowledge of iron-uptake mechanisms in *H. pylori* is still limited. Many bacteria secrete siderophores, high-affinity ferric chelators, and take up ferric iron-siderophore complexes via specific outer membrane proteins (OMPs) [51]. Although *H. pylori* does not have an identified siderophore or its specific receptor, the microorganism expresses several proteins associated with iron metabolism, including the ferric uptake regulator (Fur), high-affinity transporters of ferrous iron (FeoB) and ferric dicitrate (FecA), as well as non-heme iron-containing ferritin (Pfr) [52] (Table 1). In addition, several iron-responsive OMPs are suggested to play roles in *H. pylori* heme uptake [53,54]. Under iron-restricted conditions, *fecA* gene and *frpB* encoding iron-regulated OMP were up-regulated [34], while in iron-replete environments, *H. pylori* expresses a single *fecA3* and *frpB4* OMP [52]. Contrarily, *pfr* gene is down-regulated under iron-restricted conditions. Under iron-restricted conditions, the expression of several genes is up-regulated in a Fur-dependent manner [52,55]. *H. pylori* Fur protein is also a versatile regulator involved in many pathways essential for gastric colonization [55].

Table 1. Primary genes associated with iron uptake in *H. pylori* host infection and regulation of their expression by iron.

Gene	Function (Hypothetical)	Iron-Deplete Condition	Fur-Regulated
fur	Ferric uptake regulator	up-regulation	-
fecA	Ferric dicitrate transportor	up-regulation	Yes
feoB	Ferrous iron transportor	up-regulation	Yes
frpB	Iron-regulated OMP *	up-regulation	Yes
pfr	Iron-containing ferritin	down-regulation	Yes
ceuE	Iron-transport protein	no regulation?	No

* Outer membrane protein.

3.4.2. Bacterial Virulence Factors

A number of studies demonstrated that *H. pylori* colonizes the stomach with multiple or plural strains and that the degree, severity and phenotype of gastric pathology depends on complex interplay between various *H. pylori* virulence genes, host genetics, and environmental factors [56]. In particular, it is not known at what stage during the natural history of the infection a certain *H. pylori* strain genotype predominates the persisting infection, thereby resulting in a specific disease phenotype or outcome. It is also known that *H. pylori* shows the genetic diversity across species [57]. *H. pylori* virulence genes can be mainly categorized into three classes: those related to adhesion and colonization, those related to their virulence and ability to confer gastroduodenal mucosal injury, and others [58]. With regard to the initial stage of the colonization of *H. pylori* in the stomach, OMPs expressed on the bacterial surface are important as virulence factors and can bind to gastric epithelial cells [59]. The *H. pylori* genome has nearly 60 genes encoding the OMPs [60].

H. pylori Colonization and Adhesins

Establishment of *H. pylori* colonization in the stomach is the initial and important step for the development of the subsequent related diseases (Figure 2). *H. pylori* neutralizes the gastric mucosal local environment using its urease activity, which, thereby, enables this organism to occupy the unique biologic microaerophilic neutral pH niche at the mucosal surface underneath the strong acidic gastric environment. *H. pylori* move freely in the dense mucosal layer with a bundle of 2–6 unipolar flagella. However, these specific virulent determinants are similar across all viable *H. pylori* strains and, thus, are thought to be non-specific factor for IDA developments. On the other hand, it is suggested that genes that regulate flagellar synthesis might be involved in the regulation of other virulence factors such as adhesins [61].

Among OMPs, the members of *H. pylori* outer membrane protein (Hop) group, sialic acid-binding adhesin (SabA), and blood group antigen-binding adhesin (BabA) are some of the most frequently studied OMPs [62]. *H. pylori* attaches to the surface-adherent mucus and directly to the gastric epithelial cells with several adhesins, such as SabA and BabA [62] (Figure 2). Once *H. pylori* colonization on the epithelium is established, the bacteria release toxins, including cytotoxin-associated gene A (CagA) and vacuolating cytotoxin A (VacA), leading to gastric inflammation and injury. Risk factors of *H. pylori*-associated diseases include the presence of the *cag* pathogenicity island (*cag*PAI) encoding Type IV secretion system and CagA, *vacA* genotypes, OMPs, including BabA and SabA, and outer membrane inflammatory protein OipA [63,64].

BabA and SabA of *H. pylori* allow the bacteria to persistently colonize in the stomach via interaction with Lewis (Le) and sialylated Lewis (sLe) antigens on gastric epithelia cells, respectively [62,65,66]. It is thought that SabA adhesin plays a key role for gastric colonization in the stage of persistent infection, whereas BabA is an important adhesin in the early stage of the infection [62]. The sLe^x and sLe^a antigens are thought to be important for *H. pylori* adherence and colonization in the stomach [56]. Although these antigens are rarely present in normal gastric mucosa, gastric inflammation induced by *H. pylori* promotes up-regulation of sLe^x antigens, resulting in enhancement of especially the SabA-mediated attachment to the gastric epithelium [65]. Among sLe antigens, the main target receptor of SabA protein is sLe^x [62]. On the other hand, the majority of *H. pylori* strains express at least one type of Le antigens. Thus, *H. pylori* molecular mimicry in the form of Le antigens on the bacterial cell surface provides effective mechanisms enabling *H. pylori* colonization within the gastric mucosa, thereby effectively evading the host immune response [67]. SabA also plays a role in non-opsonic activation of human neutrophils [68].

Major Cytotoxins

Pathogen-associated molecular patterns (PAMPs), such as lipopolysaccharide (LPS) and flagella, are also the major pathogenetic factors of virulent colonizing *H. pylori* strains [69]. The cytotoxins, such as CagA, VacA and PAMPs, activate antigen-presenting cells, dendritic cells, and macrophages, resulting in stimulation of the adaptive immune response through the production of cytokines, including IL-12 and IL-23 [70].

CagA along with a type IV secretion system is thought to play an important role in the development of gastric cancer [67]. However, *H. pylori* strains can be divided into two types, those that possesses CagA and those that do not express the protein, therefore, the presence or absence of CagA is not always a key pathogenetic factor for *H. pylori*-associated disorders [67]. In a Slovenian study, the *cagA* genotype in children was associated with the degree of gastric inflammation [71]. However, *H. pylori* strains isolated from Japanese children exclusively carried the *cagA* gene, but there were no associations between this gene and the severity of gastritis or peptic ulcer disease [72]. The adherence of *H. pylori* to the gastric epithelial cells induces the expression of CagA, which is reported to be regulated by the Fur protein [73]. In a Japanese study [34], however, there was no association observed between expression of *cagA* gene and development of childhood IDA.

VacA is also an important cytotoxin as *H. pylori* virulence factors, which promotes bacterial colonization and survival in the host cells [74,75]. VacA is considered a multifunctional toxin inducing host cell damage [21,30]. VacA stimulates the regulatory T cells and promotes differentiation to effector T cells, resulting in persistent colonization of *H. pylori* in the gastric mucosa [76]. It is suggested that VacA escapes host immune defenses by differentially regulating the expression of host genes related to immune evasion [77]. It is reported that co-expression of CagA with OipA, VacA, and BabA plays synergic effects in the outcome of *H. pylori*-induced gastric pathologies and disorders [78]. It has been further suggested that VacA is synergistically involved in the pathogenesis of childhood *H. pylori*-associated IDA [34].

IDA-Specific Bacterial Factors

Studies on an association between *H. pylori*-specific genes and IDA are limited. It must be noted that expression profiles of genes related to iron metabolism can dynamically change under both iron-replete and depleted conditions. Comparative proteomic analysis suggests that particular *H. pylori* polymorphisms could promote IDA [79]. On the other hand, it was also reported that variation of *feoB* or *pfr* gene is not implicated in IDA development [13,80]. Besides these two genes, known genes related to iron uptake/regulation such as *fecA* and *fur*, were not also involved in IDA pathogenesis [34].

Neutrophil-activating protein (NAP) stimulates neutrophil adherence to the gastric mucosa and its activation, leading to a release of IL-12 and IL-23 that facilitate the Th-1 immune response [81,82]. It is reported that genetic polymorphisms in the *napA* gene may be associated with the pathogenesis of IDA [83,84] (Figure 2). Recently, a high expression of *sabA* gene in *H. pylori* has been reported to be associated with IDA in childhood and adolescence [34]. Interestingly, as previously mentioned, this study also shows that *vacA* may play a synergic role in the development of IDA. The *sabA* gene is highly divergent and regulated with complex mechanisms [62]. Although the SabA expression is thought to enable rapid response to changing conditions in the stomach by switching the "on" (functional) "off" (non-functional), its mechanism remains to be elucidated [62]. A higher salt concentration induces a higher SabA transcription level [85]. As mentioned above, SabA is an important adhesin and detectable in approximately 40% of *H. pylori* strains [67]. SabA has an ability of activating neutrophils through non-opsonic mechanism resulting in damages of the gastric epithelial cells [70]. Sab A is associated with an increased risk of atrophic gastritis and gastric cancer, although causative mechanisms to explain this disease-related association remain controversial [65]. These facts lead to the recognition that *sabA* gene is an important virulence factor in the development of childhood *H. pylori*-associated diseases, including *H. pylori*-associated IDA.

3.4.3. Host Factors

Increased Iron Demands as Acquired Factors

It is well known that children, particularly during the first five years of life, are at risk of IDA, which is mainly associated with an increased iron demand due to their rapid growth [86]. *H. pylori* acquisition mainly occurs in infants and younger children via oral–oral or fecal–oral routes. However, *H. pylori*-associated IDA rarely occurs in the early years of life. A randomized control study reported that *H. pylori* is not a cause for treatment failure of iron supplementation in children 2–5 years of age [17]. Contrarily, *H. pylori*-associated IDA frequently occurs in school-aged children, suggesting that increased iron demand due to growth spurt and/or participation in sports-related activities is also important in the pathogenesis [9,25]. Choe et al. reported that increased daily iron demand is important in *H. pylori*-associated IDA in adolescent female athletes [87]. However, sporting activity itself is reported to have no association to *H. pylori*-associated IDA/ID, although the number of female adolescents studied is small [88]. Although both pre-school and school-aged children have increased daily iron demand, *H. pylori* seems to play some causal role for IDA development in the latter but not in the former. It is strongly suggested that on underlying mechanisms of *H. pylori*-associated IDA, the infection itself is a necessary condition but not the primary etiological agent.

Host Genetic Factors

Host immune response gene polymorphism affects the susceptibility to *H. pylori* infection and the outcome of *H. pylori*-related disorders [42]. In one study of twins with *H. pylori* infection [89], it was suggested that host genetic factors are important in the development of ID or IDA. In a recent study [27], one sibling case with recurrent *H. pylori*-associated IDA showed long-term resolution after successful eradication therapy.

Toll-like receptors (TLRs) belong to the large family of pattern recognition receptors (PRRs) and are important in the innate immunity of the host [90]. Among the 10 types of TLRs identified in humans [91], TLR2 and TLR4 on the gastric epithelial and immune cells are both associated with recognition of LPS composing the cell wall of *H. pylori*, acting as a primary defense against *H. pylori* [60,92]. However, it seems that TLRs, including these two molecules can play opposite roles, either promotion or suppression of *H. pylori* infection as innate immunity [90]. TLR5 initially plays some role for the recognition of *H. pylori* flagellin, but this bacterium appears to develop mechanisms to escape such recognition for the persistent infection [90]. Although this genetic variation may be advantageous for some individuals, such variation may be less favorable outcomes for other ones that harbor certain genotypes associated with excessive immune response [93]. The LPS recognition receptor TLR4 has been shown to be associated with a higher risk of gastric cancer [90]. Thus, we believe that the roles of TLRs for *H. pylori*-associated IDA remain to be studied.

Host genetic factors that affect cytokines may determine differences in the susceptibility or risk of infected individuals to specific *H. pylori*-associated diseases [70]. It is reported that various single-nucleotide polymorphisms (SNPs) of cytokines genes, such as tumor necrosis factor (TNF)-α, IL-1β, and IL-10, are associated with the risk of precancerous gastric pathology, including atrophic gastritis and intestinal metaplasia [60], although such an association remains controversial [70]. The allelic distribution of IL-1β is one of the most popular candidate gene studied on *H. pylori* infection [59]. Polymorphism of pro-inflammatory cytokine genes encoding IL-1, IL-8, IL-10, and TNF-α is associated with increased risk of *H. pylori*-related gastric cancer and duodenal ulcer disease [58,94,95]. The expression of IL-1β gene increases in *H. pylori*-infected children with ID [96] (Figure 2). A study in Brazilian children has shown that high gastric levels of IL-1β can be the link between *H. pylori* infection and ID/IDA in childhood [41]. Increased concentration of gastric IL-1β was an independent predictor for low blood concentration of ferritin and hemoglobin. In a case–control study from Taiwan, it was reported that IL-1β gene polymorphism may influence ID risk in *H. pylori*-infected children [42]. Pediatric patients with *H. pylori* gastritis showed significantly lower levels of serum ferritin, prohepcidin, and IL-6 compared to those with *H. pylori*-negative gastritis and the healthy control [97]. In this latter study, however, *H. pylori* eradication therapy revealed no significant difference in serum ferritin, prohepcidin, or IL-6 levels.

TNF-α is involved in persistent colonization with *H. pylori* in the stomach [98]. It has been shown that specific TNF-α genotypes are at risk for duodenal ulcer and gastric cancer, but other TNF-α genotypes have a protective function against cancer development [59]. TNF-α has no association with *H. pylori*-associated ID/IDA in children [41].

4. Clinical Management Strategies

Although *H. pylori* infection once established persists almost for the host life span, an overwhelming majority of the infected persons remain clinically asymptomatic and suffer no consequences related to their infection. Despite *H. pylori* infection being the primary causative agent for gastric cancer, the microorganisms can produce detrimental or beneficial effects [49]. In a recent systematic review and meta-analysis [99,100], there is some evidence of an inverse association between atopy/allergic diseases and *H. pylori* infection. On clinical strategies, it is very important to consider that universal eradication of *H. pylori* may cause more harm than good for the host with the infection [49]. Pediatric guidelines recommend against a test-and-treat strategy in asymptomatic children, even if the purpose of the strategy is prophylaxis for of gastric cancer [6,7]. Such a consideration is necessary especially for the management of this infection in children.

The Maastricht V/Florence Consensus Report has recommended *H. pylori* testing and eradication therapy for patients with unexplained IDA [101]. On this recommendation, however, the level of evidence is very low. Such a low evidence level suggests that the data on *H. pylori*-associated IDA is insufficient, especially in the adult population. The American Gastroenterological Association (AGA) technical review identified low-quality evidence supporting *H. pylori* testing for patients with IDA [10]. This review has suggested the causal role of *H. pylori* for IDA in the select population, in particular in children, although the relationship is unclear in the majority of adult men and postmenopausal women [10]. In this issue, it has been indicated that two of three RTCs that met the inclusion criteria were in the pediatric population. AGA clinical practice guidelines suggest noninvasive *H. pylori* testing for patients with IDA without other identifiable etiology for bidirectional endoscopy, followed by treatment if positive [102]. On the other hand, in the Houston consensus conference [103], idiopathic thrombocytopenia was discussed regarding the identification of appropriate patients for *H. pylori* testing but not IDA.

The updated North American and European joint pediatric guidelines suggest *H. pylori* testing in children with refractory IDA in which other causes have been ruled out [6]. On the other hand, these guidelines strongly recommend against diagnostic testing for *H. pylori* infection as part of the initial investigation in children with IDA. Pediatric guidelines from Japan recommend eradication therapy for *H. pylori*-infected children with IDA in whom IDA is recurrent or refractory over iron supplementation therapy [7]. The level of evidence for this recommendation from the Japanese guidelines is strong. In summary, "test-and-treat" strategy in *H. pylori* infection should be considered for children and adolescents with recurrent or refractory IDA of unknown causes.

5. Perspectives

It is beyond doubt that increased iron demands play an important pathogenetic part in *H. pylori*-associated IDA in children and adolescents. On the other hand, both bacterial virulence and host genetic factors remain to be investigated. Definitive factors are also still not identified on gastric carcinogenesis by *H. pylori* infection in adults. In any case, as mentioned previously, physicians should keep *H. pylori* infection in mind as an important differential diagnosis for children with recurrent or refractory IDA.

It is indicated that *H. pylori* is an important causative factor in the vicious cycle of malnutrition and growth impairments [38], although the literature has many confounding variables and *H pylori* infection is a marker of low economic status. These authors also suggested that direct competition between *H. pylori* and the host for iron is an important contributor to IDA. In Gambia, *H. pylori* colonization in early infancy predisposes the child for subsequent development of malnutrition and growth faltering, although the effect did not persist into later childhood [104]. Furthermore, decreased growth velocity improved significantly over time once *H. pylori* eradication was successful in Colombian children [105]. However, the relationship between *H. pylori*-associated ID/IDA and growth impairment in the *H. pylori*-infected children, especially in developing countries, remains to be further characterized. Clearly, further well-designed, population-based investigations are needed on this issue.

Author Contributions: Original draft preparation, S.K.; Review and editing, B.D.G. and A.K. All authors have read and agreed to the published version of the manuscript.

Funding: This research received no external funding.

Institutional Review Board Statement: Not applicable.

Informed Consent Statement: Not applicable.

Acknowledgments: We thank Katsuhisa Hashimoto for assistance preparing the figures.

Conflicts of Interest: The authors declare no conflict of interest.

References

1. McColl, K.E. Clinical practice. *Helicobacter pylori* infection. *N. Engl. J. Med.* **2010**, *362*, 1597–1604. [PubMed]
2. Shatila, M.; Thomas, A.S. Current and future perspectives in the diagnosis and management of *Helicobacter pylori* infection. *J. Clin. Med.* **2022**, *11*, 5086. [CrossRef] [PubMed]
3. Uemura, N.; Okamoto, S.; Yamamoto, S.; Matsumura, N.; Yamaguchi, S.; Yamakido, M.; Taniyama, K.; Sasaki, N.; Schlemper, R.J. *Helicobacter pylori* infection and the development of gastric cancer. *N. Engl. J. Med.* **2001**, *345*, 784–789. [CrossRef] [PubMed]
4. Kato, S.; Sherman, P.M. What is new related to *Helicobacter pylori* infection in children and teenagers? *Arch. Pediatr. Adolesc.* **2005**, *159*, 415–421. [CrossRef] [PubMed]
5. International Agency for Research on Cancer (IARC). *Schistosomes, Liver Flukes and Helicobacter pylori*; IARC: Lyon, France, 1994; pp. 1–241.
6. Jones, N.L.; Koletzko, S.; Goodman, K.; Bontems, P.; Cadranel, S.; Casswall, T.; Czinn, S.; Gold, B.D.; Guarner, J.; Elitsur, Y.; et al. Joint ESPGHAN/NASPGHAN guidelines for the management of *Helicobacter pylori* in children and adolescents (Update 2016). *J. Pediatr. Gastroenterol. Nutr.* **2017**, *64*, 991–1003. [CrossRef]
7. Kato, S.; Shimizu, T.; Toyoda, S.; Gold, B.D.; Ida, S.; Ishige, T.; Fujimura, S.; Kamiya, S.; Konno, M.; Kuwabara, K.; et al. The updated JSPGHAN guideline for the management of *Helicobacter pylori* infection in childhood. *Pediatr. Int.* **2020**, *62*, 1315–1331. [CrossRef]
8. Razavi, A.; Bagheri, N.; Azadegan-Dehkordi, F.; Shirzad, M.; Rahimian, G.; Rafieian-Kopaei, M.; Shirzad, H. Comparative immune response in children and adults with *H. pylori* infection. *J. Immunol. Res.* **2015**, *2015*, 315957. [CrossRef]
9. Barabino, A. *Helicobacter pylori*-related iron deficiency anemia: A review. *Helicobacter* **2002**, *7*, 71–75. [CrossRef]
10. Rockey, D.C.; Altayar, O.; Falck-Ytter, Y.; Kalmaz, D. AGA technical review on gastrointestinal evaluation of iron deficiency anemia. *Gastroenterology* **2020**, *159*, 1097–1119. [CrossRef]
11. Lombard, M.; Chua, E.; O'Toole, P. Regulation of intestinal non-haem iron absorption. *Gut* **1997**, *40*, 435–439. [CrossRef]

12. Vendt, N.; Kool, P.; Teesalu, K.; Lillemäek, K.; Maaroos, H.I.; Oona, M. Iron deficiency and *Helicobacter pylori* infection in children. *Acta Paediatr.* **2011**, *100*, 1239–1243. [CrossRef] [PubMed]
13. Baggett, H.C.; Parkinson, A.J.; Muth, P.T.; Gold, B.D.; Gessener, B.D. Endemic iron deficiency associated with *Helicobacter pylori* infection among school-aged children in Alaska. *Pediatrics* **2006**, *117*, e396–e404. [CrossRef] [PubMed]
14. Janjetic, M.A.; Goldman, C.G.; Balcarce, N.E.; Rua, E.C.; González, A.B.; Fuda, J.A.; Meseri, E.I.; Torti, H.E.; Barrado, J.; Zubillaga, M.B.; et al. Iron, zinc, and copper nutritional status in children infected with *Helicobacter Pylori*. *J. Pediatr. Gastroenterol. Nutr.* **2010**, *51*, 85–89. [CrossRef] [PubMed]
15. Thankachan, P.; Muthayya, S.; Sierksma, A.; Eilander, A.; Thomas, T.; Duchateau, G.S.; Frenken, L.G.J.; Kurpad, A.V. *Helicobacter pylori* infection does not influence the efficacy of iron and vitamin B(12) fortification in marginally nourished Indian children. *Eur. J. Clin. Nutr.* **2010**, *64*, 1101–1107. [CrossRef]
16. Mendoza, E.; Camorlinga-Ponce, M.; Perez-Perez, G.; Mera, R.; Vilchis, J.; Moran, S.; Rivera, O.; Coria, R.; Torres, J.; Correa, P.; et al. Present and past *Helicobacter pylori* infection in Mexican school children. *Helicobacter* **2014**, *19*, 55–64. [CrossRef]
17. Sarker, S.A.; Mahmud, H.; Davidsson, L.; Alam, N.H.; Ahmed, T.; Alam, N.; Salam, M.A.; Beglinger, C.; Gyr, N.; Fuchs, G.J. Causal relationship of *Helicobacter pylori* with iron-deficiency anemia or failure of iron supplementation in children. *Gastroenterology* **2008**, *135*, 1534–1542. [CrossRef]
18. Ashorn, M.; Ruuska, T.; Mäkipernaa, A. *Helicobacter pylori* and iron deficiency anemia in children. *Scand. J. Gastroenterol.* **2001**, *36*, 701–705. [CrossRef]
19. Fagan, R.P.; Dunaway, C.E.; Bruden, D.L.; Parkinson, A.J.; Gessner, B.D. Controlled, household-randomized, open-label trial of the effect of treatment of *Helicobacter pylori* infection on iron deficiency anemia among children in rural Alaska: Results at 40 months. *J. Infect. Dis.* **2009**, *199*, 652–660. [CrossRef]
20. Qu, X.H.; Huang, X.L.; Xiong, P.; Zhu, C.Y.; Huang, Y.L.; Lu, L.G.; Sun, X.; Rong, L.; Zhong, L.; Sun, D.Y.; et al. Does *Helicobacter pylori* infection play a role in iron deficiency anemia? A meta-analysis. *World J. Gastroenterol.* **2010**, *16*, 886–896.
21. Hudak, L.; Jaraisy, A.; Haj, S.; Muhsen, K. An updated systematic review and meta-analysis on the association between *Helicobacter pylori* infection and iron deficiency anemia. *Helicobacter* **2017**, *22*, e12330. [CrossRef]
22. Queiroz, D.M.M.; Harris, P.R.; Sanderson, I.R.; Windle, H.J.; Walker, M.M.; Rocha, A.M.C.; Rocha, G.A.; Carvalho, S.D.; Bittencourt, P.F.S.; Castro, L.P.F.; et al. Iron status and *Helicobacter pylori* infection in symptomatic children: An international multi-centered study. *PLoS ONE* **2013**, *8*, e68833. [CrossRef] [PubMed]
23. Malfertheiner, P.; Selgrad, M. *Helicobacter pylori* infection and current clinical areas of contention. *Curr. Opin. Gastroenterol.* **2010**, *26*, 618–623. [CrossRef] [PubMed]
24. Yuan, W.; Yumin, L.; Kehu, Y.; Bin, M.; Quanlin, G.; Wang, D.; Yang, L. Iron deficiency anemia in *Helicobacter pylori* infection: Meta-analysis of randomized controlled trials. *Scand. J. Gastroenterol.* **2010**, *45*, 665–676. [PubMed]
25. DuBois, S.; Kearney, D.J. Iron-deficiency anemia and *Helicobacter pylori* infection: A review of the evidence. *Am. J. Gastroenterol.* **2005**, *100*, 453–459. [CrossRef] [PubMed]
26. Gheibi, S.; Farrokh-Eslamlou, H.R.; Noroozi, M.; Pakniyat, A. Refractory iron deficiency anemia and *Helicobacter pylori* infection in pediatrics: A review. *Iran. J. Pediatr. Hematol. Oncol.* **2015**, *15*, 50–64.
27. Kato, S.; Gold, B.D.; Kato, A. The resolution of severe iron-deficiency anemia after successful eradication of *Helicobacter pylori* in teenagers. *JPGN Rep.* **2022**, *3*, e238. [CrossRef]
28. Annibale, B.; Marignani, M.; Monarca, B.; Antonelli, G.; Marcheggiano, A.; Martino, G.; Mandelli, F.; Caprilli, R.; Delle Fave, G. Reversal of iron deficiency anemia after *Helicobacter pylori* eradication in patients with asymptomatic gastritis. *Ann. Intern. Med.* **1999**, *131*, 668–672. [CrossRef]
29. Marignani, M.; Angeletti, S.; Bordi, C.; Malagnino, F.; Mancino, C.; Delle Fave, G.; Annibale, B. Reversal of long-standing iron deficiency anemia after eradication of *Helicobacter pylori* infection. *Scand. J. Gastroenterol.* **1997**, *32*, 617–622. [CrossRef]
30. DiGirolamo, A.M.; Perry, G.S.; Gold, B.D.; Parkinson, A.; Provost, E.M.; Parvanta, I.; Grummer-Strawn, L.M. *Helicobacter pylori*, anemia, and iron deficiency: Relationship explored among Alaska native children. *Pediatr. Infect. Dis. J.* **2007**, *26*, 927–934. [CrossRef]
31. Kato, S.; Ozawa, A.; Ebina, K.; Nakagawa, H. Endoscopic ethanol injection for treatment of bleeding peptic ulcer. *Eur. J. Pediatr.* **1994**, *153*, 873–875. [CrossRef]
32. Kato, S.; Takeyama, J.; Ebina, K.; Naganuma, H. Omeprazole-based dual and triple regimens for *Helicobacter pylori* eradication in children. *Pediatrics* **1997**, *100*, e3. [CrossRef] [PubMed]
33. Kato, S.; Nishino, Y.; Ozawa, K.; Konno, M.; Maisawa, S.; Toyoda, S.; Tajiri, H.; Ida, S.; Fujisawa, T.; Iinuma, K. The prevalence of *Helicobacter pylori* in Japanese children with gastritis or peptic ulcer disease. *J. Gastroenterol.* **2004**, *39*, 734–738. [CrossRef] [PubMed]
34. Kato, S.; Osaki, T.; Kamiya, S.; Zhang, X.S.; Blaser, M.J. *Helicobacter pylori sabA* gene is associated with iron deficiency anemia in childhood and adolescence. *PLoS ONE* **2017**, *12*, e0184046. [CrossRef] [PubMed]
35. Virkkula, A.; Kivela, L.; Hiltunen, P.; Sotka, A.; Huhtala, H.; Kurppa, K.; Repo, M. Prevalence and clinical significance of *Helicobacter pylori*-negative chronic gastritis in children. *J. Pediatr. Gastroenterol. Nutr.* **2022**, *74*, 949–955. [CrossRef] [PubMed]
36. Annibale, B.; Capurso, G.; Lahner, E.; Passi, S.; Ricci, R.; Maggio, F.; Fave, G.D. Concomitant alterations in intragastric pH and ascorbic acid concentration in patients with *Helicobacter pylori* gastritis and associated iron deficiency anaemia. *Gut* **2003**, *52*, 496–501. [CrossRef] [PubMed]

37. Harris, P.R.; Serrano, C.A.; Villagran, A.; Walker, M.M.; Thomson, M.; Duarte, I.; Windle, H.J.; Crabtree, J.E. *Helicobacter pylori*-associated hypochlorhydria in children, and development of iron deficiency. *J. Clin. Pathol.* **2013**, *66*, 343–347. [CrossRef] [PubMed]
38. Windle, H.J.; Kelleher, D.; Crabtree, J.E. Childhood *Helicobacter pylori* infection and growth impairment in developing countries: A vicious cycle? *Pediatrics* **2007**, *119*, e754–e759. [CrossRef]
39. Kato, S.; Nakajima, S.; Nishino, Y.; Ozawa, K.; Minoura, T.; Konno, M.; Maisawa, S.; Toyoda, S.; Yoshimura, N.; Vaid, A.; et al. Association between gastric atrophy and *Helicobacter pylori* infection in Japanese children: A retrospective multicenter study. *Dig. Dis. Sci.* **2006**, *51*, 99–104. [CrossRef]
40. Yu, Y.; Su, L.; Wang, X.; Wang, X.; Xu, C. Association between *Helicobacter pylori* infection and pathological changes in the gastric mucosa in Chinese children. *Intern. Med.* **2014**, *53*, 83–88. [CrossRef]
41. Queiroz, D.M.M.; Rocha, A.M.C.; Melo, F.F.; Rocha, G.A.; Teixeira, K.N.; Carvalho, S.D.; Bittencourt, P.F.S.; Castro, L.P.F.; Crabtree, J.E. Increased gastric IL-1β concentration and iron deficiency parameters in *H. pylori* infected children. *PLoS ONE* **2013**, *8*, e57420. [CrossRef]
42. Chen, S.T.; Ni, Y.H.; Liu, S.H. Potential association of *IL1B* polymorphism with iron deficiency risk in childhood *Helicobacter pylori* infection. *J. Pediatr. Gastroenterol. Nutr.* **2018**, *66*, e36–e40. [CrossRef] [PubMed]
43. El-Omar, E.M.; Oien, K.; El-Nujumi, A.; Gillen, D.; Wirz, A.; Dahill, S.; Williams, C.; Ardill, J.E.; McColl, K.E. *Helicobacter pylori* infection and chronic gastric acid hyposecretion. *Gastroenterology* **1997**, *113*, 15–24. [CrossRef] [PubMed]
44. Kato, S.; Ozawa, K.; Koike, T.; Sekine, H.; Ohara, S.; Minoura, T.; Iinuma, K. Effect of *Helicobacter pylori* infection on gastric acid secretion and meal-stimulated serum gastrin in children. *Helicobacter* **2004**, *9*, 100–105. [CrossRef] [PubMed]
45. Andrews, N.C. Anemia of inflammation: The cytokine-hepcidin link. *J. Clin. Investig.* **2004**, *113*, 1251–1253. [CrossRef] [PubMed]
46. Nemeth, E.; Valore, E.V.; Territo, M.; Schiller, G.; Lichtenstein, A.; Ganz, T. Hepcidin, a putative mediator of anemia of inflammation, is a type II acute-phase protein. *Blood* **2003**, *101*, 2461–2463. [CrossRef]
47. Azab, S.F.; Esh, A.M. Serum hepcidin levels in *Helicobacter pylori*-infected children with iron-deficiency anemia: A case-control study. *Ann. Hematol.* **2013**, *92*, 1477–1483. [CrossRef]
48. Beutler, E. Hepcidin mimetics from microorganisms? A possible explanation for the effect of *Helicobacter pylori* on iron homeostasis. *Blood Cells Mol. Dis.* **2007**, *38*, 54–55. [CrossRef]
49. Miller, A.K.; Williams, S.M. *Helicobacter pylori* infection causes both protective and deleterious effects in human health and disease. *Genes Immun.* **2021**, *22*, 218–226. [CrossRef]
50. Yokota, S.; Konno, M.; Mino, E.; Sato, K.; Takahashi, M.; Fujii, N. Enhanced Fe ion-uptake activity in *Helicobacter pylori* strains isolated from patients with iron-deficiency anemia. *Clin. Infect. Dis.* **2008**, *46*, e31–e33. [CrossRef]
51. Andrews, S.C.; Robinson, A.K.; Rodríguez-Quiñones, F. Bacterial iron homeostasis. *FEMS. Microbiol. Rev.* **2003**, *27*, 215–237. [CrossRef]
52. van Vliet, A.H.; Stoof, J.; Vlasblom, R.; Wainwright, S.A.; Hughes, N.J.; Kelly, D.J.; Bereswill, S.; Bijlsma, J.J.; Hoogenboezem, T.; Vandenbrouck-Grauls, C.M.; et al. The role of the Ferric Uptake Regulator (Fur) in regulation of *Helicobacter pylori* iron uptake. *Helicobacter* **2002**, *7*, 237–244. [CrossRef] [PubMed]
53. Worst, D.J.; Otto, B.R.; de Graaff, J. Iron-repressible outer membrane proteins of *Helicobacter pylori* involved in heme uptake. *Infect. Immun.* **1995**, *63*, 4161–4165. [CrossRef] [PubMed]
54. Dhaenens, L.; Szczebara, F.; Husson, M.O. Identification, characterization, and immunogenicity of the lactoferrin-binding protein from *Helicobacter pylori*. *Infect. Immun.* **1997**, *65*, 514–518. [CrossRef] [PubMed]
55. Ernst, F.D.; Bereswill, S.; Waidner, B.; Stoof, J.; Mäder, U.; Kusters, J.G.; Kuipers, E.J.; Kist, M.; van Vliet, A.H.; Homuth, G. Transcriptional profiling of *Helicobacter pylori* Fur- and iron-regulated gene expression. *Microbiology* **2005**, *151*, 533–546. [CrossRef]
56. Sterbenc, A.; Jarc, E.; Poljak, M.; Homan, M. *Helicobacter pylori* virulence genes. *World J. Gastroenterol.* **2019**, *25*, 4870–4884. [CrossRef] [PubMed]
57. Blaser, M.J.; Berg, D.E. *Helicobacter pylori* genetic diversity and risk of human disease. *J. Clin. Investig.* **2001**, *107*, 767–773. [CrossRef]
58. Chen, Y.L.; Mo, X.Q.; Huang, G.R.; Huang, Y.Q.; Xiao, J.; Zhao, L.J.; Wei, H.Y.; Liang, Q. Gene polymorphism of pathogenic *Helicobacter pylori* in patients with different types of gastrointestinal diseases. *World J. Gastroenterol.* **2016**, *28*, 9718–9726. [CrossRef]
59. Datta De, D.; Roychoudhury, S. To be or not to be: The host genetic factor and beyond in *Helicobacter pylori* mediated gastro-duodenal diseases. *World J. Gastroenterol.* **2015**, *21*, 2883–2895. [CrossRef]
60. Zeyaullah, M.; AlShahrani, A.M.; Ahmad, I. Association of *Helicobacter pylori* infection and host cytokine gene polymorphism with gastric cancer. *Can. J. Gastroenterol. Hepatol.* **2021**, *2021*, 8810620. [CrossRef]
61. Clyne, M.; Ocroinin, T.; Suerbaum, S.; Josenhans, C.; Drumm, B. Adherence isogenic flagellum-negative mutants of *Helicobacter pylori* and *Helicobacter mustelae* to human and ferret gastric epithelial cells. *Infect. Immun.* **2000**, *68*, 4335–4339. [CrossRef]
62. Doohan, D.; Rezkitha, Y.A.A.; Waskito, L.A.; Yamaoka, Y.; Miftahussurur, M. *Helicobacter pylori* BabA-SabA key roles in the adherence phase: The synergic mechanism for successful colonization and diseases development. *Toxins* **2021**, *13*, 485. [CrossRef] [PubMed]
63. Kusters, J.G.; van Vliet, A.H.; Kuipers, E.J. Pathogenesis of *Helicobacter pylori* infection. *Clin. Microbiol. Rev.* **2006**, *19*, 449–490. [CrossRef] [PubMed]

64. de Klerk, N.; Maudsdotter, L.; Gebreegziabher, H.; Saroj, S.D.; Eriksson, B.; Eriksson, O.S.; Roos, S.; Lindén, S.; Sjölinder, H.; Jonsson, A.B. Lactobacilli reduce *Helicobacter pylori* attachment to host gastric epithelial cells by inhibiting adhesion gene expression. *Infect. Immun.* **2016**, *84*, 1526–1535. [CrossRef] [PubMed]
65. Mahdavi, J.; Sondén, B.; Hurtig, M.; Olfat, F.O.; Forsberg, L.; Roche, N.; Angström, J.; Larsson, T.; Teneberg, S.; Karlsson, K.A.; et al. *Helicobacter pylori* SabA adhesin in persistent infection and chronic inflammation. *Science* **2002**, *297*, 573–578. [CrossRef] [PubMed]
66. Sheu, B.S.; Odenbreit, S.; Hung, K.H.; Liu, C.P.; Sheu, S.M.; Yang, H.B.; Wu, J.J. Interaction between host gastric sialyl-Lewis x and *H. pylori* SabA enhances *H. pylori* density in patients lacking gastric Lewis b antigen. *Am. J. Gastroenterol.* **2006**, *101*, 36–44. [CrossRef] [PubMed]
67. Baj, J.; Forma, A.; Sitarz, M.; Portincasa, P.; Garruti, G.; Krasowska, D.; Maciejewski, R. *Helicobacter pylori* virulence factors-Mechanisms of bacterial pathogenicity in the gastric microenvironment. *Cells* **2021**, *10*, 27. [CrossRef] [PubMed]
68. Unemo, M.; Aspholm-Hurtig, M.; Ilver, D.; Bergström, J.; Borén, T.; Danielsson, D.; Teneberg, S. The sialic acid binding SabA adhesin of *Helicobacter pylori* is essential for nonopsonic activation of human neutrophils. *J. Biol. Chem.* **2005**, *280*, 15390–15397. [CrossRef]
69. Yamaoka, Y. Mechanisms of disease: *Helicobacter pylori* virulence factors. *Nat. Rev. Gastroenterol. Hepatol.* **2010**, *7*, 629–641. [CrossRef]
70. Figueiredo, C.A.; Marques, C.R.; Costa, R.S.; Silva, H.B.F.; Alcantara-Neves, N.M. Cytokines, cytokine gene polymorphisms and *Helicobacter pylori* infection: Friend or foe? *World J. Gastroenterol.* **2014**, *20*, 5235–5243. [CrossRef]
71. Homan, M.; Luzar, B.; Kocjan, B.J.; Orel, R.; Mocilnik, T.; Shrestha, M.; Kveder, M.; Poljak, M. Prevalence and clinical relevance of *cagA*, *vacA*, and *iceA* genotypes of *Helicobacter pylori* isolated from Slovenian children. *J. Pediatr. Gastroenterol. Nutr.* **2009**, *49*, 289–296. [CrossRef]
72. Azuma, T.; Kato, S.; Zhou, W.; Yamazaki, S.; Yamakawa, A.; Ohtani, M.; Fujiwara, S.; Minoura, T.; Iinuma, K.; Kato, T. Diversity of *vacA* and *cagA* genes of *Helicobacter pylori* in Japanese children. *Aliment. Pharmacol. Ther.* **2004**, *20* (Suppl. S1), 7–12. [CrossRef] [PubMed]
73. Raghwan; Chowdhury, R. Host cell contact induces Fur-dependent expression of virulence factors CagA and VacA in *Helicobacter pylori*. *Helicobacter* **2014**, *19*, 17–25.
74. Raju, D.; Hussey, S.; Ang, M.; Terebiznik, M.R.; Sibony, M.; Galindo-Mata, E.; Gupta, V.; Blanke, S.R.; Delgado, A.; Romero-Gallo, J.; et al. Vacuolating cytotoxin and variants in Atg16L1 that disrupt autophagy promote *Helicobacter pylori* infection in humans. *Gastroeterology* **2012**, *142*, 1160–1171. [CrossRef] [PubMed]
75. Basso, D.; Zambon, C.F.; Letley, D.P.; Stranges, A.; Marchet, A.; Rhead, J.L.; Schiavon, S.; Guariso, G.; Ceroti, M.; Nitti, D.; et al. Clinical relevance of *Helicobacter pylori cagA* and *vacA* gene polymorphisms. *Gastroenterology* **2008**, *135*, 91–99. [CrossRef] [PubMed]
76. Djekic, A.; Müller, A. The immunomodulator VacA promotes immune tolerance and persistent *Helicobacter pylori* infection through its activities on T-cells and antigen-presenting cells. *Toxin* **2016**, *8*, 187. [CrossRef] [PubMed]
77. Yuan, J.P.; Li, T.; Li, Z.H.; Yang, G.Z.; Hu, B.Y.; Shi, X.D.; Shi, T.L.; Tong, S.Q.; Guo, X.K. mRNA expression profiling reveals a role of *Helicobacter pylori* vacuolating toxin in escaping host defense. *World J. Gastroenterol.* **2004**, *10*, 1528–1532. [CrossRef] [PubMed]
78. Zambon, C.F.; Navaglia, F.; Basso, D.; Rugge, M.; Plebani, M. *Helicobacter pylori* babA2, cagA, and s1 vacA genes work synergistically in causing intestinal metaplasia. *J. Clin. Pathol.* **2003**, *56*, 287–291. [CrossRef]
79. Park, S.A.; Lee, H.W.; Hong, M.H.; Choi, Y.W.; Choe, Y.H.; Ahn, B.Y.; Cho, Y.J.; Kim, D.S.; Lee, N.G. Comparative proteomic analysis of *Helicobacter pylori* strains associated with iron deficiency anemia. *Proteomics* **2006**, *6*, 1319–1328. [CrossRef]
80. Choe, Y.H.; Hwang, T.S.; Kim, H.J.; Shin, S.H.; Song, S.U.; Choi, M.S. A possible relation of the *Helicobacter pylori pfr* gene to iron deficiency anemia? *Helicobacter* **2001**, *6*, 55–59. [CrossRef]
81. Amedei, A.; Cappon, A.; Codolo, G.; Cabrelle, A.; Polenghi, A.; Benagiano, M.; Tasca, E.; Azzurri, A.; D'Elios, M.M.; Del Prete, G.; et al. The neutrophil-activating protein of *Helicobacter pylori* promotes Th1 immune responses. *J. Clin. Investig.* **2006**, *116*, 1092–1101. [CrossRef]
82. D'Elios, M.M.; Amedei, A.; Cappon, A.; Del Prete, G.; de Bernard, M. The neutrophil-activating protein of *Helicobacter pylori* (HP-NAP) as an immune modulating agent. *FEMS Immunol. Med. Microbiol.* **2007**, *50*, 157–164. [CrossRef] [PubMed]
83. Yokota, S.; Toita, N.; Yamamoto, S.; Fujii, N.; Konno, M. Positive relationship between a polymorphism in *Helicobacter pylori* neutrophil-activating protein A gene and iron-deficiency anemia. *Helicobacter* **2013**, *18*, 112–116. [CrossRef] [PubMed]
84. Shan, W.; Kung, H.F.; Ge, R. Comparison of iron-binding ability between Thr70-NapA and Ser70-NapA of *Helicobacter pylori*. *Helicobacter* **2016**, *21*, 192–200. [CrossRef] [PubMed]
85. Loh, J.T.; Beckett, A.C.; Scholz, M.B.; Cover, T.L. High-salt conditions alter transcription of *Helicobacter pylori* genes encoding outer membrane proteins. *Infect. Immun.* **2018**, *86*, e00626-17. [CrossRef]
86. Thompson, J.; Biggs, B.A.; Pasricha, S.R. Effects of daily iron supplementation in 2- to 5-years-old children: Systematic review and meta-analysis. *Pediatrics* **2013**, *131*, 739–753. [CrossRef]
87. Choe, Y.H.; Kwon, Y.S.; Jung, M.K.; Kang, S.K.; Hwang, T.S.; Hong, Y.C. *Helicobacter pylori*-associated iron deficiency anemia in adolescent female athletes. *J. Pediatr.* **2001**, *139*, 100–104. [CrossRef]
88. Sandström, G.; Rödjer, S.; Kaijser, B.; Börjesson, M. *Helicobacter pylori* antibodies and iron deficiency in female adolescents. *PLoS ONE* **2014**, *9*, e113059. [CrossRef]

89. Malaty, H.M.; Engstrand, L.; Pedersen, N.L.; Graham, D.Y. *Helicobacter pylori* infection: Genetic and environmental influences. A study of twins. *Ann. Intern. Med.* **1994**, *120*, 982–986. [CrossRef]
90. Melit, L.E.; Marginean, C.O.; Marginean, C.D.; Marginean, M.O. The relationship between Tool-like receptors and *Helicobacter pylori*-related gastropathies: Still a controversial topic. *J. Immunol. Res.* **2019**, *2019*, 8197048. [CrossRef]
91. O'Neill, L.A.J.; Golenbock, D.; Bowie, A.G. The history of toll-like receptors—Redefining innate immunity. *Nat. Rev. Immunol.* **2013**, *13*, 453–460. [CrossRef]
92. Castano-Rodríguez, N.; Kaakoush, N.O.; Pardo, A.L.; Goh, K.L.; Fock, K.M.; Mitchell, H.M. Genetic polymorphisms in the toll-like receptor signaling pathway in *Helicobacter pylori* infection and related gastric cancer. *Hum. Immunol.* **2014**, *75*, 808–815. [CrossRef] [PubMed]
93. El-Omar, E.M.; Ng, M.T.; Hold, G.L. Polymorphisms in Toll-like receptor genes and risk of cancer. *Oncogene* **2008**, *27*, 244–252. [CrossRef] [PubMed]
94. El-Omar, E.M.; Rabkin, C.S.; Gammon, M.D.; Vaughan, T.L.; Risch, H.A.; Schoenberg, J.B.; Stanford, J.L.; Mayne, S.T.; Goedert, J.; Blot, W.J.; et al. Increased risk of noncardia gastric cancer associated with proinflammatory cytokine gene polymorphisms. *Gastroenterology* **2003**, *124*, 1193–1201. [CrossRef] [PubMed]
95. Furuta, T.; Shirai, N.; Takashima, M.; Xiao, F.; Sugimura, H. Effect of genotypic differences in interleukin-1 beta on gastric acid secretion in Japanese patients infected with *Helicobacter pylori*. *Am. J. Med.* **2002**, *112*, 141–143. [CrossRef]
96. Serrano, C.A.; Villagrán, A.; Toledo, H.; Crabtree, J.E.; Harris, P.R. Iron deficiency and IL1β polymorphisms in *Helicobacter pylori*-infected children. *Helicobacter* **2016**, *21*, 124–130. [CrossRef] [PubMed]
97. Emiralioglu, N.; Yenicesu, I.; Sari, S.; Egritas, O.; Poyraz, A.; Pasaoglu, O.T.; Celik, B.; Dalgic, B. An insight into the relationship between prohepcidin, iron deficiency anemia, and interleukin-6 values in pediatric *Helicobacter pylori* gastritis. *Eur. J. Pediatr.* **2015**, *174*, 903–910. [CrossRef] [PubMed]
98. Amieva, M.; Peek, R.M., Jr. Pathobiology of *Helicobacter pylori*-induced gastric cancer. *Gastroenterology* **2016**, *150*, 64–78. [CrossRef]
99. Blaser, M.J.; Chen, Y.; Reibman, J. Does *Helicobacter pylori* protect against asthma and allergy? *Gut* **2008**, *57*, 561–567. [CrossRef]
100. Lionetti, E.; Leonardi, S.; Lanzafame, A.; Garozzo, M.T.; Filippelli, M.; Tomarchio, S.; Ferrara, V.; Salpietro, C.; Pulvirenti, A.; Francavilla, R.; et al. *Helicobacter pylori* infection and atopic diseases: Is there a relationship? A systematic review and meta-analysis. *World J. Gastroenterol.* **2014**, *20*, 17635–17647. [CrossRef]
101. Malfertheiner, P.; Megraud, F.; Rokkas, T.; Gishert, J.P.; Liou, J.; Schulz, C.; Gasbarrini, A.; Hunt, R.H.; Leja, M.; O'Morain, C.; et al. Management of *Helicobacter pylori* infection: The Maastricht VI/Florence consensus report. *Gut* **2022**, *71*, 1724–1762.
102. Ko, C.W.; Siddique, S.M.; Patel, A.; Harris, A.; Sultan, S.; Altayar, O.; Falck-Ytter, Y. AGA clinical practice guidelines on the gastrointestinal evaluation of iron deficiency anemia. *Gastroenterology* **2020**, *159*, 1085–1094. [CrossRef]
103. El-Serag, H.B.; Kao, J.Y.; Kanwal, F.; Gilger, M.; LoVecchio, F.; Moss, S.F.; Crowe, S.E.; Elfant, A.; Haas, T.; Hapke, R.J.; et al. Houston consensus conference on testing for *Helicobacter pylori* infection in the United States. *Clin. Gastroenterol. Hepatol.* **2018**, *16*, 992–1002. [CrossRef] [PubMed]
104. Thomas, J.E.; Dale, A.; Bunn, J.E.G.; Harding, M.; Coward, W.A.; Cole, T.J.; Weaver, L.T. Early *Helicobacter pylori* colonization: The association with growth faltering in the Gambia. *Arch. Dis. Child.* **2004**, *89*, 1149–1154. [CrossRef] [PubMed]
105. Mera, R.M.; Correa, P.; Fontham, E.E.; Reina, J.C.; Pradilla, A.; Alzate, A.; Bravo, L.E. Effects of a new *Helicobacter pylori* infection on height and weight in Colombian children. *Ann. Epidemiol.* **2006**, *16*, 347–351. [CrossRef] [PubMed]

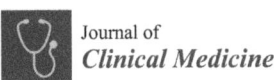

Review

Diagnosis and Treatment for Gastric Mucosa-Associated Lymphoid Tissue (MALT) Lymphoma

Shotaro Nakamura [1,2,*] and Mariko Hojo [3]

1. Department of Gastroenterology, International University of Health and Welfare, Narita 286-8686, Japan
2. Center of Gastroenterology, Takagi Hospital, Fukuoka 831-0016, Japan
3. Department of Gastroenterology, Juntendo University School of Medicine, Tokyo 113-8421, Japan
* Correspondence: shonaka@kouhoukai.org; Tel.: +81-944-87-0001; Fax: +81-944-87-9310

Abstract: Mucosa-associated lymphoid tissue (MALT) lymphoma, which was first reported in 1984, shows an indolent clinical course. However, the detailed clinicopathological characteristics of gastric MALT lymphoma have not been fully elucidated. We performed a literature search concerning the clinical features and treatment for gastric MALT lymphoma using PubMED. MALT lymphomas develop in single or multiple extranodal organs, of which the stomach is one of the most frequent sites; gastric MALT lymphoma accounts for 7% to 9% of all B-cell lymphomas, and 40% to 50% of primary gastric lymphomas. The eradication of *Helicobacter pylori* (*H. pylori*) is the first-line treatment for patients with gastric MALT lymphoma, regardless of the clinical stage. Approximately 60–90% of cases with stage I/II$_1$ disease only achieve a complete histological response via *H. pylori* eradication. In patients who do not respond to *H. pylori* eradication therapy, second-line treatments such as watch-and-wait, radiotherapy, chemotherapy, rituximab immunotherapy, and/or a combination of these are recommended. Thus, *H. pylori* plays a causative role in the pathogenesis of gastric MALT lymphoma, and *H. pylori* eradication leads to complete histological remission in the majority of cases.

Keywords: gastric lymphoma; MALT lymphoma; *Helicobacter pylori*; radiotherapy; chemotherapy; rituximab

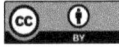

1. Introduction

Extranodal marginal zone lymphoma of mucosa-associated lymphoid tissue (MALT lymphoma) was first described by Isaacson and Wright in 1984 [1]. They reported four cases of MALT lymphoma, with one case each presenting in the stomach, salivary gland, lung, and thyroid. MALT lymphoma is a low-grade non-Hodgkin's lymphoma composed of small- to medium-sized neoplastic B cells including marginal-zone centrocyte-like cells, monocytoid cells, and scattered immunoblasts [2–9]. MALT lymphoma most frequently develops within the stomach. In most cases of gastric MALT lymphoma, *Helicobacter pylori* (*H. pylori*) is involved in the pathogenesis, and the eradication of *H. pylori* results in the complete histological response of the lymphoma in 60–90% of patients [2–9]. In the present article, the authors review the recent findings concerning the pathogenesis, diagnosis, and treatment strategies for cases of gastric MALT lymphoma.

2. Epidemiology of Gastric MALT Lymphoma

Primary gastric lymphoma (PGL) is the most frequent extranodal non-Hodgkin's lymphoma, comprising 30–40% of all extranodal lymphomas. Among the 676 cases of primary gastrointestinal lymphoma treated at our institution [10,11], the most commonly affected site was the stomach (456 cases (67%)), followed by the small and large bowels (183 cases; (27%)). The remaining 37 cases (5%) had lymphomas in both the stomach and intestines. The most frequent histologic type of gastric lymphoma was MALT lymphoma (226 cases (51%)), followed by diffuse large B-cell lymphoma (DLBCL) (170 cases (39%)).

Gastric MALT lymphoma comprises 7–9% of all B-cell lymphomas, 3–6% of all malignant neoplasms in the stomach, and 40–50% of all PGLs [2–5,10–14]. While gastric MALT lymphoma is relatively rare, its incidence has been increasing over the past 20–30 years. In a nationwide survey using the Dutch nationwide histopathology registry (PALGA), Capelle et al. identified 1419 newly diagnosed cases of gastric MALT lymphoma over a 16-year period [15]. In addition, they and other authors reported an increased risk for the metachronous development of gastric adenocarcinoma after gastric MALT lymphoma [15,16].

3. Pathogenesis of Gastric MALT Lymphoma

3.1. Helicobacter pylori

The etiological association of *H. pylori* with gastric MALT lymphoma was first reported by Wotherspoon et al. in 1991 [4]. Thereafter, several clinical and histopathologic studies showing a definite association between *H. pylori* infection and gastric MALT lymphoma were confirmed [1–7].

Approximately 80–90% of patients with gastric MALT lymphoma are infected with *H. pylori*, and 60–80% of those cases achieve remission via *H. pylori* eradication alone [5–9]. In *H. pylori*-dependent cases, the growth of lymphoma cells is driven by *H. pylori*-generated immune responses that include signaling from CD40 and CD86 through the aid of bystander T-cells [2,3]. In addition, a proliferation-inducing ligand (APRIL), which is a member of the tumor necrosis factor (TNF) superfamily and is produced by eosinophils in *H. pylori*-infected gastric mucosa, promotes the survival and proliferation of neoplastic B cells [17,18]. Interestingly, *H. pylori* eradication therapy is not only effective in *H. pylori*-positive cases but also in *H. pylori*-negative cases. In our experience, the complete remission (CR) rate of MALT lymphoma after *H. pylori* eradication therapy was 75% among *H. pylori*-positive cases, while it was 29% among *H. pylori*-negative cases [13,14].

It should be noted that t(11;18)(q21;q21)/*BIRC3-MALT1* translocation is frequent (53% or 60%) in *H. pylori*-negative gastric MALT lymphomas [19–22]. Recently, Tanaka et al. obtained gastric mucosal biopsy specimens from *H. pylori*-negative gastric MALT lymphoma patients and from control participants without *H. pylori* infection or cancer and studied their mucosal microbiota by performing 16S rRNA gene sequencing. They found that the *H. pylori*-negative gastric MALT lymphoma patients showed lower alpha diversity than the control participants ($p = 0.04$) [23]. A comparison concerning the patients' beta diversity revealed that there were significant differences in the microbes that were present in the gastric mucosa between the two groups ($p = 0.04$). They concluded that *H. pylori*-negative gastric MALT lymphoma cases exhibited altered gastric mucosal microbial compositions, and such altered microbiota might be involved in the pathogenesis of *H. pylori*-negative gastric MALT lymphoma [23].

In addition, patients with gastric MALT lymphoma have an increased risk of the metachronous development of gastric adenocarcinoma [15,16]. Palmela et al. reported that the relative risk (RR) for gastric adenocarcinoma among patients who had gastric MALT lymphoma was 4.32 (95% CI 2.64–6.67) compared to the American population. The median latency time was 5 years, and the risk was maintained thereafter [RR 4.92, 95% confidence interval (CI) 2.45–8.79] [16].

3.2. Genetic Aberrations

Genetically, MALT lymphoma is associated with the following four chromosomal translocations: t(11;18)(q21;q21)/*BIRC3-MALT1*, t(1;14)(q22;q32)/*BCL10-IGH*, t(14;18)(q32;q21)/*IGH-MALT1*, and t(3;14)(q31;q32)/*FOXP1-IGH* [2,3,11,19–22]. Especially in MALT lymphomas with t(11;18)(q21;q21)/*BIRC3-MALT1*, the resulting BIRC3-MALT1 fusion product forms self-oligomers via a non-homotypic interaction mediated by the BIRC3 moiety, leading to constitutive nuclear factor kappa B (NF-κB) activation. These oncogenic products are most likely synergic with both innate and acquired immune stimulations with respect to the activation of the NF-κB pathway [18–26].

All four above-mentioned translocations are considered to exert their oncogenic activities alongside the constitutive activation of the NF-κB pathway, which leads to the expression of several genes for cell survival and proliferation [24–28]. Among these translocations, t(11;18)(q21;q21)/*BIRC3-MALT1* is the most frequent, and is detected in 15–30% of all cases of gastric MALT lymphomas. The translocation fuses the N-terminal region of *BIRC3* to the C-terminal region of *MALT1*, generating a functional chimeric fusion protein that gains the ability to activate the NF-κB pathway [25–27]. The t(11;18) (q21;q21)/*BIRC3-MALT1* translocation is frequently associated with the absence of *H. pylori*, and cases that are positive for this translocation do not respond to *H. pylori* eradication [19–22]. Interestingly, t(11;18)(q21;q21)-positive MALT lymphomas occasionally transform into DLBCL [20,21].

The TNF-α-induced protein 3 gene (*TNFAIP3*, *A20*), which was identified as the target of 6q23 deletion in MALT lymphoma, is an important inhibitor of NF-κB [27]. Mutations or deletions of *A20* that lead to A20 protein inactivation are frequent in MALT lymphomas of the ocular adnexa, salivary glands, thyroid, and liver. A20-mediated oncogenic activities in MALT lymphoma depend on NF-κB activation triggered by TNF-α or other unidentified molecules [25–27].

4. Diagnosis of Gastric MALT Lymphoma

4.1. Endoscopic/Macroscopic Findings

To date, a standard endoscopic or macroscopic classification system for PGLs has not been established. In Western nations, PGLs are macroscopically classified as either ulcerative (34–69%), mass/polypoid (26–35%), diffuse-infiltrating (15–40%), or other types [6,7,28]. In our institute, PGLs have been classified as either superficial (41%), mass-forming (43%), diffuse-infiltrating (6%), or other types (10%). Figure 1 shows conventional and magnified endoscopic findings of superficial-type gastric MALT lymphomas. In Figure 1, the upper three photos show conventional endoscopic images, while the lower three photos are magnified endoscopic images that show a characteristic tree-like appearance (TLA) with amorphous, whitish areas. Superficial-type gastric MALT lymphoma is sometimes misdiagnosed as depressed-type early gastric cancer [6,11]. In an article by Lee et al., endoscopic findings of 122 cases of gastric MALT lymphoma were classified as either polypoid (n = 18, 15%), ulceration (n = 43, 35%), or diffuse infiltration (n = 61, 50%) types [28].

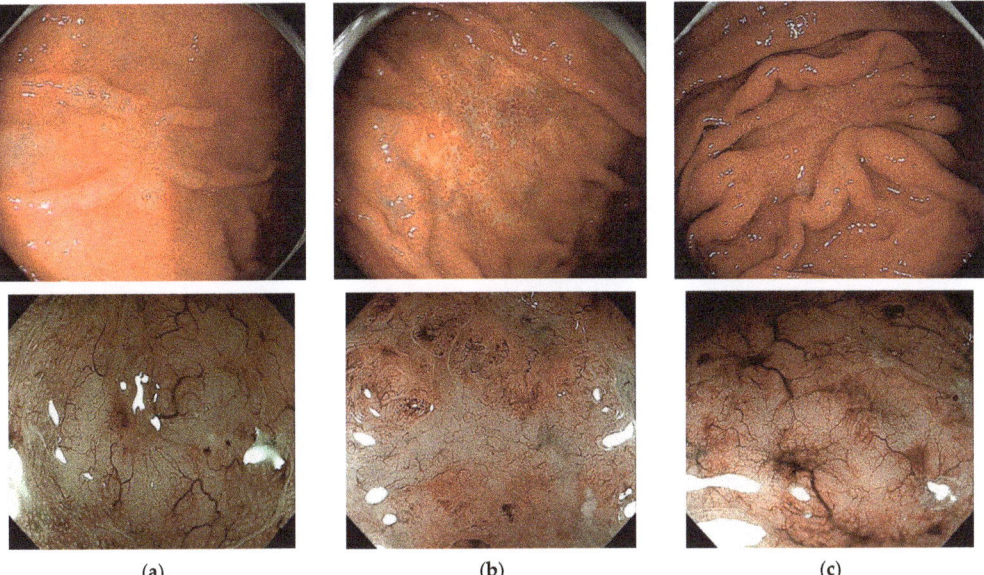

Figure 1. Endoscopic findings of superficial-type gastric MALT lymphomas in three patients (from author's original research). The upper three photos are conventional endoscopic images and lower three photos are magnified endoscopic images showing a characteristic tree-like appearance with whitish, amorphous areas. (**a**) Patient 1, (**b**) Patient 2, and (**c**) Patient 3.

4.2. Histopathology of Gastric MALT Lymphomas

A definite diagnosis of gastric MALT lymphoma is made based on the histopathologic criteria of the World Health Organization (WHO) classification system [2,3], the Consensus report of the European Gastro-Intestinal Lymphoma Study (EGILS) group [29], and the National Comprehensive Cancer Network (NCCN) guidelines [30]. Histologically, the diffuse infiltrate of atypical neoplastic lymphoid cells (centrocyte-like cells) around reactive follicles showing a marginal-zone growth pattern, which often infiltrate into gastric glands causing the destruction of epithelial cells (lymphoepithelial lesions (LELs), Figure 2), is observed in gastric MALT lymphomas [1–4]. MALT lymphoma cells immunohistochemically exhibit CD20+, CD79a+, CD5-, CD10-, CD23-, CD43+/-, and cyclin D1-. However, when large lymphoma cells are present in a solid or sheet pattern, a diagnosis of DLBCL should be made [6,7,10,11]. DLBCL usually shows high Ki-67 expression upon immunohistochemical staining [6,19,20]. The histologic diagnosis of gastric lymphomas should be confirmed by an expert hematopathologist [1–3].

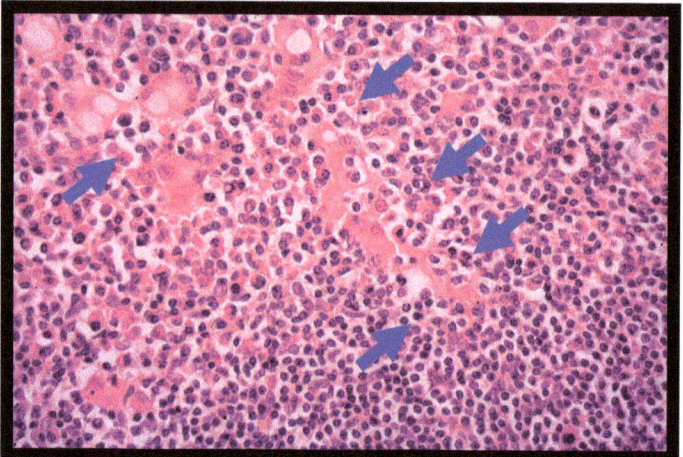

Figure 2. Histological features of gastric MALT lymphoma (H&E; X400). Diffuse infiltrate of small- to medium-sized atypical neoplastic lymphoid cells (centrocyte-like cells) around reactive follicles with a marginal zone growth pattern is shown. Lymphoepithelial lesions (LELs) (blue arrows) are also shown.

The histological features of MALT lymphoma are occasionally similar to those of reactive inflammatory conditions such as *H. pylori*-related chronic gastritis. Histologically, MALT lymphoma can be distinguished from gastritis based on the presence of a dense infiltrate of monotonous B-cells extending away from lymphoid follicles, the cytologic atypia of lymphoid cells, Dutcher bodies, and LELs in MALT lymphomas [2,3]. The Wotherspoon score is used to make a confident histologic diagnosis of gastric MALT lymphoma on examination of biopsy specimens (Table 1) [4].

Table 1. Histologic scoring system for the diagnosis of gastric MALT lymphoma (Wotherspoon score) [4].

Grade	Description	Histologic Features
0	Normal	Scattered plasma cells in mucosa; no lymphoid follicles.
1	Chronic active gastritis	Small clusters of lymphocytes in mucosa; no lymphoid follicles; no lymphoepithelial lesions.
2	Chronic active gastritis with florid lymphoid follicle formation	Prominent lymphoid follicles with surrounding mantle zone and plasma cells; no lymphoepithelial lesions.

Table 1. Cont.

Grade	Description	Histologic Features
3	Suspicious lymphoid infiltrate in mucosa, probably reactive	Lymphoid follicles surrounded by small lymphocytes that have infiltrated diffusely in the mucosa and occasionally into epithelium.
4	Suspicious lymphoid infiltrate in mucosa, probably lymphoma	Lymphoid follicles surrounded by centrocyte-like cells that have infiltrated diffusely in the mucosa and epithelium in small groups.
5	MALT lymphoma	Presence of dense diffuse infiltrate of centrocyte-like cells in the mucosa with prominent lymphoepithelial lesions.

For the diagnosis of gastrointestinal MALT lymphoma, a minimum of 10 biopsy samples should be taken, and not only from visible lesions, but also from endoscopically normal-appearing mucosa, according to the Consensus report of the EGILS group [29]. The detection of immunoglobulin light chain (κ or λ) restriction by immunohistochemistry or in situ hybridization, and analyses for clonality of the rearranged immunoglobulin genes by polymerase chain reaction (PCR), may help diagnose B-cell lymphoma [2,3]. Cytogenetic analyses using G-banding, reverse-transcription polymerase chain reaction (RT-PCR), and/or fluorescence in situ hybridization (FISH) to detect t(11;18) (q21;q21)/*BIRC3-MALT1* and/or other specific chromosomal translocations can be performed to confirm the certain diagnosis of MALT lymphoma [2,3,19–22].

4.3. Clinical Staging

Clinical staging is essential for determining the management strategy for PGLs. In general, the Lugano International Conference (Blackledge) classification system (I, II$_1$, II$_2$, IIE, or IV, Table 2) [30] and/or the Ann-Arbor staging system with its modifications by Musschoff and Radaszkiewicz (I$_1$E, I$_2$E, II$_1$E, II$_2$E, IIIE, or IV) are used for patients with gastrointestinal lymphomas. Recently, the EGILS Consensus report and the European Society of Medical Oncology (ESMO) guidelines recommended the Paris Classification system, which is a modification of the TNM system including the degree of the spread of lymphoma as assessed by endoscopic ultrasound (EUS) [29]. In our institute, we have combined the Lugano system and Paris system, as shown in our original Table 2. Esophagogastroduodenoscopy (EGD) with or without multiple biopsies, ileocolonoscopy, and balloon-assisted enteroscopy (BAE) are useful for detecting possible gastrointestinal lesions of lymphomas during a follow-up. In addition, computed tomography (CT) of the chest, abdomen, and pelvis, as well as fluorine-18 [^{18}F] fluoro-deoxyglucose positron-emission tomography (FDG-PET), should be considered [31].

Table 2. Lugano and Paris staging systems for gastrointestinal lymphomas [29,30].

Stage	Lugano System	Paris System	Tumor Extension
I	Tumor confined to GI tract (single, primary site or multiple, noncontiguous lesions)	T1m N0 M0 T1sm N0 M0 T2 N0 M0 T3 N0 M0	Mucosa Submucosa Muscularis propria Serosa
II	Tumor extending into abdomen	NA	NA
II$_1$	Local nodal involvement	T1–3 N1 M0	Perigastric lymph nodes
II$_2$	Distant nodal involvement	T1–3 N2 M0	More distant regional lymph nodes
IIE	Perforation of serosa to involve adjacent organs or tissues	T4 N0–2 M0	Invasion of adjacent structures with or without invasion of abdominal lymph nodes
IV	Disseminated extranodal involvement or concomitant supradiaphragmatic nodal involvement	T1–4 N3 M0 T1–4 N0–3 M1 T1–4 N0–3 M2 T1–4 N0–3 M0–2 BX T1–4 N0–3 M2 B1	Extra-abdominal lymph nodes and/or additional distant GI/non-GI sites BM not assessed BM not involved BM involvement

BM: bone marrow; GI: gastrointestinal; NA: not available.

Cohen et al. performed an analysis of 66 patients with MALT lymphoma to assess the usefulness of FDG-PET. They found that all extranodal lesions of MALT lymphoma located in subcutaneous tissues, breasts, lungs, and liver were detected by FDG-PET [31]. However, only 26.3% of the lesions located in the stomach and 28.6% of the lesions located in the intestinal tract were detected by FDG-PET. They evaluated the predictive value of PET in the patients and found that increased ^{18}F-FDG-uptake in extranodal lesions was associated with disease progression [31]. The gastrointestinal tract has high/heterogeneous physiologic ^{18}F-FDG-uptake. They concluded that the detection rate of extranodal MALT lymphoma lesions located in tissues with low and/or homogenous physiologic [^{18}F]FDG-uptake is excellent using [^{18}F]FDG-PET-CT.

5. Treatments for Gastric MALT Lymphoma

5.1. Helicobacter pylori Eradication

The first-line therapy for all patients with gastric MALT lymphoma is *H. pylori* eradication, regardless of the clinical stage [5–9,11–14,29,30,32–42]. *H. pylori* eradication therapy consisting of a proton-pump inhibitor, the administration of amoxicillin, and either clarithromycin or metronidazole administration for 7 days has been recommended in Japan. The histopathologic evaluation of post-treatment biopsy specimens is conducted based on the Groupe d'Etude des Lymphomes de l'Adulte (GELA) grading system (Table 3 [29]), because the Wotherspoon score (Table 1), which is applied for the initial diagnosis, is no longer adequate for assessing the response to treatment during follow-up [29,42]. Among patients with stage I/II$_1$ disease, *H. pylori* eradication therapy resulted in complete histologic response (ChR) in 60–90% of cases [5,7–13,32,33,35–41]. However, it should be noted that antibiotic resistance has been the critical factor responsible for treatment failure. In particular, a recent increase in clarithromycin resistance induces treatment failure in *H. pylori* eradication in a considerable number of infected patients.

Table 3. GELA histologic grading system for post-treatment evaluation of gastric MALT lymphoma [29].

Score	Lymphoid Infiltrate	LEL	Stromal Changes	Clinical Significance
Complete histologic response (ChR)	Absent or scattered plasma cells and small lymphoid cells in LP	Absent	Normal or empty LP and/or fibrosis	Complete remission
Probable minimal residual disease (pMRD)	Aggregates of lymphoid cells or lymphoid nodules in LP/MM and/or SM	Absent	Empty LP and/or fibrosis	Complete remission
Responding residual disease (rRD)	Dense, diffuse, or nodular, extending around glands in LP	Focal or absent	Focal empty LP and/or absent	Partial remission
No change (NC)	Dense, diffuse, or nodular	Present, may be absent	No changes	Stable or progressive disease

GELA: Groupe d'Etude des Lymphomes de l'Adulte; LEL: lymphoepithelial lesion; LP: lamina propria; MALT: mucosa-associated lymphoid tissue; MM: muscularis mucosae; SM: submucosa.

In a systematic review of 32 published clinical studies including 1408 patients with gastric MALT lymphoma by Zullo et al., the CR rate after *H. pylori* eradication therapy was 78% [33]. The factors associated with resistance to *H. pylori* eradication therapy included the absence of an *H. pylori* infection, an advanced clinical stage, a proximal location of the lymphoma in the stomach, an endoscopic non-superficial type, deep invasion in the gastric wall, and t(11;18)/*BIRC3-MALT1* translocation [11,12,19–22,25–28,30,31,33–37,40–45]. In addition, Zullo et al. [34] also performed a pooled-data analysis of 315 patients who did not respond to *H. pylori* eradication therapy. The most frequent second-line therapy was radiotherapy (112 patients), followed by surgery (80 patients) and chemotherapy (68 patients). The patients who underwent radiotherapy had a similar remission rate as those who underwent surgical resection (97% vs. 93%; $p = 0.2$) and a significantly higher remission rate than those who underwent chemotherapy (97% vs. 85%; $p = 0.007$).

We conducted a retrospective multicenter study of 420 Japanese patients with gastric MALT lymphoma to assess the long-term clinical outcome after successful *H. pylori* eradication [36]. As a result, CR was achieved in 77% (323/420) of patients solely via *H. pylori* eradication. During the follow-up period (mean 6.5 years and median 6.04 years), treatment failure was seen in only 37 patients (9%) (relapse in 10 of 323 responders; progressive disease (PD) in 27 of 97 non-responders). The long-term prognosis was excellent; the probabilities of freedom from treatment failure, overall survival, and event-free survival after 10 years were 90%, 95%, and 86%, respectively. In addition, we performed another literature review of 32 published articles regarding the efficacy of *H. pylori* eradication in gastric MALT lymphoma cases in our same paper [36], which revealed that *H. pylori* eradication therapy led to CR of gastric MALT lymphoma in 1793 (73%) of 2451 patients.

Subsequently, we performed a prospective multicenter study to evaluate the clinical efficacy of *H. pylori* eradication therapy in 108 Japanese patients with *H. pylori*-infected gastric MALT lymphoma in 34 hospitals (December 2010–February 2016) [45]. As a result, the CR of lymphoma was achieved in 84 (87%) of the 97 patients (11 patients dropped out of the study). Second-line treatments (radiotherapy, rituximab, or gastrectomy) were needed for 10 (10%) of the 97 patients. During the follow-up period (2–45 months; median 5.3 months), three patients died of causes unrelated to lymphoma. The overall survival probability was 97%.

5.2. Treatment Strategies for Patients with Gastric MALT Lymphoma Who Do Not Respond to Helicobacter pylori Eradication

There is no consensus on the treatment strategy for patients with gastric MALT lymphoma who do not respond to *H. pylori* eradication therapy. While patients with PD or a clinically evident relapse can undergo oncologic treatment, for patients with persistent histologic lymphoma without PD (responding residual disease (rRD) or no change (NC)), a "watch-and-wait" strategy is recommended for up to 24 months after *H. pylori* eradication therapy. Thereafter, the decision of whether to continue the "watch-and-wait" strategy or to start oncologic treatment is made on a case-by-case basis [11,37].

As for the second-line oncologic treatment, radiotherapy, immunotherapy (e.g., rituximab), and/or chemotherapy are recommended. While radiotherapy and chemotherapy both have a curative potential in localized (stage I/II$_1$) gastric MALT lymphoma, radiotherapy (30–40 Gy/15–20 fractions) is generally preferred and is highly effective (response rate of 93–100%) [43,44].

Chemotherapy and/or rituximab immunotherapy are also effective, and these systemic treatments are suitable for cases with histologic transformation into DLBCL, cases with disseminated disease, and those with advanced stages [46,47]. Although rituximab plus cyclophosphamide, doxorubicin, vincristine, and prednisolone (R-CHOP) chemotherapy is relatively toxic for indolent MALT lymphoma, the rituximab plus cyclophosphamide, vincristine, and prednisolone (R-COP) regimen seems to be well-tolerated and effective [45,48–50].

Oral alkylating agents, such as cyclophosphamide or chlorambucil, employed as a sole treatment are also well-tolerated and effective, and resulted in CR in 75% of patients, although relapse was observed in 28% of patients [27,41]. Recently, the combination of rituximab and chlorambucil [48], fludarabine [49], and bendamustine [50,51] provided excellent responses in patients with MALT lymphoma of various organs, including gastric MALT lymphoma cases.

In summary, the treatment strategies for patients with gastric MALT lymphoma should be based on the modified version of the ESMO guidelines [29,43,47,51]. For all patients in stages I$_1$–IIE, *H. pylori* eradication should be the first-line treatment. In patients with stage IV, *H. pylori* eradication also should be performed if the infection is present.

6. Risk for Other Malignancies

It has been reported that patients with gastric MALT lymphoma had a higher risk of synchronous and/or metachronous gastric cancers than healthy control subjects [15,16]. In a Dutch epidemiological study covering the period from 1991–2006 by Capelle et al. [15], new gastric cancers developed in 34 (2.4%) of 1419 patients with gastric MALT lymphoma. The risk of gastric cancer was 16.6 times higher in patients with gastric MALT lymphoma aged 45–59 years than in the Dutch population ($p < 0.001$). They concluded that the risk of gastric cancer in patients with gastric MALT lymphoma is six times higher than that in the Dutch population and recommended that patients with gastric MALT lymphoma should be monitored in thorough follow-ups.

In a US population-based study (National Cancer Institute Surveillance, Epidemiology and End Results 13 (SEER) database 1992–2012), Palmela et al. [16] reported that gastric cancer developed in 20 (0.91%) of 2195 patients with gastric MALT lymphoma, with a relative risk of 4.32 (95% CI 2.64–6.67) compared to the rest of the American population. They concluded that gastric MALT lymphoma is associated with an increased risk of metachronous gastric adenocarcinoma. It should be noted that the risk for gastric cancer was still present beyond 5 years of follow-up [16].

7. Discussion

In 1984, Isaacson and Wright reported the first four cases of MALT lymphoma, with one case each arising in the stomach, salivary gland, lung, and thyroid, which was published in the international medical journal *Cancer* [1]. Since then, a large number of clinical studies on the diagnosis and treatment of gastric MALT lymphoma have been published. In 1993, Wotherspoon et al. first reported that *H. pylori* eradication with antibiotic treatment resulted in the complete histological regression of gastric MALT lymphoma in five of six *H. pylori*-infected gastric MALT lymphoma patients [5]. It has been established that *H. pylori* eradication is the first-line treatment for gastric MALT lymphomas. A meta-analysis by Zullo et al. concerning 1408 patients with gastric MALT lymphoma from 32 published studies revealed that after *H. pylori* eradication, 1091 patients (77%) achieved CR, while 43 patients (1.7%) developed progressive disease (PD) and 78 patients (3.1%) experienced a relapse [34]. Thus, treatment failure occurred in only 121 (8.6%) of the 1408 patients.

We performed another meta-analysis of 2451 patients with gastric MALT lymphoma who underwent *H. pylori* eradication therapy from 32 published studies [37]. As a result, 1793 patients (73%) achieved CR after *H. pylori* eradication. Forty-three patients (1.8%) developed PD, while seventy-eight patients (3.2%) suffered a relapse. Thus, only 121 (4.9%) of the 2451 patients experienced treatment failure.

While *H. pylori* eradication therapy is widely accepted as the first-line treatment of gastric MALT lymphoma, the National Comprehensive Cancer Network (NCCN) [30] and ESMO [31,43] guidelines slightly differ regarding which patients should receive antibiotic treatment. NCCN considers *H. pylori* eradication as the first-line therapy of choice for those with early stage lymphoma (Lugano I_1, I_2, or II_1), an *H. pylori*-positive status, and concomitant negativity or unknown status of t(11;18) translocation [30]. Conversely, the ESMO guidelines recommend *H. pylori* eradication therapy for all patients with gastric MALT lymphoma regardless of the stage, translocation status, and *H. pylori* positivity [31,43].

The role of eradication therapy in *H. pylori*-negative MALT lymphoma remains controversial. Since *H. pylori*-negative MALT lymphoma is increasing worldwide, we should discuss it more deeply. Xie et al. [44] performed a meta-analysis regarding the efficacy of modified eradication therapy for *H. pylori*-negative gastric MALT lymphoma concerning 14 studies with 148 patients. As a result, the overall response rate was 0.38 (95% confidence interval (CI): 0.29–0.47). They concluded that their modified *H. pylori* eradication therapy is also effective for patients with *H. pylori*-negative MALT lymphoma.

For patients with gastric MALT lymphoma who do not respond to *H. pylori* eradication therapy and who do not develop PD, a "watch-and-wait" strategy without additional treatment may be adopted. We previously reported that the watch-and-wait strategy resulted in no change in 20% of non-responders with gastric MALT lymphoma after eradication therapy [35]. In addition, more than half of the relapsed cases with gastric MALT lymphoma under the watch-and-wait strategy achieved CR. Thus, we recommend the watch-and-wait strategy for asymptomatic non-responders with early-stage gastric MALT lymphoma. When the clinical stage of patients progresses during the follow-up period, medical treatments including *H. pylori* eradication with or without oncological treatment should be considered. Continuous single-agent chemotherapy with cyclophosphamide or chlorambucil has been useful as a monotherapy [11,41]. However, patients with t(11;18)(q21;q21) translocation may not respond to oral single- or multi-agent immuno/chemotherapy such as rituximab, cladribine, and others.

Non-responders to *H. pylori* eradication therapy have been reported to comprise 17–61% of patients with gastric MALT lymphoma [7–9,27,28,48]. As a second-line treatment for such non-responders, radiotherapy (RT) and/or imuno- or chemotherapy should be recommended. Of these, RT at a moderate dose (total 30–36 Gy) is highly effective, although it has been associated with rare acute or late toxicity [51]. Yahalom et al. treated 178 patients with *H. pylori*-independent gastric MALT lymphoma with RT with a median dose of 30 Gy over 20 fractions; consequently, 95% of the patients achieved a complete histologic response [44].

8. Conclusions

Nowadays, *H. pylori* eradication therapy is widely accepted as the first-line treatment for patients with gastric MALT lymphoma. To date, a large number of patients with gastric MALT lymphoma have been successfully treated with *H. pylori* eradication therapy. However, there is no consensus regarding the treatment strategies for patients with gastric MALT lymphoma who do not respond to *H. pylori* eradication therapy. In these patients, second-line treatments including a "watch-and-wait" strategy, radiotherapy, chemotherapy, rituximab immunotherapy, or a combination of these should be tailored in consideration of the extent of lymphoma and the clinical stage in each patient.

It is of interest that gastric MALT lymphoma is the only malignancy for which antibiotics are the first choice of treatment with a curative intent [11,41]. Despite recent advances in our understanding of the pathogenesis of gastric MALT lymphoma, there are many unanswered questions. Thus, further clinicopathological and molecular research studies are necessary in order to clarify the detailed mechanisms in the development of gastric MALT lymphoma and the long-term clinical course of patients with said disease.

Author Contributions: Conceptualization, writing, original draft preparation, review, and editing by S.N. and M.H. All authors have read and agreed to the published version of the manuscript.

Funding: This research received no external funding.

Institutional Review Board Statement: Not applicable.

Informed Consent Statement: Not applicable.

Conflicts of Interest: The authors (S.N. and M.H.) declare no conflicts of interest.

References

1. Isaacson, P.; Wright, D.H. Extranodal malignant lymphoma arising from mucosa-associated lymphoid tissue. *Cancer* **1984**, *53*, 2515–2524. [CrossRef] [PubMed]
2. Cook, J.R.; Isaacson, P.G.; Chott, A.; Nakamura, S.; Muller-Hermelink, H.K.; Harris, N.L.; Swerdlow, S.H. Extranodal marginal zone lymphoma of mucosa-associated lymphoid tissue (MALT lymphoma). In *WHO Classification of Tumours of Haematopoietic and Lymphoid Tissues*, 4th ed.; Swerdlow, S.H., Campo, E., Harris, N.L., Eds.; IARC: Lyon, France, 2008; pp. 214–217.
3. Nakamura, S.; Müller-Hermelink, H.K.; Delabe, J. Lymphoma of the stomach. In *WHO Classification of Tumours of the Digestive System*, 4th ed.; Bosman, F.T., Carnerio, F., Hruban, R.H., Theise, N.D., Eds.; IARC: Lyon, France, 2010; pp. 69–73.
4. Wotherspoon, A.C.; Ortiz-Hidalgo, C.; Falzon, M.R.; Isaacson, P.G. Helicobacter pylori-associated gastritis and primary B-cell gastric lymphoma. *Lancet* **1991**, *338*, 1175–1176. [CrossRef] [PubMed]
5. Wotherspoon, A.; Diss, T.; Pan, L.; Isaacson, P.; Doglioni, C.; Moschini, A.; de Boni, M. Regression of primary low-grade B-cell gastric lymphoma of mucosa-associated lymphoid tissue type after eradication of Helicobacter pylori. *Lancet* **1993**, *342*, 575–577. [CrossRef] [PubMed]
6. Nakamura, S.; Akazawa, K.; Yao, T.; Tsuneyoshi, M. Primary gastric lymphoma. A clinicopathologic study of 233 cases with special reference to evaluation with the MIB-1 index. *Cancer* **1995**, *76*, 1313–1324. [CrossRef] [PubMed]

7. Nakamura, S.; Yao, T.; Aoyagi, K.; Iida, M.; Fujishima, M.; Tsuneyoshi, M. Helicobacter pylori and primary gastric lymphoma. A histopathologic and immunohistochemical analysis of 237 patients. *Cancer* **1997**, *79*, 3–11. [CrossRef]
8. Bayerdorffer, E.; Miehlke, S.; Neubauer, A.; Stolte, M. Gastric MALT-lymphoma and Helicobacter pylori infection. *Aliment. Pharmacol. Ther.* **1997**, *11*, 89–94. [CrossRef]
9. Ryu, K.D.; Kim, G.H.; Park, S.O.; Lee, K.J.; Moon, J.Y.; Jeon, H.K.; Baek, D.H.; Lee, B.E.; Song, G.A. Treatment Outcome for gastric mucosa-associated jymphoid tissue lymphoma according to *Helicobacter pylori* infection status: A single-center experience. *Gut Liver* **2014**, *8*, 408–414. [CrossRef]
10. Nakamura, S.; Matsumoto, T.; Iida, M.; Yao, T.; Tsuneyoshi, M. Primary gastrointestinal lymphoma in Japan: A clinicopathologic analysis of 455 patients with special reference to its time trends. *Cancer* **2003**, *97*, 2462–2473. [CrossRef]
11. Nakamura, S.; Matsumoto, T. Gastrointestinal lymphoma: Recent advances in diagnosis and treatment. *Digestion* **2013**, *87*, 182–188. [CrossRef]
12. Nakamura, S.; Matsumoto, T. Gastrointestinal lymphomas: Recent topics in diagnosis and treatment. *J. Jpn Soc. Gastroenterol.* **2017**, *114*, 1833–1938. (In Japanese)
13. Nakamura, S.; Matsumoto, T.; Suekane, H.; Nakamura, S.; Matsumoto, H.; Esaki, M.; Yao, T.; Iida, M. Long-term clinical outcome of *Helicobacter pylori* eradication for gastric mucosa-associated lymphoid tissue lymphoma with a reference to second-line treatment. *Cancer* **2005**, *104*, 532–540. [CrossRef]
14. Nakamura, S.; Matsumoto, T.; Ye, H.; Nakamura, S.; Suekane, H.; Matsumoto, H.; Yao, T.; Tsuneyoshi, M.; Du, M.-Q.; Iida, M. *Helicobacter pylori*-negative gastric mucosa-associated lymphoid tissue lymphoma: A clinicopathologic and molecular study with reference to antibiotic treatment. *Cancer* **2006**, *107*, 2770–2778. [CrossRef]
15. Capelle, L.; de Vries, A.; Looman, C.; Casparie, M.; Boot, H.; Meijer, G.; Kuipers, E. Gastric MALT lymphoma: Epidemiology and high adenocarcinoma risk in a nation-wide study. *Eur. J. Cancer* **2008**, *44*, 2470–2476. [CrossRef]
16. Palmela, C.; Fonseca, C.; Faria, R.; Baptista, R.B.; Ribeiro, S.; Ferreira, A.O. Increased risk for metachronous gastric adenocarcinoma following gastric MALT lymphoma—A US population-based study. *United Eur. Gastroenterol. J.* **2016**, *5*, 473–478. [CrossRef]
17. Blosse, A.; Peru, S.; Levy, M.; Marteyn, B.; Floch, P.; Sifré, E.; Giese, A.; Prochazkova-Carlotti, M.; Martin, L.A.; Dubus, P.; et al. APRIL-producing eosinophils are involved in gastric MALT lymphomagenesis induced by Helicobacter sp infection. *Sci. Rep.* **2020**, *10*, 1–10. [CrossRef]
18. Shi, F.; Xue, R.; Zhou, X.; Shen, P.; Wang, S.; Yang, Y. Teliacicept as a BLyS/APRIL dual inhibitor for autoimmune disease. *Immunopharmacol. Immunotoxicol.* **2021**, *43*, 666–673. [CrossRef]
19. Ye, H.; Liu, H.; Raderer, M.; Chott, A.; Ruskone-Fourmestraux, A.; Wotherspoon, A.; Dyer, M.; Chuang, S.-S.; Dogan, A.; Isaacson, P.G.; et al. High incidence of t(11;18)(q21;q21) in *Helicobacter pylori*-negative gastric MALT lymphoma. *Blood* **2002**, *101*, 2547–2550. [CrossRef]
20. Huang, X.; Zhang, Z.; Liu, H.; Ye, H.; Chuang, S.-S.; Wang, J.; Lin, S.; Gao, Z.; Du, M.-Q. T(11;18)(q21;q21) in gastric MALT lymphoma and diffuse large B-cell lymphoma of Chinese patients. *Hematol. J.* **2003**, *4*, 342–345. [CrossRef]
21. Chuang, S.-S.; Lee, C.; Hamoudi, R.A.; Liu, H.; Lee, P.-S.; Ye, H.; Diss, T.C.; Dogan, A.; Isaacson, P.G.; Du, M.-Q. High frequency of t(11;18) in gastric mucosa-associated lymphoid tissue lymphomas in Taiwan, including one patient with high-grade transformation. *Br. J. Haematol.* **2002**, *120*, 97–100. [CrossRef]
22. Nakamura, S.; Ye, H.; Bacon, C.; Goatly, A.; Liu, H.; Banham, A.; Ventura, R.; Matsumoto, T.; Iida, M.; Ohji, Y.; et al. Clinical impact of genetic aberrations in gastric MALT lymphoma: A comprehensive analysis using interphase fluorescence in situ hybridisation. *Gut* **2007**, *56*, 1358–1363. [CrossRef]
23. Tanaka, T.; Matsuno, Y.; Torisu, T.; Shibata, H.; Hirano, A.; Umeno, J.; Kawasaki, K.; Fujioka, S.; Fuyuno, Y.; Moriyama, T.; et al. Gastric microbiota in patients with Helicobacter pylori-negative gastric MALT lymphoma. *Medicine* **2021**, *100*, e27287. [CrossRef] [PubMed]
24. Sagaert, X.; Van Cutsem, E.; De Hertogh, G.; Geboes, K.; Tousseyn, T. Gastric MALT lymphoma: A model of chronic inflammation-induced tumor development. *Nat. Rev. Gastroenterol. Hepatol.* **2010**, *7*, 336–346. [CrossRef] [PubMed]
25. Du, M.Q. MALT lymphoma: A paradigm of NF-κB dysregulation. *Semin. Cancer Biol.* **2016**, *39*, 49–60. [CrossRef] [PubMed]
26. Du, M.-Q. MALT lymphoma: Genetic abnormalities, immunological stimulation and molecular mechanism. *Best Pract. Res. Clin. Haematol.* **2017**, *30*, 13–23. [CrossRef] [PubMed]
27. Chanudet, E.; Huang, Y.; Ichimura, K.; Dong, G.; Hamoudi, R.; Radford, J.; Wotherspoon, A.C.; Isaacson, P.G.; Ferry, J.; Du, M.-Q. A20 is targeted by promoter methylation, deletion and inactivating mutation in MALT lymphoma. *Leukemia* **2009**, *24*, 483–487. [CrossRef] [PubMed]
28. Lee, C.M.; Lee, D.H.; Ahn, B.K.; Hwang, J.J.; Yoon, H.; Park, Y.S.; Shin, C.M.; Kim, N. Correlation of endoscopic findings of gastric mucosa-associated lymphoid tissue lymphoma with recurrence after complete remission. *Clin. Endosc.* **2017**, *50*, 51–57. [CrossRef]
29. Ruskone-Fourmestraux, A.; Fischbach, W.; Aleman, B.M.P.; Boot, H.; Du, M.Q.; Megraud, F.; Montalban, C.; Raderer, M.; Savio, A.; Wotherspoon, A.; et al. EGILS consensus report. Gastric extranodal marginal zone B-cell lymphoma of MALT. *Gut* **2011**, *60*, 747–758. [CrossRef]
30. In Proceedings of the 5th International Conference on Malignant Lymphoma, Part Proceedings, Lugano, Switzerland, 9–12 June 1994; Volume 5, pp. 1–163.
31. Cohen, D.; Perry, C.; Hazut-Krauthammer, S.; Kesler, M.; Herishanu, Y.; Luttwak, E.; Even-Sapir, E.; Avivi, I. Is there a role for [^{18}F]FDG PET-CT in staging MALT lymphoma? *Cancers* **2022**, *14*, 750. [CrossRef]

32. Stathis, A.; Chini, C.; Bertoni, F.; Proserpio, I.; Capella, C.; Mazzucchelli, L.; Pedrinis, E.; Cavalli, F.; Pinotti, G.; Zucca, E. Long-term outcome following *Helicobacter pylori* eradication in a retrospective study of 105 patients with localized gastric marginal zone B-cell lymphoma of MALT type. *Ann. Oncol.* **2009**, *20*, 1086–1093. [CrossRef]
33. Zullo, A.; Hassan, C.; Cristofari, F.; Andriani, A.; De Francesco, V.; Ierardi, E.; Tomao, S.; Stolte, M.; Morini, S.; Vaira, D. Effects of *Helicobacter pylori* eradication on early stage gastric mucosa–associated lymphoid tissue lymphoma. *Clin. Gastroenterol. Hepatol.* **2010**, *8*, 105–110. [CrossRef]
34. Zullo, A.; Hassan, C.; Andriani, A.; Cristofari, F.; Bassanelli, C.; Spinelli, G.P.; Tomao, S.; Morini, S. Treatment of low-grade gastric MALT-lymphoma unresponsive to *Helicobacter pylori* therapy: A pooled-data analysis. *Med. Oncol.* **2010**, *27*, 291–295. [CrossRef]
35. Gisbert, J.P.; Calvet, X. Review article: Common misconceptions in the management of Helicobacter pylori-associated gastric MALT-lymphoma. *Aliment. Pharmacol. Ther.* **2011**, *34*, 1047–1062. [CrossRef]
36. Nakamura, S.; Sugiyama, T.; Matsumoto, T.; Iijima, K.; Ono, S.; Tajika, M.; Tari, A.; Kitadai, Y.; Matsumoto, H.; Nagaya, T.; et al. Long-term clinical outcome of gastric MALT lymphoma after eradication of *Helicobacter pylori*: A multicentre cohort follow-up study of 420 patients in Japan. *Gut* **2011**, *61*, 507–513. [CrossRef]
37. Nakamura, S.; Matsumoto, T. *Helicobacter pylori* and gastric mucosa-associated lymphoid tissue lymphoma: Recent progress in pathogenesis and management. *World J. Gastroenterol.* **2013**, *19*, 8181–8187. [CrossRef]
38. Guo, Q.; Guo, S.; Zhang, Y. Treatment of gastric MALT lymphoma with a focus on *Helicobacter pylori* eradication. *Int. J. Hematol.* **2013**, *97*, 735–742. [CrossRef]
39. Zucca, E.; Bergman, C.C.; Ricardi, U.; Thieblemont, C.; Raderer, M.; Ladetto, M. Gastric marginal zone lymphoma of MALT type: ESMO Clinical Practice Guidelines for diagnosis, treatment and follow-up. *Ann. Oncol.* **2013**, *24*, vi144–vi148. [CrossRef]
40. Xie, Y.-L.; He, C.-Y.; Wei, S.-Q.; Guan, W.-J.; Jiang, Z. Clinical efficacy of the modified *Helicobacter pylori* eradication therapy for *Helicobacter pylori*-negative gastric mucosa-associated lymphoid tissue lymphoma: A meta analysis. *Chin. Med. J.* **2020**, *133*, 1337–1346. [CrossRef]
41. Choi, Y.J.; Kim, N.; Paik, J.H.; Kim, J.M.; Lee, S.H.; Park, Y.S.; Hwang, J.-H.; Kim, J.-W.; Jeong, S.-H.; Lee, D.H.; et al. Characteristics of *Helicobacter pylori*-positive and *Helicobacter pylori*-negative gastric mucosa-associated lymphoid tissue lymphoma and their influence on clinical outcome. *Helicobacter* **2013**, *18*, 197–205. [CrossRef]
42. Bergman, C.C.; Wotherspoon, A.C.; Capella, C.; Motta, T.; Pedrinis, E.; Pileri, S.A.; Bertoni, F.; Conconi, A.; Zucca, E.; Ponzoni, M.; et al. Gela histological scoring system for post-treatment biopsies of patients with gastric MALT lymphoma is feasible and reliable in routine practice. *Br. J. Haematol.* **2012**, *160*, 47–52. [CrossRef]
43. Zucca, E.; Conconi, A.; Martinelli, G.; Bouabdallah, R.; Tucci, A.; Vitolo, U.; Martelli, M.; Pettengell, R.; Salles, G.; Sebban, C.; et al. Final results of the IELSG-19 randomized trial of mucosa-associated lymphoid tissue lymphoma: Improved event-free and progression-free survival with rituximab plus chlorambucil versus either chlorambucil or rituximab monotherapy. *J. Clin. Oncol.* **2017**, *35*, 1905–1912. [CrossRef]
44. Yahalom, J.; Xu, A.J.; Noy, A.; Lobaugh, S.; Chelius, M.; Chau, K.; Portlock, C.; Hajj, C.; Imber, B.S.; Straus, D.J.; et al. Involved-site radiotherapy for *Helicobacter pylori*–independent gastric MALT lymphoma: 26 years of experience with 178 patients. *Blood Adv.* **2021**, *5*, 1830–1836. [CrossRef] [PubMed]
45. Sugizaki, K.; Tari, A.; Kitadai, Y.; Oda, I.; Nakamura, S.; Yoshino, T.; Sugiyama, T. Anti-*Helicobacter pylori* therapy in localized gastric mucosa-associated lymphoid tissue lymphoma: A prospective, nationwide, multicenter study in Japan. *Helicobacter* **2018**, *23*, e12474. [CrossRef] [PubMed]
46. Levitt, M.; Gharibo, M.; Strair, R.; Schaar, D.; Rubin, A.; Bertino, J. Accelerated R-COP: A Pilot Study for the Treatment of Advanced Low Grade Lymphomas that Has a High Complete Response Rate. *J. Chemother.* **2009**, *21*, 434–438. [CrossRef] [PubMed]
47. Fischbach, W. Gastric MALT lymphoma—Update on diagnosis and treatment. *Best Pract. Res. Clin. Gastroenterol.* **2014**, *28*, 1069–1077. [CrossRef]
48. Cencini, E.; Fabbri, A.; Lauria, F.; Bocchia, M. Long-term efficacy and toxicity of rituximab plus fludarabine and mitoxantrone (R-FM) for gastric marginal zone lymphoma: A single-center experience and literature review. *Ann. Hematol.* **2018**, *97*, 821–829. [CrossRef]
49. Morigi, A.; Argnani, L.; Lolli, G.; Broccoli, A.; Pellegrini, C.; Nanni, L.; Stefoni, V.; Coppola, P.E.; Carella, M.; Casadei, B.; et al. Bendamustine-rituximab regimen in untreated indolent marginal zone lymphoma: Experience on 65 patients. *Hematol. Oncol.* **2020**, *38*, 487–492. [CrossRef]
50. Alderuccio, J.P.; Arcaini, L.; Watkins, M.P.; Beaven, A.W.; Shouse, G.; Epperla, N.; Spina, M.; Stefanovic, A.; Sandoval-Sus, J.; Torka, P.; et al. An international analysis evaluating frontline bendamustine with rituximab in extranodal marginal zone lymphoma. *Blood Adv.* **2022**, *6*, 2035–2044. [CrossRef]
51. Zucca, E.; Arcaini, L.; Buske, C.; Johnson, P.; Ponzoni, M.; Raderer, M.; Ricardi, U.; Salar, A.; Stamatopoulos, K.; Thieblemont, C.; et al. Marginal zone lymphomas: ESMO clinical practice guidelines for diagnosis, treatment and follow-up. *Ann. Oncol.* **2020**, *31*, 17–29. [CrossRef]

Disclaimer/Publisher's Note: The statements, opinions and data contained in all publications are solely those of the individual author(s) and contributor(s) and not of MDPI and/or the editor(s). MDPI and/or the editor(s) disclaim responsibility for any injury to people or property resulting from any ideas, methods, instructions or products referred to in the content.

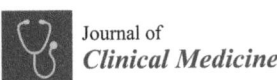

Review

Expectations for the Dual Therapy with Vonoprazan and Amoxicillin for the Eradication of *H. pylori*

Takahisa Furuta [1,*], Mihoko Yamade [2], Tomohiro Higuchi [2], Satoru Takahashi [2], Natsuki Ishida [2], Shinya Tani [2], Satoshi Tamura [2], Moriya Iwaizumi [3], Yasushi Hamaya [2], Satoshi Osawa [4] and Ken Sugimoto [2]

1. Furuta Clinic for Internal Medicine, 1963-15 Mitsuke, Iwata, Shizuoka 438-0086, Japan
2. First Department of Medicine, Hamamatsu University School of Medicine, 1-20-1 Handayama, Higashi-ku, Hamamatsu 431-3192, Japan
3. Clinical Laboratories, Hamamatsu University School of Medicine, 1-20-1 Handayama, Higashi-ku, Hamamatsu 431-3192, Japan
4. Endoscopic and Photodynamic Medicine, Hamamatsu University School of Medicine, 1-20-1 Handayama, Higashi-ku, Hamamatsu 431-3192, Japan
* Correspondence: tafuruta@fd6.so-net.ne.jp; Tel.: +81-538-31-4105; Fax: +81-538-31-4106

Abstract: Vonoprazan (VPZ) inhibits gastric acid secretion more potently than proton pump inhibitors. Recently, attention has been focused on the dual therapy with VPZ and amoxicillin (AMOX) for the eradication of *H. pylori*. The dual VPZ/AMOX therapy attains the sufficient eradication rate with lowering the risk of adverse events in comparison with the triple therapy and quadruple therapy. Therefore, the dual VPZ/AMOX therapy is considered a useful eradication regimen for *H. pylori* infection.

Keywords: *H. pylori*; dual therapy; vonoprazan (VPZ); amoxicillin (AMOX); clarithromycin (CAM)

1. Introduction

One of the first-line eradication regimens for *H. pylori* has long been a triple therapy with proton pump inhibitor (PPI), amoxicillin (AMOX), and clarithromycin (CAM). However, with the recent increase in CAM-resistant strains of *H. pylori*, the eradication rates of PPI/AMOX/CAM therapy have been declining [1], which is a global problem. The reported incidences of CAM-resistance strains of *H. pylori* are approximately 25–32% [2–4]. In addition, since the effects of PPIs are influenced by the genetic polymorphism of CYP2C19, which is the main metabolic enzyme of PPIs, it has been pointed out that the eradication rates in the CYP2C19 extensive metabolizers are lower in comparison with other metabolizers [5,6]. In order to recover the eradication rates of the first-line eradication therapy, bismuth or non-bismuth quadruple therapies are being used, which are recommended especially in areas with high CAM-resistance rates [7]. Although the eradication rates of quadruple therapy are high, multiple drugs must be taken and the frequency of side effects is high.

There have been some reports of dual therapy with PPIs and AMOX as listed in Table 1 [5,8–25]. Originally, eradication therapy for *H. pylori* started with classical triple therapy followed by the dual therapy. However, the eradication rates of the dual therapy have varied as shown in Table 1. After the triple therapy for 1 week was developed [14], the dual therapy with PPI and AMOX was no longer the main therapy for *H. pylori* infection.

Vonoprazan (VPZ) has been clinically available since 2015. VPZ inhibits gastric acid secretion more potently than PPIs [26]. The eradication rate of the triple therapy with VPZ 20 mg bid, CAM 200 mg bid, and AMOX 750 mg bid was reported 92.6%, which was significantly higher than that of the triple therapy with lansoprazole 30 mg and the same doses of CAM and AMOX [27]. Interestingly, in this report, the eradication rate by the triple therapy with VPZ, CAM, and AMOX in patients infected with CAM-resistant strains

of *H. pylori* was 82.0%, suggesting that the dual therapy with VPZ and AMOX for 1 week can attain the eradication rate higher than 80.0%. Then, the attention has recently been focused on the dual therapy with VPZ and AMOX.

Table 1. Lists of reports of dual therapy with PPI and AMOX.

Author	Year	Dosing Scheme of AMOX	Dosing Scheme of PPI	Duration	n	Eradication Rate (%) (ITT)
Furuta [8]	2001	500 mg qid	RPZ 10 mg qid	14 days	17	100.0%
Tai [9]	2019	750 mg qid	EPZ 40 mg tid	14 days	120	91.7%
Shirai [10]	2007	500 mg qid	RPZ 10 mg qid	14 days	66	90.9%
Bayerdorffer [11]	1995	750 mg tid	OPZ 40 mg tid	14 days	139	90.6%
Furuta [12]	2010	500 mg qid	RPZ 10 mg qid	14 days	49	87.8%
Miehlke [13]	2003	750 mg qid	OPZ 40 mg qid	14 days	38	83.8%
Furuta [5]	2001	500 mg tid	RPZ 10 mg bid	14 days	97	81.4%
Schwartz [14]	1998	1000 mg tid	LPZ 30 mg tid	14 days	51	77%
Miehlke [15]	2006	1000 mg tid	OPZ 40 mg tid	14 days	72	70%
Miyoshi [16]	2001	500 mg tid	OPZ 20 mg bid	14 days	98	66.3%
Nishizawa [17]	2012	500 mg qid	RPZ 10 mg qid	14 days	46	63.0%
Moiyoshi [16]	2001	500 mg tid	RPZ 10 mg tid	14 days	101	62.4%
Isomoto [18]	2003	1000 mg bid	RPZ 20 mg bid	14 days	63	59%
Wong [19]	2000	1000 mg bid	LPZ 30 mg bid	14 days	75	57%
Attumi [20]	2014	1000 mg bid	Dexlansoprazole 120 mg bid	14 days	13	53.8%
Schwartz [14]	1998	1000 mg tid	LPZ 30 mg bid	14 days	49	53%
Koizumi [21]	1998	500 mg tid	OPZ 20 mg qd	14 days	25	52%
Furuta [22]	1998	500 mg qid	OPZ 20 mg qd	14 days	62	50%
Bell [23]	1995	500 mg tid	OPZ 40 mg qd	14 days	60	46%
Cottrill [24]	1997	1000 mg bid	OPZ 40 mg qd	14 days	85	44%
Kagaya [25]	2000	750 mg bid	LPZ 30 mg qd	14 days	24	43%

Abbreviations: PPI = proton pump inhibitor, EPZ = esomeprazole, LPZ = lansoprazole, OPZ = omeprazole, RPZ = rabeprazole, qd = once daily, bid = twice daily, tid = three times daily qid = four times daily.

2. Gastric Acid Secretion Required for the Dual Therapy with Amoxicillin

AMOX exerts its antibacterial action by binding to penicillin-binding protein (PBP) and inhibiting the synthesis of bacterial cell wall. According to a report examining the relationship between PBP expression in *H. pylori* and pH, *H. pylori* does not proliferate and PBP expression is low at around pH 3.0 [28]. However, at pH 7.4, *H. pylori* proliferates vigorously and the expression of PBP also increases, indicating that the number of targets of AMOX increases, and it is thought that AMOX becomes more effective. In addition, inhibition of gastric acid secretion leads to stabilization of antibacterial drugs in the stomach and increases their concentration in gastric juice [29], which greatly contributes to the success of eradication.

There is a report examining the relationship among the success or failure of eradication by triple therapy, CAM-resistance of *H. pylori* and intragastric pH [30]. When the mean 24-h intragastric pH is less than 4.5 and when the percent time for intragastric pH < 4.0 is longer than 40%, eradication will fail even if *H. pylori* strain is sensitive to CAM (Figure 1 blue area). In contrast, when the mean 24-h intragastric pH exceeds 5, CAM-susceptible bacteria can be successfully eradicated (Figure 1 yellow area). Interestingly, if the mean 24-h intragastric pH in the stomach is higher than 6.5 and the percent time for intragastric pH < 4.0 is 5% or less (pink part in Figure 1), in other words, if the pH 4 holding time ratio (pH 4 HTR) is 95% or more and if the mean 24 h intragastric pH is no less than 6.5, CAM-resistant strains can be eradicated. Therefore, it is suggested that eradication of *H. pylori* can be attained by a single antibiotic, such as AMOX, when the intragastric pH is strictly controlled to be neutral.

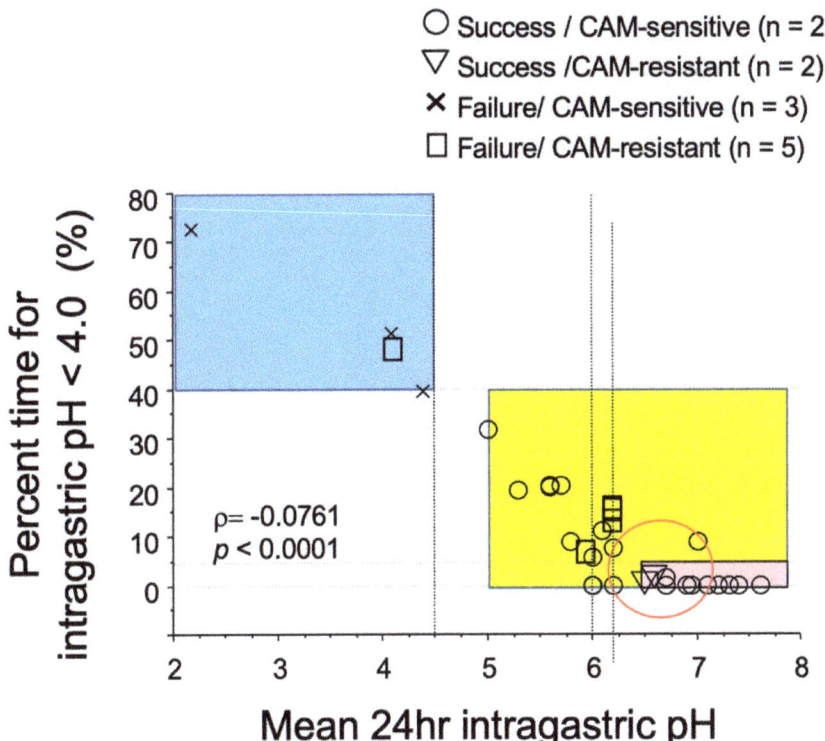

Figure 1. Relationship of success or failure of eradication of *H. pylori* by the triple therapy with PPI, amoxicillin, and clarithromycin (CAM) with CAM-resistance, 24 h intragastric pH, and percent time for intragastric pH < 4.0. When the mean intragastric pH is less than 4.5 and the percent time for intragastric pH < 4.0 was longer than 40% (blue area), eradication of *H. pylori* fails in patients infected with not only CAM-resistant strains (□) but also CAM-sensitive strains (×) of *H. pylori*. When 24 h intragastric pH is higher than 5.0 (yellow area), eradication of *H. pylori* succeeds for CAM-sensitive strains (○) of *H. pylori*. When the mean intragastric pH is no less than 6.5 and the percent time for intragastric pH < 4.0 is less than 5% (pink area), eradication of *H. pylori* succeeds in patients infected with CAM-resistant strains (∇) as well as CAM-sensitive strains (○) of *H. pylori*. Modified [30].

The relationship between dosing schemes of PPI and eradication rates of the dual therapies with PPI and AMOX listed in Table 1 is plotted in Figure 2. As the dosing frequency of PPI increases, the eradication rates increase. Because the acid inhibitory effect of PPI is enhanced by the divided dosing [31], the eradication rates with dual therapy with PPI and AMOX increase with the grade of acid inhibition.

Kagami et al. [32] compared the acid inhibitory effects of VPZ and EPZ and found that 95% of pH 4 HTR could be achieved by VPZ 20 mg once daily and that 100.0% of pH 4 HTR and 6.8 of the mean 24 h intragastric pH could be attained by VPZ 20 mg twice daily, but not EPZ (Figure 3). Moreover, the acid inhibitory action of VPZ was not influenced by CYP2C19 polymorphism, meaning that the gastric acid inhibition required for eradication of the *H. pylori* by the dual therapy with AMOX can be achieved by VPZ 20 mg twice a day irrespective of CYP2C19 polymorphism.

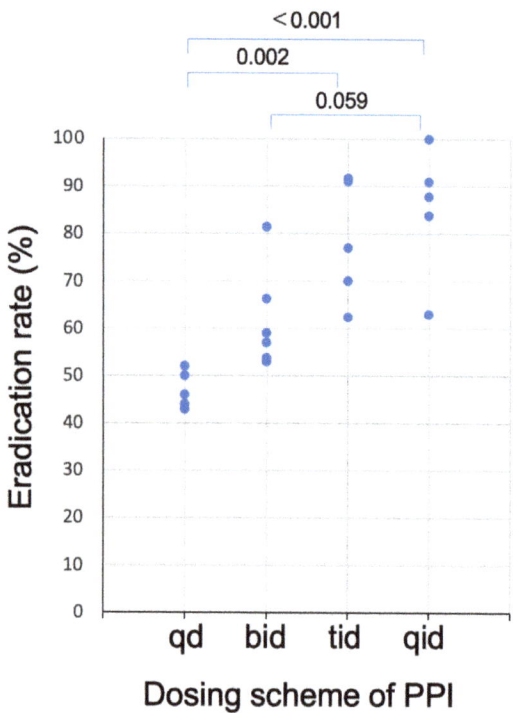

Figure 2. Plots of the eradication rates of studies of dual therapy with PPI and amoxicillin as a function of dosing schemes of PPI listed in Table 1. Eradication rates of regimen with three (tid) or four (qid) times daily dosing of PPI was significantly higher than those with once (qd) or twice (bid) daily dosing.

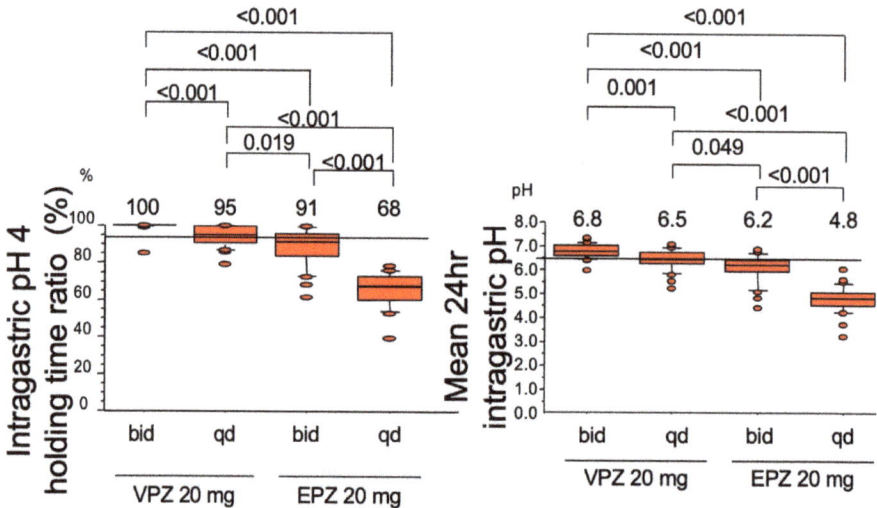

Figure 3. Intragastric pH 4 holding time ratio (**Left** panel) and mean 24 h intragastric pH (**Right** panel) attained by the twice (bid) or once (qd) daily dosing of 20 mg of vonoprazan (VPZ) or esomeprazole (EPZ) on day 7. VPZ 20 mg twice daily can attain both the intragastric pH 4 holding time ratio 100.0% and the mean 24 h intragastric pH 6.8.

3. Antibacterial Effect and Optimal Dosing Scheme of Amoxicillin

The relationship between the eradication rates and dosing scheme of AMOX is shown in Figure 4. When AMOX was dosed twice daily, the eradication rates were all less than 60%. To attain eradication rates higher than 90.0%, at least 3 times daily dosing seems necessary for AMOX in the dual therapy. Because the antibacterial effect of AMOX is time-dependent [33] and because it has no post antibiotic effect [34], its antibacterial activity depends on the percent time above MIC (%T > MIC) [35]. Since the plasma half-life of AMOX is as short as around 1 h, it will decrease below MIC in a few hours after dosing, and therefore, it is necessary to be dosed 3–4 times a day for AMOX to be effective. This is the reason why results of the twice-daily dosing regimens of AMOX are insufficient. In contrast, in reports that achieved high eradication rates, AMOX was administered 3–4 times daily when PPI was also administered at high doses 3–4 times a day.

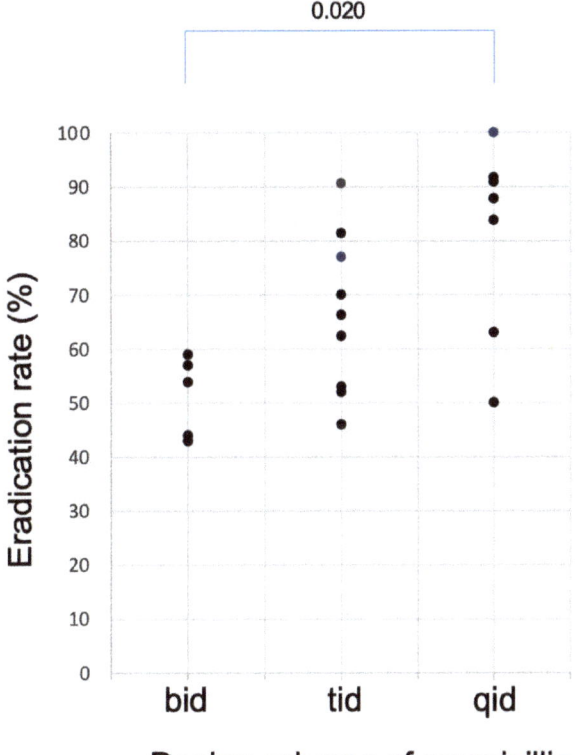

Figure 4. Plots of the eradication rates of studies of dual therapy with PPI and amoxicillin listed in Table 1 as a function of dosing schemes of amoxicillin. Eradication rates higher than 90.0% can be attained when amoxicillin was dosed at least three time daily (tid).

There was no significant correlation between the total daily dose of AMOX and eradication rates in the regimens listed in Table 1 ($p = 0.414$)

Accordingly, to attain the sufficient eradication rates by the dual therapy with AMOX and an acid inhibitor, it is considered necessary to administer AMOX in 3 or more divided doses under the potent acid inhibition that can be attained by the higher doses of PPI dosed 3 or 4 times daily or VPZ 20 mg twice daily. Because the acid inhibitory effect of PPI is influenced by CYP2C19 polymorphism, but not for VPZ, VPZ is ideal and should be used for the dual therapy.

It is obvious that the time above the MIC obtained with 3 doses of AMOX 500 mg is longer than the time above the MIC obtained with 2 doses of AMOX 750 mg (Figure 5). Furthermore, since the MIC is lowered by strongly suppressing gastric acid, it is speculated that the time above the MIC will be even longer when an ultra-potent acid inhibitor, such as VPZ, is used.

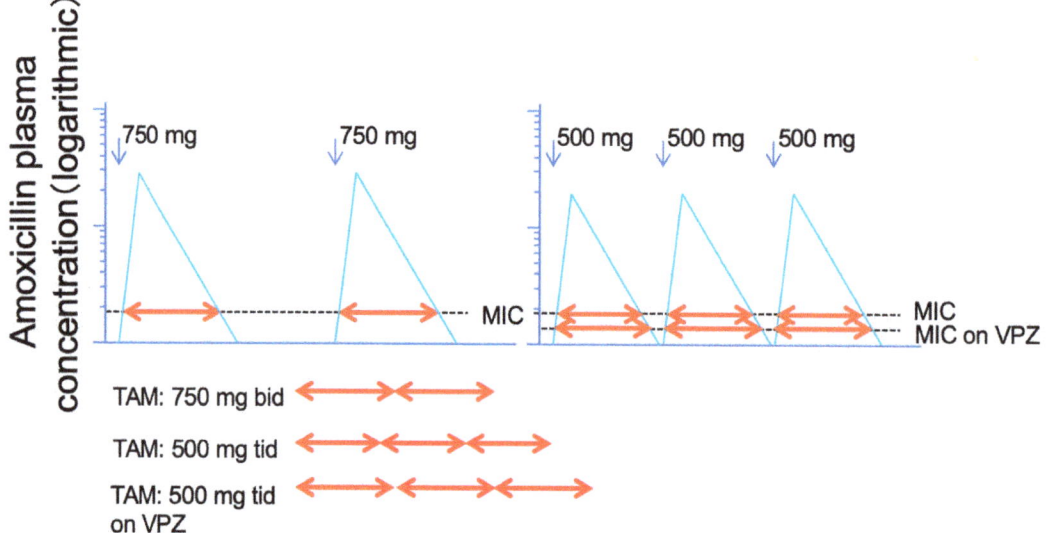

Figure 5. Logarithmic model of Time above MIC (T > MIC) of plasma level of amoxicillin 750 mg dosed twice and 500 mg three times daily. The total of T > MIC of amoxicillin 500 mg three times daily is longer than that of 750 mg twice daily. By using the vonoprazan, MIC is expected to be lowered, resulting in the further elongation of T > MIC of amoxicillin.

4. Eradication Rates of Dual Therapy with Vonoprazan and Amoxicillin

The eradication rate reported in the first study of the dual therapy with VPZ and AMOX was 92.9%, which was identical to that of the triple therapy with VPZ, AMOX, and CAM [36]. In this report, there were no statistically significant differences in adverse events between dual therapy and triple therapy, but tended to be less with dual therapy. Therefore, it was considered that the dual VPZ/AMOX therapy could be a regimen for the first-line eradication therapy.

Since this report, there have been several studies on the dual therapy with VPZ and AMOX as listed in Table 2 [37–45]. Although the sufficient eradication rate could be attained by the first study [36], the eradication rates of the dual VPZ/AMOX therapies varies by different dosing schemes of AMOX and treatment periods as in the cases of PPIs.

As the duration of the treatment period, Lin et al. [42] reported that the dual VPZ/AMOX therapies for 7 days could not achieve an acceptable eradication rates (58.3% and 60.7%). Hu et al. [45] compared the 7 day and 10 day regimen with different AMOX dosing schemes and found that none of the 7 or 10 day regimens could attain the sufficient eradication rates. However, they reported that a 14 day regimen could attained a sufficient eradication rate (89.1%) [37]. However, studies by Suzuki et al. [38] Gotoda et al. [39] and Sue et al. [40], which were all from Japan, demonstrated that 7 days seemed a sufficient treatment period for the dual VPZ/AMMOX therapy. The optimal treatment periods for the dual VPZ/AMOX therapy seem to differ among different regions and ethnic groups.

Table 2. Lists of reports of dual therapy with VPZ and AMOX.

Author	Year	Dosing Scheme of AMOX	Dosing Scheme of VPZ	Duration	n	Eradication Rate (%) (ITT)
Furuta [36]	2019	500 mg tid	20 mg bid	7 days	56	92.9%
Suzuki [38]	2020	750 mg bid	20 mg bid	7 days	168	84.5%
Gotoda [39]	2020	750 mg bid	20 mg bid	7 days	60	85.0%
Sue [40]	2022	500 mg qid	20 mg bid	7 days	20	90.0%
Lin [42]	2022	750 mg qid	20 mg bid	7 days	84	58.3%
Lin [42]	2022	500 mg qid	20 mg bid	7 days	61	60.7%
Hu [45]	2022	1000 mg bid	20 mg bid	7 days	24	66.7%
Hu [45]	2022	1000 mg bid	20 mg bid	10 days	37	89.2%
Hu [45]	2022	1000 mg tid	20 mg bid	7 days	21	81.0%
Hu [45]	2022	1000 mg tid	20 mg bid	10 days	37	81.1%
Qian [41]	2022	750 mg qid	20 mg bid	10 days	125	93.4%
Qian [41]	2022	1000 mg bid	20 mg bid	10 days	125	85.1%
Hu [37]	2022	1000 mg bid	20 mg bid	14 days	55	89.1%
Hu [37]	2022	1000 mg tid	20 mg bid	14 days	55	87.3%
Zuberi [44]	2022	1000 mg bid	20 mg bid	14 days	92	93.5%
Chey [46]	2022	1000 mg tid	20 mg bid	14 days	324	78.5%
Gao [43]	2022	1000 mg tid/750 mg qid	10 mg bid	14 days	43	95.3%
Gao [43]	2022	1000 mg tid/750 mg qid	20 mg bid	14 days	143	91.6%

Abbreviations: VPZ = vonoprazan AMOX = amoxicillin, bid = twice daily, tid = three times daily, qid = 4 times daily.

Qian et al. [41] compared two types of ten-day dual VPZ/AMOX therapies with bismuth-containing quadruple therapy. The dual therapy with VPZ 20 mg bid and AMOX 750 mg qid attained the 93.4% of eradication rate, which was as high as that of the quadruple therapy (90.9%). Interestingly, the incidence of side effects of the dual therapy was significantly lower than that of the quadruple therapy. Zuberi [44] also reported that dual VPZ/AMOX therapy provides an acceptable and higher eradication rate (93.5%) with fewer adverse events in comparison with the triple therapy with omeprazole, CAM, and AMOX. Gao [43] reported that the dual VPZ/AMOX therapies were useful as the rescue therapy. However, the eradication rate of the report by Chey [46] was 78.5%, although the regimen was almost the same as that of study of Gao [43]. Accordingly, the optimal dosing schemes of the dual VPZ/AMOX therapy remains to be determined. The best regimens of the dual VPZ/AMOX therapy should be developed for each region and ethnicity.

5. Merits of the Dual Therapy with Vonoprazan and Amoxicillin

One of merits of the dual VPZ/AMOX therapy is to reduce the incidence of adverse events. As noted above, the incidence of adverse events observed in the dual therapies was lower in comparison with the triple therapy and quadruple therapy [36,41].

Pharmacologically, the greatest advantage of the dual therapy is that fewer drugs are used, reducing the risk of drug–drug interactions. CAM, which is often used in triple therapy, is a potent inhibitor of CYP3A4 and p-glycoprotein [47]. CAM has been reported to increase plasma levels of drugs metabolized and transported by these enzymes [29]. However, CAM is not involved in the dual VPZ/AMOX therapy. Therefore, the risk of drug–drug interactions related to CAM can be avoided. Of course, AMOX and VPZ are not without risk of interaction. VPZ has also been reported to affect the antiplatelet effects of Clopidogrel and Prasugrel [48], and has also been reported to affect CYPs [49]. Therefore, it cannot be said that the dual VPZ/AMOX is completely safe. However, it is considered safer than triple therapy from the viewpoint of drug–drug interactions. CAM also has an arrhythmia risk [50]. Therefore, dual therapy with VPZ and AMOX is particularly useful in patients with a risk of arrythmia, such as QT prolongation.

6. Dual Therapy with Vonoprazan and Amoxicillin with Reference to Clarithromycin Susceptibility

Suzuki et al. investigated influence of the CAM resistance in the comparative study of the dual therapy with VPZ 20 mg bid + AMOX 750 mg bid for 1 week and the triple therapy with VPZ 20 mg bid + CAM 20 mg bid + AMOX 750 mg bid for 1 week. In their study in patients infected with CAM-sensitive strains of *H. pylori*, the eradication rates of the dual and triple therapies were 85.5% and 95.1%, respectively. However, in patients infected with CAM-resistant strains of *H. pylori*, the respective eradication rates were 92.3% and 76.2% ($p < 0.05$). In other words, CAM has a negative effect on patients infected with CAM-resistant strains of *H. pylori*. There are many possible reasons, but one possible explanation is the pharmacodynamic antagonism between CAM and APMC.

In other bacteria, the combination of AMOX and CAM has been reported to be antagonistic [51,52]. The target of AMOX is PBP as noted above, which is the enzyme involved in biosynthesis of bacterial cell wall. When *H. pylori* grows, the expression of PBP is enhanced, which means that the expression of target of AMOX is increased, resulting in the bactericidal effect of AMOX being enhanced. In contrast, when the growth of *H. pylori* is inhibited, the expression of PBP is decreased. In this situation, the bactericidal effect of AMOX is decreased because the expression of target of AMOX is decreased. CAM is known as the inhibitor of rRNA, indicating that CAM inhibits the protein synthesis including PBP. Then, the sensitivity to AMOX is decreased by CAM.

However, if the patient is infected with CAM-sensitive strains, there is no problem because they can be killed by CAM. However, in cases infected with CAM-resistant strains of *H. pylori*, there might be some problems. MIC ranges of CAM-resistant strains of *H. pylori* are very wide (e.g., from 1 μg/mL to >32 μg/mL). In cases infected with CAM-weakly resistant strains of *H. pylori*, CAM will work halfway. Although *H. pylori* strains cannot be killed by CAM, the inhibitory effect of CAM on rRNA may affect the subsequent protein synthesis including PBP, leading to the reduced sensitivity to AMOX [53]. This seems to be the reason why the eradication rates attained by a PPI, AMOX, and CAM were reportedly very low in patients infected with CAM-resistant strains of *H. pylori* [54,55], although AMOX-resistant strains of *H. pylori* are rare.

7. Strategy for Patients Allergic to Penicillin

The dual therapy with VPZ and AMOX cannot be used for patients allergic to penicillin. Gao et al. [56] performed dual therapy with VPZ 20 mg bid and tetracycline 500 mg tid (body weight < 70 kg) or 500 mg qid (body weight ≥ 70 kg) for 14 days in patients who were allergic to penicillin or who had failed before. The eradication rate was 93.5%. Therefore, it is suggested that if one antibacterial agent with high susceptibility is selected besides AMOX, *H. pylori* eradication can be achieved with dual therapy with VPZ plus single effective antibacterial agent.

8. Conclusions

As mentioned above, the greatest merit of the dual VPZ/AMOX therapy is to reduce the risk of adverse events without lowering the eradication rates. In this regimen, CAM is not used, indicating the risk reduction of drug–drug interactions, arrhythmia, and other adverse events caused by CAM. The regimen is simple. There is also a report of the effective dual therapy with VPZ and single antimicrobial agent other than AMOX, such as tetracycline.

Now that we have vonoprazan in our hands, it is expected that eradication therapy will be reconstructed into a simpler regimen, such as dual therapy with VPZ and one antibacterial agent with high susceptibility (i.e., AMOX) in the optimal dosing scheme. It is also expected that we can break away from the stereotype of using multiple antibiotics to eradicate *H. pylori*.

Unfortunately, the use of VPZ is not widespread worldwide. It is hoped that VPZ will become widely available around the world in the future, and new drugs with similar effects will be developed, leading to the simplification of eradication regimens in many countries.

Author Contributions: Conceptualization, T.F., M.Y., T.H., S.T. (Satoru Takahashi). Validation, S.O., M.I., Y.H. Formal analysis, S.T. (Satoshi Tamura), S.T. (Shinya Tani), N.I. Investigation, T.F., M.Y., T.H., S.T. (Satoru Takahashi). Resources T.F.; data curation Writing—original draft preparation: T.F. Writing—review and editing: M.Y., T.H., S.T. (Satoru Takahashi), S.O., M.I., S.T. (Shinya Tani), S.T. (Satoshi Tamura). Visualization, T.F. Supervision K.S. All authors have read and agreed to the published version of the manuscript.

Funding: This research received no external funding.

Institutional Review Board Statement: Not applicable.

Informed Consent Statement: Not applicable.

Data Availability Statement: We have used the published data.

Conflicts of Interest: The authors declare no conflict of interest.

Abbreviations

AMOX = amoxicillin, CAM = clarithromycin, CYP = cytochrome P450, EPZ = esomeprazole, RPZ = rabeprazole, T>MIC = time above MIC, VPZ = vonoprazan.

References

1. Sasaki, M.; Ogasawara, N.; Utsumi, K.; Kawamura, N.; Kamiya, T.; Kataoka, H.; Tanida, S.; Mizoshita, T.; Kasugai, K.; Joh, T. Changes in 12-Year First-Line Eradication Rate of *Helicobacter pylori* Based on Triple Therapy with Proton Pump Inhibitor, Amoxicillin and Clarithromycin. *J. Clin. Biochem. Nutr.* **2010**, *47*, 53–58. [CrossRef] [PubMed]
2. Fasciana, T.; Calà, C.; Bonura, C.; Di Carlo, E.; Matranga, D.; Scarpulla, G.; Manganaro, M.; Camilleri, S.; Giammanco, A. Resistance to clarithromycin and genotypes in *Helicobacter pylori* strains isolated in Sicily. *J. Med. Microbiol.* **2015**, *64*, 1408–1414. [CrossRef] [PubMed]
3. Tsuda, M.; Watanabe, Y.; Oikawa, R.; Watanabe, R.; Higashino, M.; Kubo, K.; Yamamoto, H.; Itoh, F.; Kato, M. Clinical evaluation of a novel molecular diagnosis kit for detecting *Helicobacter pylori* and clarithromycin-resistant using intragastric fluid. *Helicobacter* **2022**, *27*, e12933. [CrossRef] [PubMed]
4. Sue, S.; Ogushi, M.; Arima, I.; Kuwashima, H.; Nakao, S.; Naito, M.; Komatsu, K.; Kaneko, H.; Tamura, T.; Sasaki, T.; et al. Vonoprazan- vs. proton-pump inhibitor-based first-line 7-day triple therapy for clarithromycin-susceptible *Helicobacter pylori*: A multicenter, prospective, randomized trial. *Helicobacter* **2018**, *23*, e12456. [CrossRef]
5. Furuta, T.; Shirai, N.; Takashima, M.; Xiao, F.; Hanai, H.; Nakagawa, K.; Sugimura, H.; Ohashi, K.; Ishizaki, T. Effects of genotypic differences in CYP2C19 status on cure rates for *Helicobacter pylori* infection by dual therapy with rabeprazole plus amoxicillin. *Pharmacogenetics* **2001**, *11*, 341–348. [CrossRef]
6. Furuta, T.; Shirai, N.; Takashima, M.; Xiao, F.; Hanai, H.; Sugimura, H.; Ohashi, K.; Ishizaki, T.; Kaneko, E. Effect of genotypic differences in CYP2C19 on cure rates for *Helicobacter pylori* infection by triple therapy with a proton pump inhibitor, amoxicillin, and clarithromycin. *Clin. Pharmacol. Ther.* **2001**, *69*, 158–168. [CrossRef]
7. Malfertheiner, P.; Megraud, F.; O'morain, C.A.; Gisbert, J.P.; Kuipers, E.J.; Axon, A.T.; Bazzoli, F.; Gasbarrini, A.; Atherton, J.; Graham, D.Y.; et al. Management of *Helicobacter pylori* infection-the Maastricht V/Florence Consensus Report. *Gut* **2017**, *66*, 6–30. [CrossRef]
8. Furuta, T.; Shirai, N.; Xiao, F.; Takashita, M.; Sugimoto, M.; Kajimura, M.; Ohashi, K.; Ishizaki, T. High-dose rabeprazole/amoxicillin therapy as the second-line regimen after failure to eradicate *H. pylori* by triple therapy with the usual doses of a proton pump inhibitor, clarithromycin and amoxicillin. *Hepatogastroenterology* **2003**, *50*, 2274–2278.
9. Tai, W.-C.; Liang, C.-M.; Kuo, C.-M.; Huang, P.-Y.; Wu, C.-K.; Yang, S.-C.; Kuo, Y.-H.; Lin, M.-T.; Lee, C.-H.; Hsu, C.-N.; et al. A 14 day esomeprazole- and amoxicillin-containing high-dose dual therapy regimen achieves a high eradication rate as first-line anti-Helicobacter pylori treatment in Taiwan: A prospective randomized trial. *J. Antimicrob. Chemother.* **2019**, *74*, 1718–1724. [CrossRef]
10. Shirai, N.; Sugimoto, M.; Kodaira, C.; Nishino, M.; Ikuma, M.; Kajimura, M.; Ohashi, K.; Ishizaki, T.; Hishida, A.; Furuta, T. Dual therapy with high doses of rabeprazole and amoxicillin versus triple therapy with rabeprazole, amoxicillin, and metronidazole as a rescue regimen for *Helicobacter pylori* infection after the standard triple therapy. *Eur. J. Clin. Pharmacol.* **2007**, *63*, 743–749. [CrossRef]

11. Bayerdörffer, E.; Miehlke, S.; Mannes, G.A.; Sommer, A.; Höchter, W.; Weingart, J.; Heldwein, W.; Klann, H.; Simon, T.; Schmitt, W.; et al. Double-blind trial of omeprazole and amoxicillin to cure *Helicobacter pylori* infection in patients with duodenal ulcers. *Gastroenterology* **1995**, *108*, 1412–1417. [CrossRef] [PubMed]
12. Furuta, T.; Sugimoto, M.; Kodaira, C.; Nishino, M.; Yamade, M.; Uotani, T.; Ikuma, M.; Shirai, N. The dual therapy with 4 times daily dosing of rabeprazole and amoxicillin as the 3rd rescue regimen for eradication of *H. pylori*. *Hepatogastroenterology* **2010**, *57*, 1314–1319. [PubMed]
13. Miehlke, S.; Kirsch, C.; Schneider-Brachert, W.; Haferland, C.; Neumeyer, M.; Bastlein, E.; Papke, J.; Jacobs, E.; Vieth, M.; Stolte, M.; et al. A Prospective, Randomized Study of Quadruple Therapy and High-Dose Dual Therapy for Treatment of *Helicobacter pylori* Resistant to Both Metronidazole and Clarithromycin. *Helicobacter* **2003**, *8*, 310–319. [CrossRef] [PubMed]
14. Schwartz, H.; Krause, R.; Sahba, B.; Haber, M.; Weissfeld, A.; Rose, P.; Siepman, N.; Freston, J. Triple versus dual therapy for eradicating *Helicobacter pylori* and preventing ulcer recurrence: A randomized, double-blind, multicenter study of lansoprazole, clarithromycin, and/or amoxicillin in different dosing regimens. *Am. J. Gastroenterol.* **1998**, *93*, 584–590. [CrossRef]
15. Miehlke, S.; Hansky, K.; Schneider-Brachert, W.; Kirsch, C.; Morgner, A.; Madisch, A.; Kuhlisch, E.; Bästlein, E.; Jacobs, E.; Bayerdörffer, E.; et al. Randomized trial of rifabutin-based triple therapy and high-dose dual therapy for rescue treatment of *Helicobacter pylori* resistant to both metronidazole and clarithromycin. *Aliment. Pharmacol. Ther.* **2006**, *24*, 395–403. [CrossRef]
16. Miyoshi, M.; Mizuno, M.; Ishiki, K.; Nagahara, Y.; Maga, T.; Torigoe, T.; Nasu, J.; Okada, H.; Yokota, K.; Oguma, K.; et al. A randomized open trial for comparison of proton pump inhibitors, omeprazole versus rabeprazole, in dual therapy for *Helicobacter pylori* infection in relation to CYP2C19 genetic polymorphism. *J. Gastroenterol. Hepatol.* **2001**, *16*, 723–728. [CrossRef]
17. Nishizawa, T.; Suzuki, H.; Maekawa, T.; Harada, N.; Toyokawa, T.; Kuwai, T.; Ohara, M.; Suzuki, T.; Kawanishi, M.; Noguchi, K.; et al. Dual therapy for third-line *Helicobacter pylori* eradication and urea breath test prediction. *World J. Gastroenterol.* **2012**, *18*, 2735–2738. [CrossRef]
18. Isomoto, H.; Inoue, K.; Furusu, H.; Enjoji, A.; Fujimoto, C.; Yamakawa, M.; Hirakata, Y.; Omagari, K.; Mizuta, Y.; Murase, K.; et al. High-dose rabeprazole-amoxicillin versus rabeprazole-amoxicillin-metronidazole as second-line treatment after failure of the Japanese standard regimen for *Helicobacter pylori* infection. *Aliment. Pharmacol. Ther.* **2003**, *18*, 101–107. [CrossRef]
19. Wong, B.; Xiao, S.; Hu, P.; Qian, S.; Huang, N.; Li, Y.; Manan, C.; Lesmana, L.; Carpio, R.; Perez, J.Y.; et al. Comparison of lansoprazole-based triple and dual therapy for treatment of *Helicobacter pylori*-related duodenal ulcer: An Asian multicentre double-blind randomized placebo controlled study. *Aliment. Pharmacol. Ther.* **2000**, *14*, 217–224. [CrossRef]
20. Attumi, T.A.; Graham, D.Y. High-Dose Extended-Release Lansoprazole (Dexlansoprazole) and Amoxicillin Dual Therapy for *Helicobacter pylori* Infections. *Helicobacter* **2014**, *19*, 319–322. [CrossRef]
21. Koizumi, W.; Tanabe, S.; Hibi, K.; Imaizumi, H.; Ohida, M.; Okabe, H.; Saigenji, K.; Okayasu, I. A prospective randomized study of amoxycillin and omeprazole with and without metronidazole in the eradication treatment of *Helicobacter pylori*. *J. Gastroenterol. Hepatol.* **1998**, *13*, 301–304. [CrossRef] [PubMed]
22. Furuta, T.; Ohashi, K.; Kamata, T.; Takashima, M.; Kosuge, K.; Kawasaki, T.; Hanai, H.; Kubota, T.; Ishizaki, T.; Kaneko, E. Effect of genetic differences in omeprazole metabolism on cure rates for *Helicobacter pylori* infection and peptic ulcer. *Ann. Intern. Med.* **1998**, *129*, 1027–1030. [CrossRef] [PubMed]
23. Bell, G.D.; Bate, C.M.; Axon, A.T.R.; Tildesley, G.; Kerr, G.D.; Green, J.R.B.; Emmas, C.E.; Taylor, M.D. Addition of metronidazole to omeprazole/amoxicillin dual therapy increases the rate of *Helicobacter pylori* eradication: A double-blind, randomized trial. *Aliment. Pharmacol. Ther.* **1995**, *9*, 513–520. [CrossRef] [PubMed]
24. Cottrill, M.R.B.; Kinnon, C.M.C.; Mason, I.; Chesters, S.A.; Slatcher, G.; Copeman, M.B.; Turbitt, M.L. Two omeprazole-based *Helicobacter pylori* eradication regimens for the treatment of duodenal ulcer disease in general practice. *Aliment. Pharmacol. Ther.* **1997**, *11*, 919–927. [CrossRef]
25. Kagaya, H.; Kato, M.; Komatsu, Y.; Mizushima, T.; Sukegawa, M.; Nishikawa, K.; Hokari, K.; Takeda, H.; Sugiyama, T.; Asaka, M. High-dose ecabet sodium improves the eradication rate of *Helicobacter pylori* in dual therapy with lansoprazole and amoxicillin. *Aliment. Pharmacol. Ther.* **2000**, *14*, 1523–1527. [CrossRef]
26. Sakurai, Y.; Mori, Y.; Okamoto, H.; Nishimura, A.; Komura, E.; Araki, T.; Shiramoto, M. Acid-inhibitory effects of vonoprazan 20 mg compared with esomeprazole 20 mg or rabeprazole 10 mg in healthy adult male subjects—A randomised open-label cross-over study. *Aliment. Pharmacol. Ther.* **2015**, *42*, 719–730. [CrossRef]
27. Murakami, K.; Sakurai, Y.; Shiino, M.; Funao, N.; Nishimura, A.; Asaka, M. Vonoprazan, a novel potassium-competitive acid blocker, as a component of first-line and second-line triple therapy for *Helicobacter pylori* eradication: A phase III, randomised, double-blind study. *Gut* **2016**, *65*, 1439–1446. [CrossRef]
28. Marcus, E.A.; Inatomi, N.; Nagami, G.T.; Sachs, G.; Scott, D.R. The effects of varying acidity on *Helicobacter pylori* growth and the bactericidal efficacy of ampicillin. *Aliment. Pharmacol. Ther.* **2012**, *36*, 972–979. [CrossRef]
29. Furuta, T.; Graham, D.Y. Pharmacologic Aspects of Eradication Therapy for *Helicobacter pylori* Infection. *Gastroenterol. Clin. N. Am.* **2010**, *39*, 465–480. [CrossRef]
30. Sugimoto, M.; Furuta, T.; Shirai, N.; Kodaira, C.; Nishino, M.; Ikuma, M.; Ishizaki, T.; Hishida, A. Evidence that the Degree and Duration of Acid Suppression are Related to *Helicobacter pylori* Eradication by Triple Therapy. *Helicobacter* **2007**, *12*, 317–323. [CrossRef]

31. Sugimoto, M.; Furuta, T.; Shirai, N.; Kajimura, M.; Hishida, A.; Sakurai, M.; Ohashi, K.; Ishizaki, T. Different dosage regimens of rabeprazole for nocturnal gastric acid inhibition in relation to cytochrome P450 2C19 genotype status. *Clin. Pharmacol. Ther.* **2004**, *76*, 290–301. [CrossRef]
32. Kagami, T.; Sahara, S.; Ichikawa, H.; Uotani, T.; Yamade, M.; Sugimoto, M.; Hamaya, Y.; Iwaizumi, M.; Osawa, S.; Miyajima, H.; et al. Potent acid inhibition by vonoprazan in comparison with esomeprazole, with reference to CYP2C19 genotype. *Aliment. Pharmacol. Ther.* **2016**, *43*, 1048–1059. [CrossRef] [PubMed]
33. Craig, W.A. State-of-the-Art Clinical Article: Pharmacokinetic/Pharmacodynamic Parameters: Rationale for Antibacterial Dosing of Mice and Men. *Clin. Infect. Dis.* **1998**, *26*, 1–10, quiz 11–12. [CrossRef] [PubMed]
34. Craig, W.A. Interrelationship between pharmacokinetics and pharmacodynamics in determining dosage regimens for broad-spectrum cephalosporins. *Diagn. Microbiol. Infect. Dis.* **1995**, *22*, 89–96. [CrossRef] [PubMed]
35. Craig, W.A. Choosing an antibiotic on the basis of pharmacodynamics. *Ear Nose Throat J.* **1998**, *77* (Suppl. S6), 7–11. [PubMed]
36. Furuta, T.; Yamade, M.; Kagami, T.; Uotani, T.; Suzuki, T.; Higuchi, T.; Tani, S.; Hamaya, Y.; Iwaizumi, M.; Miyajima, H.; et al. Dual Therapy with Vonoprazan and Amoxicillin Is as Effective as Triple Therapy with Vonoprazan, Amoxicillin and Clarithromycin for Eradication of *Helicobacter pylori*. *Digestion* **2019**, *101*, 743–751. [CrossRef]
37. Hu, Y.; Xu, X.; Liu, X.-S.; He, C.; Ouyang, Y.-B.; Li, N.-S.; Xie, C.; Peng, C.; Zhu, Z.-H.; Xie, Y.; et al. Fourteen-day vonoprazan and low- or high-dose amoxicillin dual therapy for eradicating *Helicobacter pylori* infection: A prospective, open-labeled, randomized non-inferiority clinical study. *Front. Immunol.* **2022**, *13*, 1049908. [CrossRef]
38. Suzuki, S.; Gotoda, T.; Kusano, C.; Ikehara, H.; Ichijima, R.; Ohyauchi, M.; Ito, H.; Kawamura, M.; Ogata, Y.; Ohtaka, M.; et al. Seven-day vonoprazan and low-dose amoxicillin dual therapy as first-line *Helicobacter pylori* treatment: A multicentre randomised trial in Japan. *Gut* **2020**, *69*, 1019–1026. [CrossRef]
39. Gotoda, T.; Kusano, C.; Suzuki, S.; Horii, T.; Ichijima, R.; Ikehara, H. Clinical impact of vonoprazan-based dual therapy with amoxicillin for *H. pylori* infection in a treatment-naive cohort of junior high school students in Japan. *J. Gastroenterol.* **2020**, *55*, 969–976. [CrossRef]
40. Sue, S.; Kondo, M.; Sato, T.; Oka, H.; Sanga, K.; Ogashiwa, T.; Matsubayashi, M.; Kaneko, H.; Irie, K.; Maeda, S. Vonoprazan and high-dose amoxicillin dual therapy for *Helicobacter pylori* first-line eradication: A single-arm, interventional study. *JGH Open* **2023**, *7*, 55–60. [CrossRef]
41. Qian, H.-S.; Li, W.-J.; Dang, Y.-N.; Li, L.-R.; Xu, X.-B.; Yuan, L.; Zhang, W.-F.; Yang, Z.; Gao, X.; Zhang, M.; et al. Ten-Day Vonoprazan-Amoxicillin Dual Therapy as a First-Line Treatment of *Helicobacter pylori* Infection Compared with Bismuth-Containing Quadruple Therapy. *Am. J. Gastroenterol.* **2022**, *118*, 627–634. [CrossRef] [PubMed]
42. Lin, Y.; Xu, H.; Yun, J.; Yu, X.; Shi, Y.; Zhang, D. The efficacy of vonoprazan combined with different dose amoxicillin on eradication of *Helicobacter pylori*: An open, multicenter, randomized clinical study. *Ann. Transl. Med.* **2022**, *10*, 987. [CrossRef] [PubMed]
43. Gao, W.; Teng, G.; Wang, C.; Xu, Y.; Li, Y.; Cheng, H. Eradication rate and safety of a "simplified rescue therapy": 14-day vonoprazan and amoxicillin dual regimen as rescue therapy on treatment of *Helicobacter pylori* infection previously failed in eradication: A real-world, retrospective clinical study in China. *Helicobacter* **2022**, *27*, e12918. [PubMed]
44. Zuberi, B.F.; Ali, F.S.; Rasheed, T.; Bader, N.; Hussain, S.M.; Saleem, A. Comparison of Vonoprazan and Amoxicillin Dual Therapy with Standard Triple Therapy with Proton Pump Inhibitor for *Helicobacter pylori* eradication: A Randomized Control Trial. *Pak. J. Med. Sci.* **2022**, *38*, 965–969. [CrossRef]
45. Hu, Y.; Xu, X.; Ouyang, Y.B.; He, C.; Li, N.S.; Xie, C.; Peng, C.; Zhu, Z.H.; Xie, Y.; Shu, X.; et al. Optimization of vonoprazan-amoxicillin dual therapy for eradicating *Helicobacter pylori* infection in China: A prospective, randomized clinical pilot study. *Helicobacter* **2022**, *27*, e12896. [CrossRef]
46. Chey, W.D.; Mégraud, F.; Laine, L.; López, L.J.; Hunt, B.J.; Howden, C.W. Vonoprazan Triple and Dual Therapy for *Helicobacter pylori* Infection in the United States and Europe: Randomized Clinical Trial. *Gastroenterology* **2022**, *163*, 608–619. [CrossRef]
47. Zhou, S.; Chan, S.Y.; Goh, B.C.; Chan, E.; Duan, W.; Huang, M.; McLeod, H.L. Mechanism-Based Inhibition of Cytochrome P450 3A4 by Therapeutic Drugs. *Clin. Pharmacokinet.* **2005**, *44*, 279–304. [CrossRef]
48. Kagami, T.; Yamade, M.; Suzuki, T.; Uotani, T.; Hamaya, Y.; Iwaizumi, M.; Osawa, S.; Sugimoto, K.; Umemura, K.; Miyajima, H.; et al. Comparative study of effects of vonoprazan and esomeprazole on anti-platelet function of clopidogrel or prasugrel in relation to CYP2C19 genotype. *Clin. Pharmacol. Ther.* **2017**, *103*, 906–913. [CrossRef]
49. Wang, Y.; Wang, C.; Wang, S.; Zhou, Q.; Dai, D.; Shi, J.; Xu, X.; Luo, Q. Cytochrome P450-Based Drug-Drug Interactions of Vonoprazan In Vitro and In Vivo. *Front. Pharmacol.* **2020**, *11*, 53. [CrossRef]
50. Kang, Y.; Kim, Y.-J.; Shim, T.S.; Jo, K.-W. Risk for cardiovascular disease in patients with nontuberculous mycobacteria treated with macrolide. *J. Thorac. Dis.* **2018**, *10*, 5784–5795. [CrossRef]
51. Drago, L.; Nicola, L.; Rodighiero, V.; Larosa, M.; Mattina, R.; De Vecchi, E. Comparative evaluation of synergy of combinations of beta-lactams with fluoroquinolones or a macrolide in *Streptococcus pneumoniae*. *J. Antimicrob. Chemother.* **2011**, *66*, 845–849. [CrossRef] [PubMed]
52. Medscape. Drug Interaction Checker. Available online: https://reference.medscape.com/drug-interactionchecker (accessed on 3 March 2023).

53. Furuta, T.; Yamade, M.; Kagami, T.; Suzuki, T.; Higuchi, T.; Tani, S.; Hamaya, Y.; Iwaizumi, M.; Miyajima, H.; Umemura, K.; et al. Influence of clarithromycin on the bactericidal effect of amoxicillin in patients infected with clarithromycin-resistant strains of *H. pylori*. *Gut* **2020**, *69*, 2056. [CrossRef] [PubMed]
54. Murakami, K.; Sato, R.; Okimoto, T.; Nasu, M.; Fujioka, T.; Kodama, M.; Kagawa, J.; Sato, S.; Abe, H.; Arita, T. Eradication rates of clarithromycin-resistant *Helicobacter pylori* using either rabeprazole or lansoprazole plus amoxicillin and clarithromycin. *Aliment. Pharmacol. Ther.* **2002**, *16*, 1933–1938. [CrossRef] [PubMed]
55. Kawabata, H.; Habu, Y.; Tomioka, H.; Kutsumi, H.; Kobayashi, M.; Oyasu, K.; Hayakumo, T.; Mizuno, S.; Kiyota, K.; Nakajima, M.; et al. Effect of different proton pump inhibitors, differences in CYP2C19 genotype and antibiotic resistance on the eradication rate of *Helicobacter pylori* infection by a 1-week regimen of proton pump inhibitor, amoxicillin and clarithromycin. *Aliment. Pharmacol. Ther.* **2003**, *17*, 259–264. [CrossRef]
56. Gao, W.; Xu, Y.; Liu, J.; Wang, X.; Dong, X.; Teng, G.; Liu, B.; Dong, J.; Ge, C.; Ye, H.; et al. A real-world exploratory study on the feasibility of vonoprazan and tetracycline dual therapy for the treatment of *Helicobacter pylori* infection in special populations with penicillin allergy or failed in previous amoxicillin-containing therapies. *Helicobacter* **2023**, *28*, e12947. [CrossRef]

Disclaimer/Publisher's Note: The statements, opinions and data contained in all publications are solely those of the individual author(s) and contributor(s) and not of MDPI and/or the editor(s). MDPI and/or the editor(s) disclaim responsibility for any injury to people or property resulting from any ideas, methods, instructions or products referred to in the content.

MDPI
St. Alban-Anlage 66
4052 Basel
Switzerland
www.mdpi.com

Journal of Clinical Medicine Editorial Office
E-mail: jcm@mdpi.com
www.mdpi.com/journal/jcm

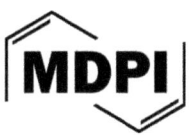

Disclaimer/Publisher's Note: The statements, opinions and data contained in all publications are solely those of the individual author(s) and contributor(s) and not of MDPI and/or the editor(s). MDPI and/or the editor(s) disclaim responsibility for any injury to people or property resulting from any ideas, methods, instructions or products referred to in the content.